Clinical Physiology of
the Lung

For Philippa

Clinical Physiology of The Lung

KENNETH B. SAUNDERS

M.A. M.D. M.R.C.P.

Senior Lecturer in Medicine,
Honorary Consultant Physician and
Postgraduate Subdean,
Middlesex Hospital and Medical School,
London W1

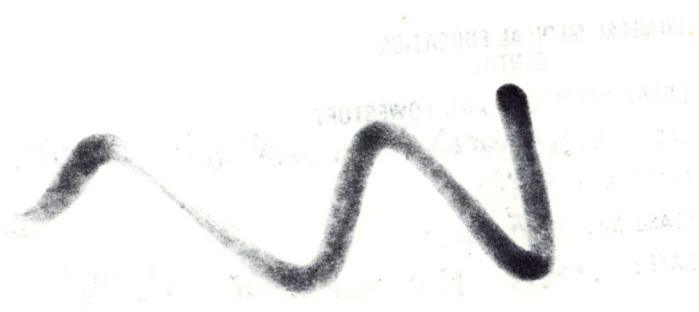

Blackwell Scientific Publications

OXFORD LONDON EDINBURGH
MELBOURNE

© 1977 by Blackwell Scientific Publications
Osney Mead, Oxford
8 John Street, London WC1N 2ES
9 Forrest Road, Edinburgh
P.O. Box 9, North Balwyn, Victoria, Australia

First published 1977

British Library Cataloguing in Publication Data
Saunders, Kenneth B
  Clinical physiology of the lung.

    1. Lungs – Diseases   2. Physiology, Patho-
                logical   I Title

616.2′4′07   RC756

ISBN 0–632–00046–5

Distributed in the U.S.A. by
J. B. Lippincott Company, Philadelphia
and in Canada by
J. B. Lippincott Company of
Canada Ltd, Toronto

Printed and bound in Great Britain by
William Clowes & Sons Limited,
London, Beccles and Colchester

Contents

Chapter 1. Introduction

WHAT IS CLINICAL PHYSIOLOGY?

The invention of the term clinical physiology is recent and confusing. If physiology is the 'science of *normal* functions and phenomena of living things' (*Concise Oxford Dictionary*), whereas the word clinical means 'of or at the sick-bed', the combination of the two words is meaningless, and in this respect the accusation that clinical physiology is neither clinical or physiologic has some smattering of truth.

Historically, physiology has for more than a century been a highly-regarded academic discipline, whereas clinical medicine had until the middle of this century (and even later) been regarded, by physiologists, as a curious practice conducted intuitively by well meaning people with poor understanding of scientific method. A defensive position was taken by doctors who began to apply scientific method to clinical work with the introduction of the term 'clinical science', but that discipline is still regarded with some reserve by the more senior professional physiologists and the more conservative medical practitioners.

There are several reasons why this schism between medicine and physiology remains to some extent, some understandable which are recounted below and some silly which are here ignored.

To the clinician physiologists appear to spend much time studying the properties of isolated tissues obtained from bizarre forms of animal life. As I understand it, this is because physiologists tend to be more interested in the basic mechanisms of nature (Greek—*physis*) than in species differences. Thus if a scientist publishes work on sodium transport in the bladder of an obscure South American toad, this probably does not imply any particular intellectual or emotional interest in the workings of the aforesaid toad. It is more likely to reflect the fact that the bladder in that animal appears to have been conveniently arranged by the Almighty for the study of sodium transport.

In designing experiments on a complex organism, two polar approaches can be detected. First, the experimental preparation may be left intact or almost so, in which case many interacting mechanisms will be affected by the simplest experimental intervention. The results of such experiments are difficult to interpret, and therefore frequently require difficult methods of data handling, signal analysis and statistics. Alternatively, the experimental preparation may be so simplified by skilful manipulation that the results may be relatively simply interpreted. In my view the major achievements of the British School of Physiology have been made in the latter way. In clinical medicine this extreme approach is almost always impossible. It is no wonder that clinical experiments often seem to physiologists to be poorly designed and overinterpreted.

It might be hoped that the combined knowledge obtained from simpler animal preparations would serve to illumine the mechanisms obtaining in man, and so it does—in normal man. In diseased man we need information from diseased animals. If in normal animals species differences make extrapolation to human physiology difficult, finding animal models for human diseases presents an even greater problem. Moreover the ethical implications of giving diseases to animals are being progressively more closely examined, and the use of large numbers of primates for this purpose rightly condemned.

Therefore most important information about human disease will continue to be found from the study of sick people. The study of function disturbed by disease may for want of a better phrase be called 'clinical physiology'. Since only clinicians can do or supervise this work, it behoves clinicians to get on with it, which raises another problem.

SOME HISTORICAL CONSIDERATIONS

In the early years of this century scientists such as Haldane and Krogh made enormous advances in respiratory physiology, particularly with respect to the gas exchanging functions of lung and blood. There was little application to clinical medicine, mainly because there was no access to arterial blood in man and no practical routine method of measuring blood gases. After the second world war there was a second series of important advances associated with such names as Comroe, Cournand, Fenn, Otis and Rahn from the United States, together with technical achievements such as arterial puncture, blood gas electrodes and body plethysmography, which allowed this knowledge to be applied to patients.

Initially the techniques and numerical ability required were too demanding for all but a few clinicians, a fact which reflected on their training rather than on their intelligence, but by the late 1950's the potential of respiratory physiology applied to medicine was clear.

While an enormous amount of information had been rapidly added to the pre-war literature it was still then easy to take a broad interest in the entire field of respiratory physiology. Moreover in the early 1960's a newly qualified doctor wishing to make his career in chest medicine could read the relevant section of a standard physiology text-book, followed by *The Lung*, by Comroe and his colleagues, followed by the *Journal of Applied Physiology* for the previous year, and could then go to any scientific meeting on respiration and understand most of what he heard. After six months preliminary reading he was well in the field.

This is no longer true. There has been a vast expansion of technique and theory in the past 15 years. Comroe's *The Lung* is sadly unrevised. Articles in the *Journal of Applied Physiology* or *Respiration Physiology* now require from the reader even more previous knowledge over and above that provided by undergraduate textbooks. It is small wonder that talented young physicians settle for practice or research at a very superficial level, or go in depth into a corner of the subject so restricted that they become rapidly bored.

PURPOSE AND STYLE OF THIS BOOK

This book is designed first to bridge the gap between undergraduate curricula and more advanced and comprehensive textbooks of respiratory physiology, and second to enable the reader to understand some difficult but basic ideas which underlie present work so that he may begin to understand the advancing fringes of the subject. It is intended therefore primarily for future professionals in chest medicine. It may also be of use to undergraduates who wish to pursue the implications of respiratory physiology in unusual depth, and possibly, if taken in very judicious doses, might aid in preparation for Higher Examinations.

It is not comprehensive, selection being made on the basis partly of relevance to common clinical problems, and partly of gaps in the author's knowledge. For example, I have not discussed a large body of work which describes the autonomic control of airway calibre in relation to lung volume (much of it from Widdecomb's laboratory), and the concept of matching deadspace to ventilation thereby, since the control system postulated, fascinating though it is, has not been shown to play an important part in furthering efficient gas exchange. In contrast, I have also not discussed disturbances of respiratory control due to cerebral disease, for example the work from Plum's group, because my knowledge of basic neurophysiology is insufficient to allow me to take the subject at a proper postgraduate level. The first omission is purposeful, the second forced, and both are regretted. On the other hand I have not shirked the more difficult concepts such as transient analysis, dynamic compression of airways, the pleural pressure gradient, or the $O_2 - CO_2$ diagram, where they appear to be basic to future understanding of function.

Comroe's *The Lung* was the first book in the field to take a primarily numerical approach to the explanation of physiologic mechanisms, in the sense that each step in the argument was accompanied by a worked example using realistic numbers. An alternative approach, best used perhaps by John West, is to describe the behaviour of a system at first intuitively by words and pictures, and subsequently to add the numerical detail. While I personally prefer the first method, the range of mathematical techniques now required is quite wide and would deter many readers. I have therefore restricted details of equations and their derivation to those techniques which are used routinely in lung function laboratories (e.g. determination of airways resistance and transfer factor), with which future professionals must certainly be acquainted.

I have endeavoured to show how systems theory has advanced the study of respiratory control in the past few years, but I have not used any differential equations or operational mathematics. Since the whole point of systems theory is that it is a numerical subject, this is rather like going in for a sword-fight without being allowed to take the scabbard off the sword. None-the-less, I hope it will give readers who are not particularly numerate some idea of the potentialities.

Although the book has been written almost entirely from primary sources, I have not given all the references used, but when the subject is particularly complicated like the control of respiration, the documentation is a little more detailed. In general I have referred to the literature of the 1970's, omitting earlier classical references not through lack of respect but because they may be found usually in the introductions of the references quoted.

Chapters 6 to 8 refer to some common respiratory diseases and to respiratory failure. The basic concepts of previous chapters are not only taken up therein, but extended. It seems simpler, for example, to consider details of elastic recoil pressure and bronchial collapsibility in the context of the disease emphysema. This does mean that Chapters 6 to 8 cannot be taken separately by the reader, but are only intelligible on the basis of an understanding of preceding chapters.

I am bored with the great debate on whether we should use hydrion concentration or pH, and on which is the best acid-base diagram. As a clinician I find it convenient to use a diagram on which I can plot the variables measured, namely pH and P_{CO_2}. When thinking about the Haldane effect I find the Davenport pH-bicarbonate diagram most helpful, but when considering the ionic composition of brain extracellular fluid I find $[H^+]$ easier. I have therefore stuck to pH in the chapter on acid-base chemistry in the blood, but later use $[H^+]$ and finally in Chapter 5 purposefully intermingle the two notations. The reader may decide for himself which he prefers in the end.

The introduction of SI units has certainly posed a problem. Since the bulk of the important work on applied respiratory physiology is still published in North American and other literature in traditional units, and since it is hoped that the reader will refer to some of the references given, and since the purpose of this book is to teach, it is written in traditional units with SI units in parentheses, except when they would clutter up an otherwise simple calculation, when the SI units are omitted altogether and without regret.

Finally I am aware that the use of the English language in this book might raise eyebrows in the Athenaeum, should a copy ever be opened in those quarters. As a pupil and an addicted reader I have always been grateful to teachers who have varied their style, especially if it is occasionally lightened. This is what I have tried to do.

Chapter 2. Lung Mechanics

INTRODUCTION TO LUNG MECHANICS

Consider the spring-block model shown in Fig. 2.1. A block of wood, resting on a surface, is attached to a wall by a spring. If a force F is applied to move the block a distance l, three different sorts of work will need to be done.

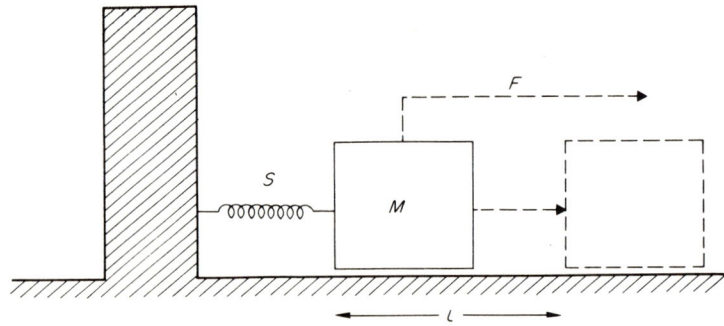

Fig. 2.1. The spring-block model. A mass M attached to a wall by a spring S, to be moved a distance l by force F.

1   The spring will be stretched. The required force F_1 will depend on a spring constant K and the distance that the block is moved, l, so that $F_1 = K \cdot l$.

2   To overcome the frictional resistance between the block and the surface on which it lies, a force F_2 must be applied, which depends on a constant of resistance R, and the rate of change of position, or velocity dl/dt, so that $F_2 = R \cdot dl/dt$.

3   Finally a third force F_3 is needed to overcome inertive forces (the extra effort needed to get it moving), depending on the mass of the block M, and the rate of change of velocity or acceleration d^2l/dt^2, so that $F_3 = M \cdot d^2l/dt^2$.

    The total force required is thus

$$F = F_1 + F_2 + F_3 = \underset{\text{elastic}}{K \cdot l} + \underset{\text{resistive}}{R \cdot dl/dt} + \underset{\substack{\text{inertive} \\ \text{components}}}{M \cdot d^2l/dt^2} \qquad (2.1)$$

    If you prefer not to think in terms of derivatives, but rather in terms of velocity v and acceleration a, then

$$F = K \cdot l + R \cdot v + M \cdot a \qquad (2.2)$$

Beware, however: you possibly do not understand the meaning of the words velocity and acceleration.

Fortunately, when we transfer to a lung model, we may ignore the third inertive term in most circumstances, for both the mass of gas in the lung and the acceleration of gas during normal breathing are small. Little harm will come if we take as our final equation from the spring-block model

$$F = K.l + R.dl/dt \qquad (2.3)$$

K is a spring constant and its corresponding term in pulmonary physiology is elastance E; we generally prefer to think in terms of compliance C which is the reciprocal of elastance $(K \equiv E = 1/C)$. Distance l become lung volume V. Resistance R is the same in both systems. Velocity, dl/dt, becomes rate of change of volume, or volume flow rate dV/dt, which is often written $\dot{V}$. Finally we now use not force, but force per unit area, or pressure P.

Thus, for the lung,

$$P = V/C + R\dot{V} \qquad (2.4)$$

In words, at any moment during breathing, a pressure across the lung is required to overcome elastic forces (V/C) and resistive forces $(R\dot{V})$.

Compliance C is expressed as volume change per unit increase in pressure distending the lung, in L/cmH_2O or L/kPa. The elastic properties of the lung reside not only in the tissues, but also in a lipoprotein surface-active material which lines the alveolar surface (p. 33).

Resistance R is expressed as pressure per unit flow in cmH_2O per L/sec (or $kPa/(L/sec)$). Depending on the technique used, we may refer to
1 airways resistance, which refers to the resistance to gas flow through all tubes between alveolus and mouth;
2 lung resistance which is airways resistance plus resistance to movement of lung tissues; or
3 total respiratory resistance which is lung resistance plus resistance to movement of tissues in the chest wall.

Time constants

Take a system with pure compliance, a 'perfect balloon' distended within a plethysmograph by a negative pressure outside the balloon, rather like the lungs within the chest (Fig. 2.2). Assume that it has zero volume at zero distending pressure. Distend the balloon with $-5\,cmH_2O\,(-0.5\,kPa)$. Then make a step change in distending pressure from -5 to $-10\,cmH_2O\,(-0.5$ to $-1.0\,kPa)$. The response in balloon volume is instantaneous. Balloon A (initial volume 10 ml) distends by 10 ml. It has a compliance of $10\,ml/5\,cmH_2O$, or $2\,ml/cmH_2O\,(20\,ml/kPa)$, which is relatively lower

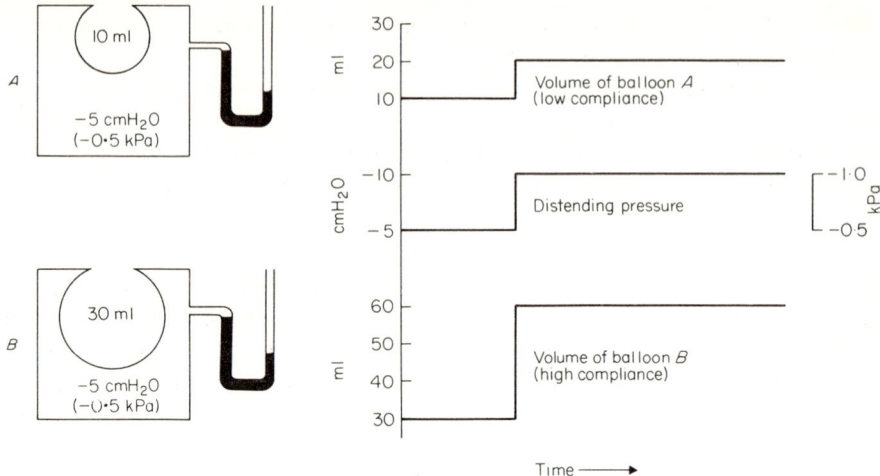

Fig. 2.2. A system with compliance. Effect of a step change in distending pressure on two balloons of different compliance.

(stiffer) than for balloon B (initial volume 30 ml), which has a compliance of 30/5 or 6 ml/cmH$_2$O (60 ml/kPa).

Now add a resistance to the model, as in Fig. 2.3. Again apply a step change in distending pressure from −5 to −10 cmH$_2$O (−0·5 to −1·0 kPa). The response in balloon volume is no longer instantaneous, and the time course of filling depends on the magnitude of compliance and resistance. Balloons A2 and B2, which have a high resistance to gas inflow, fill much more slowly than balloons A1 and B1.

Note that all balloons eventually reach the volume determined by their compliance (*cf.* Fig. 2.2). Some reach that volume quicker than others. Compliance determines 'how far there is to go'. Resistance determines 'how fast the system gets there'.

Note also the relative completion of filling at one second after the step.

Balloon A1 has 'inspired' 10 ml into an original volume of 10 ml, and has diluted 'alveolar gas' by 10/20 or 50%.

Balloon A2 has inspired about 6 ml into an original volume of 10 ml; a dilution of 6/16 or 37%.

Balloon B1 has inspired about 25 ml into an original volume of 30 ml; a dilution of 25/55 or 45%.

Balloon B2 has inspired about 12 ml into an original volume of 30 ml; a dilution of 12/40 or 30%.

If these four balloons were alveoli, and time for inhalation were limited as it is in tidal breathing a change in distending pressure would lead to an

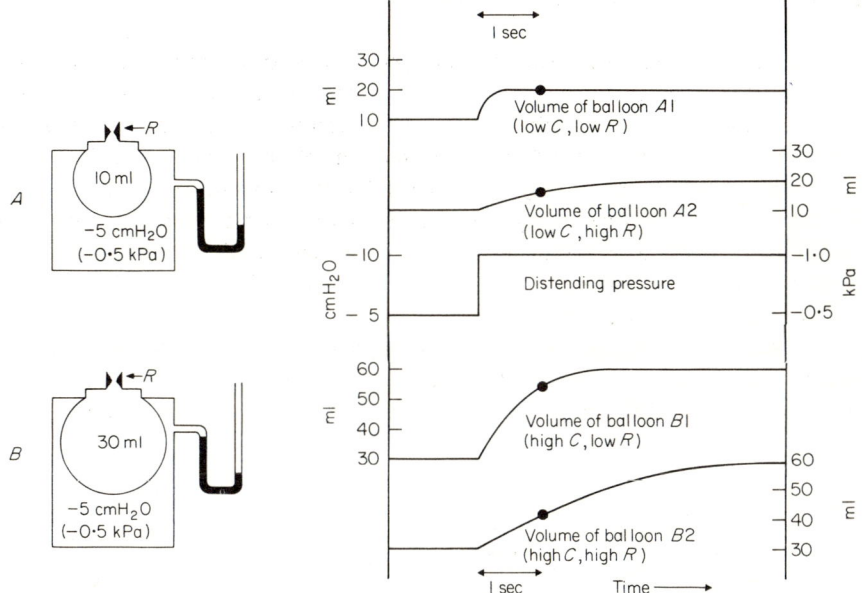

Fig. 2.3. A system with compliance and resistance. Effect of a step change in distending pressure on two balloons of different compliance, where resistance to gas inflow is also varied. C = compliance, R = resistance.

unfortunately uneven distribution of ventilation. A balloon with low compliance and low resistance ($A1$) would get more than its fair share. A balloon with high compliance and high resistance ($B2$) would be unfairly deprived.

In a system with a large number of different balloons, or alveoli, each connected to a large number of different resistances, or airways, what are the conditions required for ventilation to be evenly distributed? The mathematical solution is that for each individual alveolus-airway system, the product of resistance and compliance should be identical. This makes good intuitive sense. A high-compliance alveolus (starts larger—long way to go) must be connected to a low resistance airway (get there quicker); a low-compliance alveolus (starts smaller—not far to go) needs a high resistance airway (should take more time) so that both may inspire gas in appropriate proportion.

The product of resistance (cmH_2O per L/sec or kPa/(L/sec)) and compliance (L/cmH_2O or L/kPa) is a number with the dimension of seconds. It is called a time constant. For ventilation to be perfectly evenly distributed, time constants of all pathways should be identical. This is surprisingly close to the truth for the normal lung, and leads us to the question of static and dynamic compliance.

PULMONARY COMPLIANCE

Compliance defines the relation between distending pressure and lung volume. A compliant person is one whose character is easily moulded and whose actions are easily modified. Increased compliance in a lung implies that it may be more easily distended; decreased compliance, that it is stiffer.

Volume change may be easily measured with a spirometer, but it is more difficult to measure distending (pleural) pressure. Direct needle puncture of the pleural cavity is possible, but too risky. Fortunately, provided that the subject is in the upright position, changes in oesophageal pressure closely follow changes in pleural pressure.

A balloon is placed in mid-oesophagus and a differential pressure transducer measures the difference between oesophageal and mouth pressure—the distending pressure (Fig. 2.4). The subject takes a full

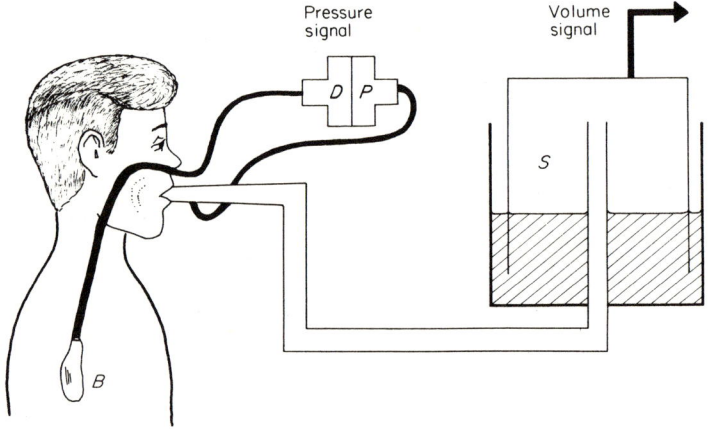

Fig. 2.4. Circuitry for measuring static compliance. B = oesophageal balloon, DP = differential pressure gauge, S = spirometer.

inspiration and exhales into the spirometer, stopping flow at intervals of a few hundred ml. Points from resulting pressure and volume plateaus may then be plotted as in Fig. 2.5. Residual volume must be separately measured to relate volume change to absolute lung volume rather than to vital capacity. Note that the relation is not linear—there is no single value (slope) for compliance which applies over the entire vital capacity. It is usual to take the best fitting line which applies over the tidal volume range in the vital capacity.

If one ml of air were pumped into the isolated lung of an elephant, a negligible change in distending pressure would occur; if the same volume were pumped into the lung of a rat it would cause a much larger pressure change. This does not imply that rat lung is intrinsically stiffer than elephant lung, but

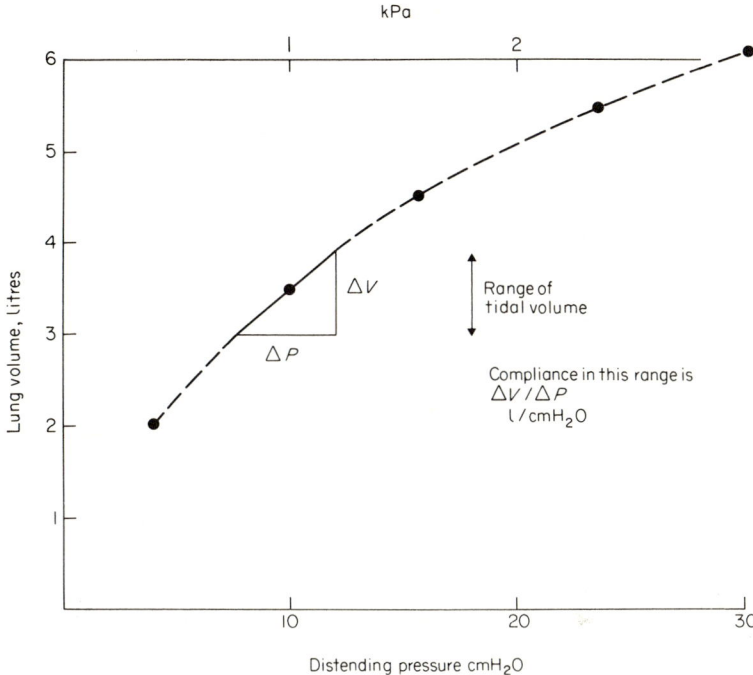

Fig. 2.5. Relation between lung volume and distending pressure, and calculation of static compliance.

merely follows from the fact that rat lung is smaller. If the compliance of the lungs in a human subject were 0.2 L/cmH$_2$O (2.0 L/kPa), and 5 cmH$_2$O (0.5 kPa) distending pressure were applied, 1.0 L would enter the lung. Suppose now that a tracheal divider were first inserted so that air could not enter or leave the left lung. Again 5 cmH$_2$O (0.5 kPa) distending pressure is applied; since only one lung can expand, only about 0.5 l will enter the lungs. Apparent compliance is $0.5/5$ or 0.1 L/cmH$_2$O (1.0 L/kPa). Is one lung then twice as stiff as two lungs? Obviously not—it is half the size, though. A measurement of compliance is meaningless unless accompanied by a statement of the volume at which it is measured.

We have so far been discussing 'static compliance', that is measurements of compliance made during breath-holding. It is also possible to measure compliance during tidal breathing, and this is called 'dynamic compliance'. Recordings of tidal volume, flow at the mouth, and oesophageal pressure are required (Fig. 2.6). We take measurements at points of no flow, at cross-over between inspiration and expiration (points *A* and *B*). At these points no force is needed to overcome resistance, for nothing is moving, and the pressures

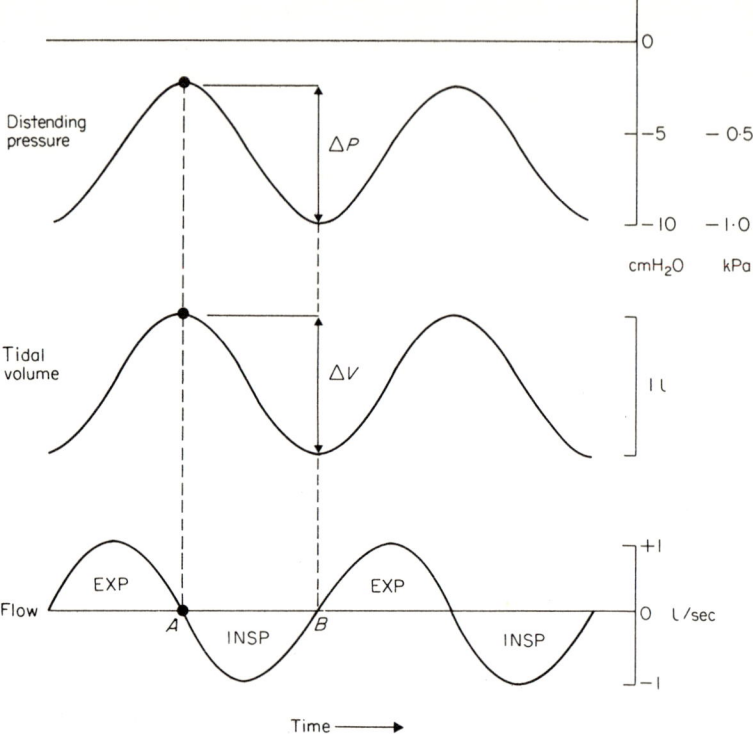

Fig. 2.6. Schematic recordings of distending pressure, tidal volume, and flow at the mouth for calculation of dynamic compliance. Records are made rather sinusoidal for clarity of presentation, but are not so in real life.

recorded are those needed to distend the lung to those two particular end-inspiratory and end-expiratory volumes. From equation 2.4, since $\dot{V}=0$, at those points, $P = V/C$, or $C = V/P$. Compliance is then calculated as $\Delta V/\Delta P$ from Fig. 2.6.

In a normal subject, dynamic and static compliance are the same, and dynamic compliance does not vary with breathing frequency. The mathematical condition which is required for this to occur is again that time constants for all pathways should be the same. If there is inequality of time constants, dynamic compliance will decrease, or the lung will appear to get stiffer, as breathing rate increases.

Thus the range of time constants within the lung determines not only the evenness of distribution of inspired gas, but also the apparent elastic behaviour of the lung during tidal breathing. This discussion applies to the compliance of the lung, and excludes the elastic properties of the chest wall, which also has compliance of a similar magnitude, about $0.1-0.2$ L/cmH$_2$O ($1-2$ L/kPa); but chest wall compliance is of less clinical importance.

Finally, what structures in the lung account for its elastic behaviour? Obviously, elastic and collagenous connective tissue; less obviously, the lipid film of surfactant material which lines the alveoli (p. 33).

AIRWAYS RESISTANCE

The respiratory system has different types of resistance; viscous (frictional) resistance of the chest wall to movement, viscous resistance of lung tissue, and, most importantly, airways resistance, or resistance to gas flow in tubes. 'Lung resistance' refers to airways resistance plus lung tissue resistance. 'Total respiratory resistance' refers to lung resistance plus chest wall resistance.

Clinically, we are mainly interested in airways resistance: to calculate it we need measurements of driving pressure and of flow through the system of branching tubes. (Resistance equals driving pressure divided by flow.) Flow can be measured at the mouth by breathing through a pneumotachygraph. Driving pressure is alveolar pressure, and cannot be directly measured. It can be derived in two ways.

Rohrer established the basic rule of respiratory mechanics, which is that alveolar pressure (Palv) is the sum of the pleural pressure (Ppl) and elastic recoil pressure of the lung (Pel).

$$Palv = Ppl + Pel \qquad\qquad (2.5)$$

Pel is always defined as positive; it always tends to make the lung smaller. Ppl may be, and usually is, negative, when it tends to expand the lung; but may be positive during expiration, when both Ppl and Pel are working together to diminish lung volume.

In inspiration, Ppl is clearly negative, and Palv, the sum of Ppl and Pel, is also negative. In quiet expiration, Ppl is still negative, but less so, and the sum of Ppl and Pel is positive. In forced expiration, both Ppl and Pel are positive, and Palv therefore markedly positive.

Pleural pressure, Ppl, can be measured continuously by the oesophageal balloon technique. If we knew Pel we could, by addition, obtain alveolar pressure (equation 2.5), and use it with a flow measurement to calculate resistance. Pel cannot be obtained during tidal breathing, but can be separately measured by the method used to estimate static compliance. An initial experiment relates each value of lung volume to a value of pleural pressure *under static conditions*, when Ppl $= -P$el, for Palv is then zero (equation 2.5). Then in a second procedure, simultaneous measurements are made of oesophageal pressure, lung volume changes, and flow at the mouth, during tidal breathing. Selected points of oesophageal pressure (equivalent to

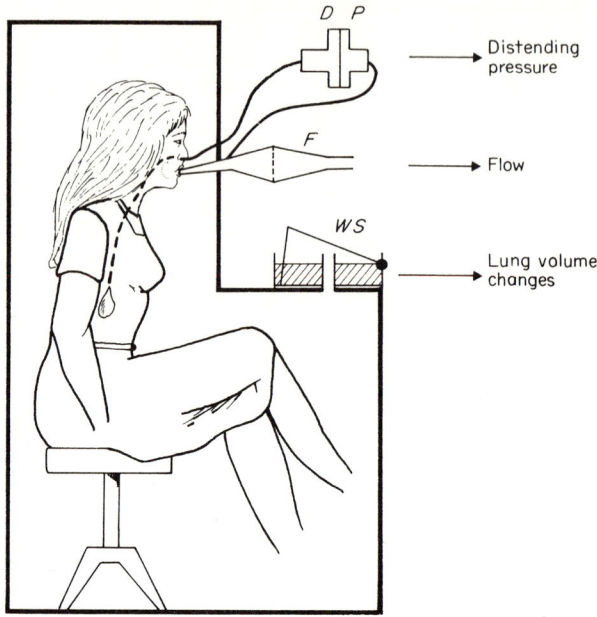

Fig. 2.7. Circuitry for measuring airways resistance with a constant-pressure plethysmograph [1]. DP = differential pressure gauge, F = flow-meter or pneumotachygraph, WS = wedge spirometer.

Ppl) are taken, and to these values are added the values of Pel previously found appropriate to the relevant lung volume. The values of alveolar pressure thus obtained may then be divided by the instantaneous flow to obtain resistance.

One might think that a spirometer would be suitable to measure lung volume changes, but this is not strictly so, for during breathing gas is compressed and expanded in the chest. This must be so, for to obtain gas flow, say in expiration, alveolar pressure must be positive with regard to atmospheric pressure. If alveolar pressure is relatively positive, alveolar gas must be relatively compressed. Therefore a better way of measuring lung volume changes is with a constant-pressure whole body plethysmograph [1] (Fig. 2.7).

The subject sits inside the box, but breathes air from outside it through a flowmeter F. The volume changes in the chest are reflected and measured by the wedge spirometer WS. Oesophageal pressure is detected by pressure gauge DP.

While this method of measuring airways resistance is relatively easy to understand, for Rohrer's equation is a simple one, it is not widely used in

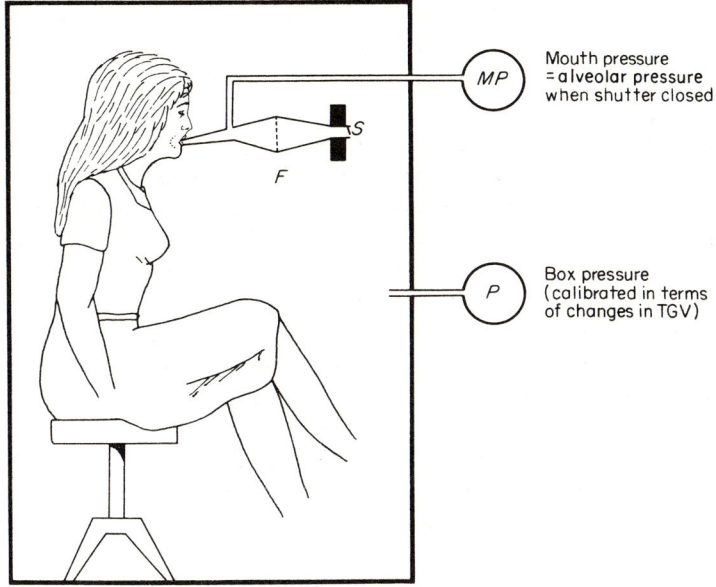

Fig. 2.8. Circuitry for measuring airways resistance with a constant-volume plethysmograph [2, 3]. MP = mouth pressure gauge, F = flow-meter or pneumotachygraph, S = shutter, P = box pressure gauge.

routine pulmonary investigation, for it requires the subject to swallow a balloon, and the necessary calculations from the recordings are tedious. There are also considerable technical problems which are not discussed here.

The second method of measuring airways resistance is more practical for clinical use, and requires a constant-volume type of whole-body plethysmograph [2, 3] (Fig. 2.8). Here the subject breathes air from inside the box, through a flowmeter F. Pressure changes within the box are measured by the sensitive pressure transducer P, and mouth pressure, by a tapping from the mouthpiece, with pressure gauge MP. The airway may be occluded by a shutter S.

Curiously, in order to determine airways resistance—we shall first measure the thoracic gas volume TGV. While the subject is breathing through the mouthpiece and flowmeter, the airway is closed by the shutter. The subject continues to make breathing movements against the shutter for a few seconds. (Some find this manoeuvre difficult.) During these breathing movements, since airflow at the mouth is blocked, air in the chest is alternately compressed and expanded. Contrariwise, air outside the chest but inside the closed plethysmograph is alternately expanded and compressed. Volume changes in the chest are equal and opposite to volume changes outside the chest, but inside the box. Volume changes outside the chest, but inside the box, are reflected by a pressure signal from the box pressure gauge P. This pressure gauge can be calibrated in terms of volume by injecting into the box known amounts of air, say 50 ml, from a syringe, and recording the accompanying pressure change. Thus the pressure signal during the compression manoeuvre can be interpreted as volume change in the box, outside the chest, which is equal and opposite to the volume changes of the gas within the chest.

At the same time, the mouth pressure gauge is recording pressure changes due to the compression and expansion of gas in chest and airways up to the closed shutter. Since there is no flow, pressure throughout this mass of gas is assumed to be identical everywhere at any given moment: in this somewhat odd manoeuvre, the mouth pressure equals alveolar pressure. We now have two continuous measurements, one of changing volume and the other of changing pressure, in a mass of gas in chest and airways during compression and expansion. Problem: what is the volume of that gas?

Boyle's law states that in a mass of gas, pressure P multiplied by volume V is a constant.

$$P.V = k \tag{2.6}$$

or

$$P = k/V \tag{2.7}$$

This is the equation of a hyperbola, shown in Fig. 2.9 for two values of k. The first derivative of this function is

$$dP/dV = -k/V^2 = (-1/V).(k/V) \tag{2.8}$$

But what is k/V? It is P (equation 2.7). Therefore

$$dP/dV = -P/V$$

or

$$V = -P/(dP/dV) \tag{2.9}$$

The first derivative dP/dV describes 'the slope of the curve', as in Fig. 2.9, where line AB is the slope of the curve at point C.

Return now to our subject in the plethysmograph, breathing against the shutter, compressing and expanding his thoracic gas volume. Plot the simultaneous values of P and V by feeding both mouth pressure and box pressure into an X-Y oscilloscope. The trace will appear to be a straight line (Fig. 2.10). The function on the oscilloscope is in fact the graphical expression of Boyle's law. It is a very tiny segment of a very big hyperbola (e.g. box D, Fig. 2.9). Since it is a very small segment, it resembles (or cannot be distinguished by eye from) a straight line. Its slope $\Delta P/\Delta V$ is a very good approximation to the slope dP/dV of the derivative at a certain point defined by the values P_1—

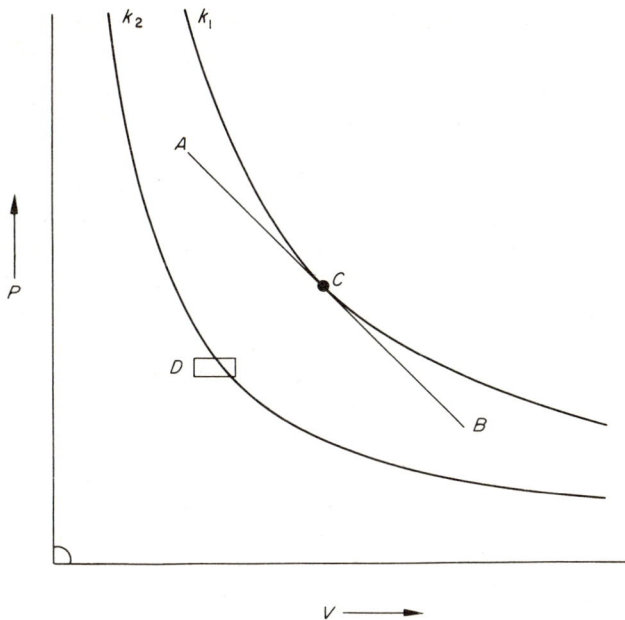

Fig. 2.9. Graph of two hyperbolas $PV = k_1$ and $PV = k_2$. P = pressure, V = volume. Line AB is tangent to graph at point C, equivalent to 'slope' or first derivative of the function at that point. D—see text.

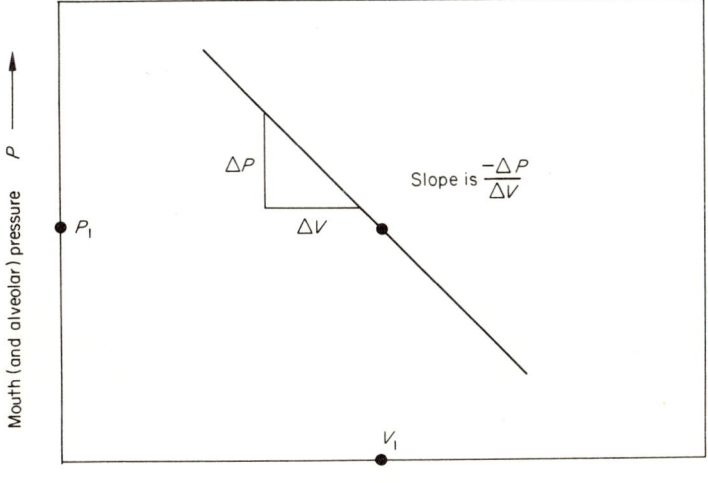

Fig. 2.10. Relation between alveolar pressure P and thoracic gas volume V as seen on oscilloscope screen. P_1 is atmospheric pressure, V_1 is the thoracic gas volume 'around which' the subject has panted.

the atmospheric pressure, and V_1—thoracic gas volume "around which" the subject is panting. Since we can measure both P_1 the atmospheric pressure, and $\Delta P/\Delta V$ from the oscilloscope face, and can make the excellent approximation that $\Delta P/\Delta V = dP/dV$, we can calculate from equation 2.9 the relevant thoracic gas volume.

For the measurement of airways resistance, in a second manoeuvre, the subject in the box breathes through the unoccluded flowmeter. During tidal breathing there are obviously changes in lung volume, but in addition there are, even without the shutter, changes in volume due to compression and expansion, which reflect the changes in alveolar pressure necessary to drive flow. The shifting of tidal volume from inside to outside the chest, in the box, creates no change in box pressure; but the compression and expansion of alveolar gas during breathing does so, and these box pressure changes are again displayed on the X-axis of the oscilloscope, against flow on the Y-axis (Fig. 2.11). (The subject is asked to pant shallowly at about 2 breaths per second, to avoid major pressure changes from warming of inspired gas, and to keep the laryngeal aperture as constant as possible.) In a normal subject, a slightly looped but generally linear response is obtained. The following calculations assume that a perfect straight line is obtained; in practice it is usual to measure the best-fitting slope, by eye, over 0 to 0.5 L/sec in

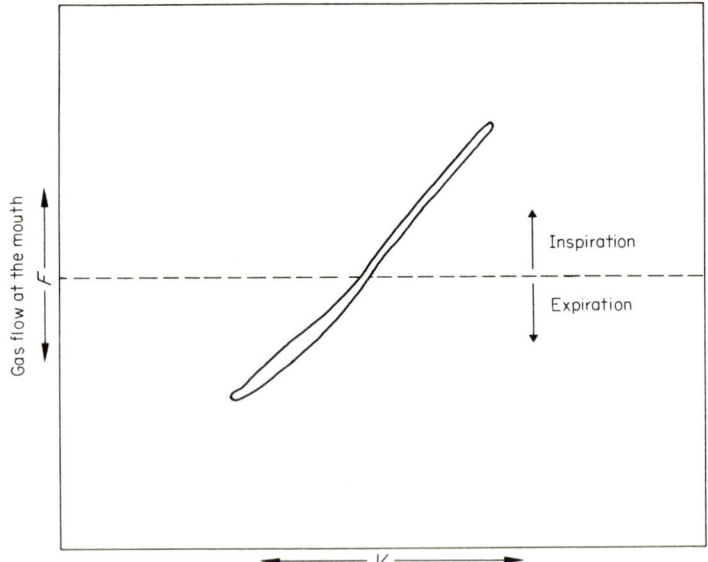

Thoracic gas volume change due to compression/expansion

Fig. 2.11. Relation between gas flow at the mouth and thoracic gas volume change as seen on oscilloscope screen. Airways resistance is derived from the measurement of slope of the inspiratory phase.

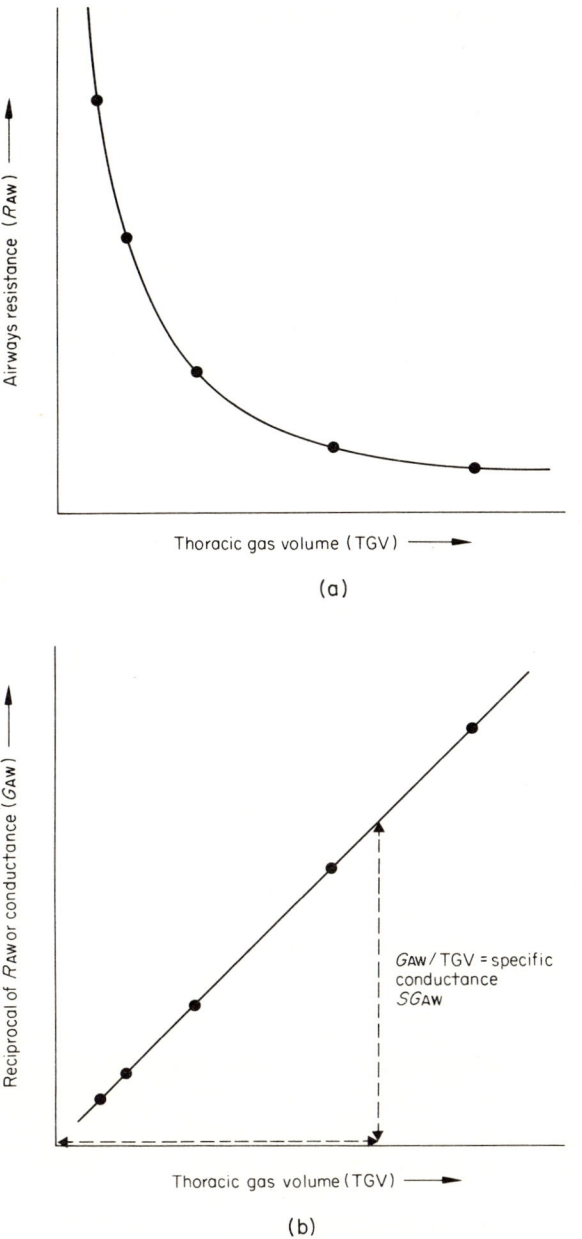

Fig. 2.12. (a) Hyperbolic relation between airways resistance and thoracic gas volume. (b) Linear relation between reciprocal of airways resistance, or conductance, and thoracic gas volume. Slope of this line, provided the line passes through zero, is specific conductance G_{AW}/TGV.

inspiration. The slope, $\Delta F/\Delta V$, relates flow F to thoracic gas volume changes caused by compression and expansion.

We now divide the slope from the first thoracic gas volume (shutter) manoeuvre, $\Delta P/\Delta V$, by the new slope $\Delta F/\Delta V$, and obtain $\Delta P/\Delta F$, which is the slope of the relation between alveolar pressure and flow—or, in a linear system, resistance.

This conclusion often appears somewhat magical. Another way of looking at it is this.

Manoeuvre 1. Breathe against shutter. Mouth pressure equals alveolar pressure, since there is no flow. Obtain relation between box pressure and alveolar pressure; i.e. *calibrate* box pressure in terms of alveolar pressure.

Manoeuvre 2. Breathe through pneumotachygraph. Obtain relation between flow and box pressure, *which has just been calibrated* in terms of alveolar pressure. Substitute calibration factor and obtain relation between alveolar pressure and flow, which is airways resistance.

Specific conductance

Since airways are distensible, they become wider on inspiration and narrower on expiration. Airways resistance varies with lung volume, therefore (Fig. 2.12a), with a roughly hyperbolic relation.

Since the relation is nearly hyperbolic, when the reciprocal of airways resistance, or conductance, is plotted against volume, a straight or nearly straight line is obtained (Fig. 2.12b). The slope of this line is conductance over thoracic gas volume, or GAW/TGV which is called specific conductance, SGAW. It is constant for that particular lung, and is a useful number for making comparisons between different subjects with varying lung volumes. While the use of specific conductance is a reasonable attempt to correct for the effect of lung volume on airways resistance, it is far from perfect, for its use in comparisons assumes that the conductance/volume relation is a straight line which passes through zero, which does not quite occur in normal subjects and is even less true in patients with airways obstruction.

DYNAMIC COMPRESSION, COLLAPSIBILITY AND FLUTTER

The following three sections owe much to an excellent review by Pride [4].

Heretofore we have been considering airways resistance as a number which describes the resistive properties of the airways of the lung, according to the relation

resistance = pressure/flow

(Compare Ohm's Law $R = E/I$.)

One might suspect that an attempt to describe by a single number the resistive properties of an assymetrically branching series of elastic tubes during all possible respiratory manoeuvres would be naive. One would be correct.

Since airways are elastic their size, and resistance, will vary with lung volume. They will expand on inspiration and get smaller on expiration. This first phenomenon holds true under static conditions—during breath-holding the airways at total lung capacity are wider than at residual volume. Thus a single number for resistance can apply at the most to a single specific lung volume.

There is another reason why airways are narrower on expiration, and wider on inspiration, but this only occurs under dynamic conditions, i.e. when gas is flowing.

In Fig. 2.13a is shown a chamber into or out of which air may be made to flow by movement of a piston. Air enters or leaves via an airway which is

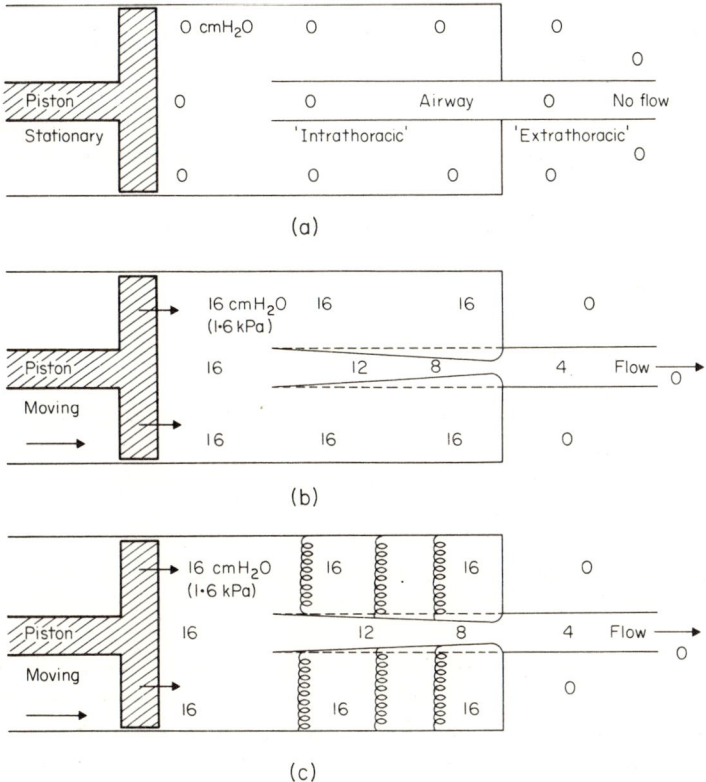

Fig. 2.13. Dimensions of an airway suspended within a rigid chamber: (a) under static conditions; (b) when gas is forced out of the chamber by movement of the piston; (c) when gas is forced out of the chamber but the walls of the airway are supported by springs.

partly inside the chamber ('intrathoracic') and partly outside ('extrathoracic'). In this instance the piston is at rest, and there is no gas flow. Pressure both outside and inside the chamber is atmospheric, taken as reference zero.

In Fig. 2.13b the piston moves to expel air from the chamber, putting up the pressure inside it to 16 cmH$_2$O (1·6 kPa). There is now a pressure gradient down the airway, which is generating flow, and also a transmural pressure gradient across the tube, which tends to narrow the airway. This tendency of the airway to narrow during expiration is called dynamic compression. The degree of narrowing which occurs will depend on two things, the ability of the airway wall to withstand distortion (collapsibility), and the degree to which the airways are supported by the connective and elastic tissue of the lung parenchyma. We have previously drawn the airway as unsupported in the middle of the chamber. In Fig. 2.13c it is shown as supported by springs connecting it to the chamber wall. The stronger (stiffer) the springs, the less the airway will narrow. By analogy in the lung, the greater the elastic recoil the less the airways will narrow in expiration.

If the airway wall were very weak and floppy, and the supporting springs very compliant, the airway might close altogether. This would not be a stable state, for if the airway closes flow stops; if flow stops the flow gradient disappears; if the flow gradient disappears the transmural gradient also vanishes—and the airway opens. Flow would then restart, the gradients would reappear, and the tube would collapse again. This alternate opening and closing of the tube would repeat itself rather rapidly, and is a type of instability known as flutter.

EQUAL PRESSURE POINTS

The previous diagram showed a chamber into which passed a single tube, like an airway. In Fig. 2.14a there is also an elastic balloon-like structure which has compliance like the alveolar part of the lung parenchyma. This model has a pressure outside the alveolus-airway, created by the piston in producing flow, which is equivalent to pleural pressure Ppl. The alveolar balloon exerts elastic recoil pressure Pel. $Palv$, by Rohrer's equation 2.5 is $Ppl + Pel$. Note that in this application Ppl is positive, implying that we are dealing with forced expiration.

Take Ppl equal to 10 cmH$_2$O (Fig. 2.14b), Pel equal to 5 cmH$_2$O, and $Palv$ therefore $10 + 5 = 15$ cmH$_2$O (1·5 kPa). During flow a pressure gradient down the tube is established. At some point the pressure inside the tube will equal the pressure outside (the equal pressure point or EPP [5]). Note that it must occur where pressure inside the tube equals Ppl, and that therefore the pressure gradient between alveolus and EPP equals Pel. The airway downstream from the EPP is dynamically compressed.

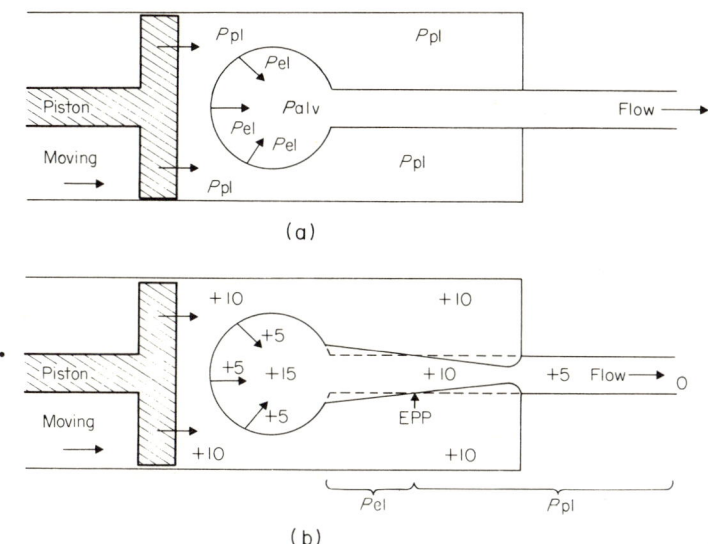

Fig. 2.14. Compare with Fig. 2.13. An elastic alveolar compartment is added. (a) Ppl = pleural (distending) pressure, which is here positive, tending to compress the alveolus, as in forced expiration. Pel = elastic recoil pressure of the lung. $Palv$ = alveolar pressure, equal to $Ppl + Pel$. (b) Figures substituted; $Ppl = 10$, $Pel = 5$, $Palv = 10 + 5 = 15$ cmH$_2$O (1·5 kPa). EPP = equal pressure point.

ISOVOLUME PRESSURE-FLOW CURVES AND MAXIMUM EXPIRATORY FLOW-VOLUME CURVES

We have previously seen that even during quiet breathing a value of airways resistance can only apply at one specific lung volume. During forced expiration, where dynamic compression occurs, the relation of lung volume to apparent airways resistance will be complex, yet it is important to understand it, for the manoeuvre of forced expiration underlies the most commonly used tests of lung function in patients with airways obstruction.

The most illuminating way to examine the problem is to construct iso-volume pressure-flow curves. The subject performs vital capacity manoeuvres with varying degrees of force and rate, with continuous measurement of flow at the mouth and of alveolar pressure (which is again pleural pressure plus separately measured elastic recoil pressure). The values for flow are taken for points of equal lung volume, say 50% VC, from each vital capacity manoeuvre, and plotted against the corresponding values for alveolar

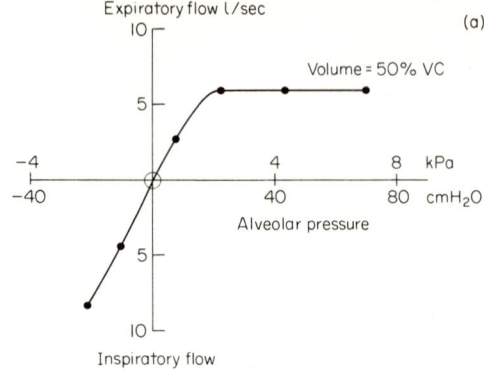

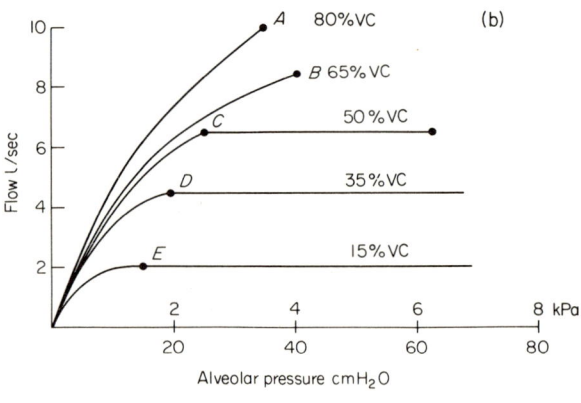

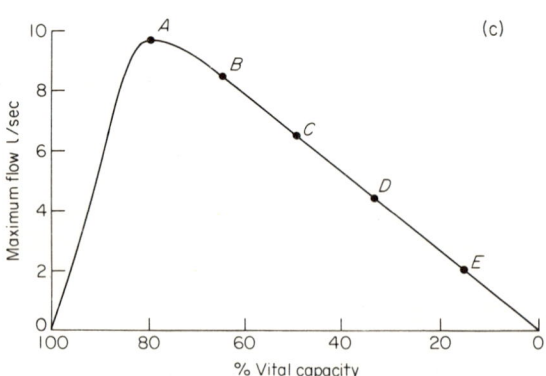

Fig. 2.15. (a) Relation between alveolar pressure and flow at a constant volume of 50% vital capacity. (b) Iso-volume pressure-flow curves at varying volumes. (c) Maximum expiratory flow volume curve. Points *A–E* are replotted from Fig. 2.15b.

pressure, as in Fig. 2.15a. It can be seen that above a certain positive alveolar pressure, here 25 cmH$_2$O (2·5 kPa), further increases in driving pressure do not cause further increases in flow but that a flow plateau is formed. What is happening is that increases in pressure are being matched by increases in resistance due to dynamic compression, so that flow cannot further increase. This phenomenon does not occur at high lung volumes in the upper third of vital capacity in normal subjects (Fig. 2.15b). At 80% and 65% of VC a flow plateau is not obtained.

The information about maximum flow at varying lung volumes shown in Fig. 2.15b may be summarised by replotting as in Fig. 2.15c where maximum flow is plotted against the lung volume at which it was obtained. This display of data may be conveniently obtained in continuous form by asking the subject to expire with maximal force, putting the flow signal into the X-axis, and volume signal into the Y-axis of an X-Y recorder. The volume signal may be simply derived from a spirometer or from integration of the flow signal, but if so will not distinguish changes in lung volume due to compression of gas within the lung, which may be considerable if airways obstruction is severe. It is therefore more precise to obtain the volume signal by plethysmography (p. 14). The plot is called a maximum expiratory flow-volume curve (MEFV curve). Note that the left hand third of the curve is effort dependent—at these volumes, the greater Palv, the greater the flow (Fig. 2.15b, points A, B). The right hand two-thirds of the curve is to a large extent effort independent, for maximum flows will be obtained provided that Palv exceeds 25 cmH$_2$O (2·5 kPa) (Fig. 2.15b, points C, D, E), a pressure obtainable by only moderate effort.

One advantage of studying the lungs under conditions of dynamic compression during forced expiration is that flow is then governed by the gradient between the alveolus and the compressed segment, which in normal man is in the segmental or lobar bronchi. Events downstream of the narrowed segment (like events downstream of a sluice) do not effect the flow through it (or over the sluice). In particular since maximum flow reaches a plateau and does not increase with alveolar pressure after sluice conditions are reached (Fig. 2.15a) and since the driving pressure above the compressed segment of the airway equals the elastic recoil pressure of the lung Pel at the relevant volume (Fig. 2.14b), then the resistance of the airways upstream of the EPP, Rus, can be calculated at a given volume as

$$Rus = Pel/\dot{V}_{max} \qquad\qquad\qquad (2.10)$$

where $\dot{V}_{max}$ is the maximum expiratory flow under sluice conditions.

Since the 'upstream' airways approximate to the intrapulmonary airways, the measurement of Rus is one way of attempting to detect abnormalities in intrapulmonary, as opposed to extrapulmonary resistance.

Rewriting the equation as

$$\dot{V}_{max} = Pel/Rus \tag{2.11}$$

it is seen that the elastic recoil pressure of the lung is an important determinant of maximum expiratory flow. The larger the value of Pel (the stiffer the lung), the greater the possible maximum flow. Another determinant of maximum flow which is not shown in equation 2.11 and is far less easy to quantitate, is collapsibility of airways of the compressed segment.

SUMMARY

While the reader may justifiably feel that the deeper he gets into this subject the worse it gets, the following conclusions are usefully summarised at this point.
1   Airways resistance may be conveniently measured by the Dubois technique of whole body plethysmography (p. 15).
2   Airways resistance varies with lung volume. A reasonable attempt may be made to correct for this by expressing the results as specific conductance.
3   During forced expiration, dynamic compression of airways occurs at the level of segmental bronchi in normal man.
4   This has the effect of creating sluice conditions for flow whereby maximum flow is determined (i) by the resistance of upstream intrapulmonary airways, (ii) surprisingly, by Pel, and (iii) by collapsibility of airways.
5   One advantage is that maximum flow rates over the lower two-thirds of the vital capacity are effort-independent provided a moderate threshold of effort is surpassed.
6   The MEFV curve, over the lower the two-thirds of the vital capacity, is relatively effort-independent, and should reflect events in intrapulmonary rather than extrapulmonary airways.

PEAK EXPIRATORY FLOW RATE AND FORCED EXPIRATORY VOLUME

Peak expiratory flow rate is represented by point A on the MEFV curve (Fig. 2.15c). It is in the effort-dependent part of the curve, and since sluice conditions are not achieved must reflect events in both extra- and intrapulmonary airways. The rapidity and convenience of the measurement with a Wright peak flowmeter is such that it has great clinical importance (p. 205).

Forced expiratory volume in one second (FEV_1) is probably the most widely used measurement of respiratory mechanical function. Flow during the initial part of the forced expiration is in the effort-dependent part of the MEFV curve, but later sluice conditions are reached. Here the value of FEV_1

is determined by the maximum flow attainable and hence by the elastic recoil pressure of the lung and the resistance of the intrapulmonary airways (equation 2.11). It is much less affected by abnormalities in the extrapulmonary airways. Thus, while the FEV_1 is a fairly sensitive measure of abnormal pulmonary mechanics, an abnormal FEV_1 does not necessarily imply pure intrinsic airways disease.

LAMINAR AND TURBULENT FLOW: CONVECTIVE ACCELERATION: THE EFFECT OF GAS DENSITY

Up to this point we have been assuming that flow through the tubes is laminar and is governed by Poiseuille's equation (see below). In laminar or orderly flow, the velocity of molecules in the centre of the stream is faster than at the edges, setting up a parabolic velocity profile. Volume flow rate will increase proportionally to driving pressure (Fig. 2.16a) and the resistance to flow through the tube may properly be quoted as a unique number which applies to all flow rates. Under conditions of turbulent or disorderly flow a bigger increase in driving pressure is required to produce a given increase in flow (Fig. 2.16b). The relation between pressure and flow is curvilinear, and no unique number for resistance exists.

In the first section of this chapter we referred briefly to acceleration, noting that during normal breathing inertive effects could reasonably be ignored. There are two types of acceleration [6]. The first is 'local', referring, as in the first section, to rate of change of either velocity or volume flow with time. This is the sort of acceleration which occurs when you press the accelerator of a motor car. The second is 'convective' acceleration, which occurs when the boundaries of a flow path converge.

The total cross-section of the airways is much larger at the level of terminal and respiratory bronchioles than at the trachea, and if the total cross-sectional area of the airways is plotted as a function of airway generation or of distance from the mouth, the result is rather like a trumpet or even a tin-tack (p. 89). Since each generation of airways is in series with the next up to the mouth, volume flow rate (in L/sec) at the alveolar end will equal volume flow rate at the mouth, but the gas will have to be pushed through a much narrower total channel at large bronchial and tracheal levels than at the alveolar end of the stream, where the total cross-section of all respiratory bronchioles is much greater than the tracheal cross-section. Therefore the linear velocity (in cm/sec) of gas molecules will be much higher at the tracheal end than at the alveolar end. This effect, due to the natural dimensions of the branching airways, will be accentuated when large airways are dynamically compressed during forced expiration. In summary, gas molecules are accelerated as they move towards the mouth and are squeezed into a narrower tube. Naturally a

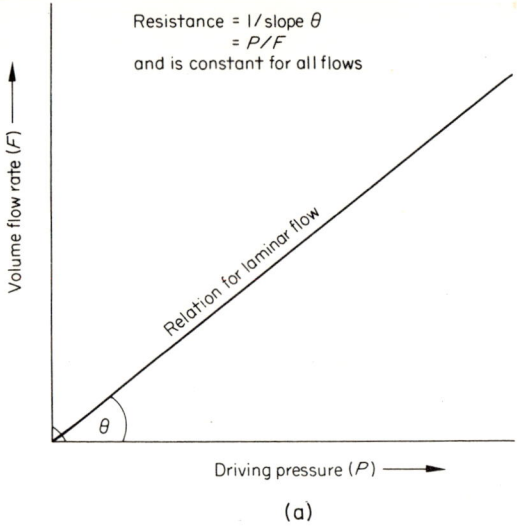

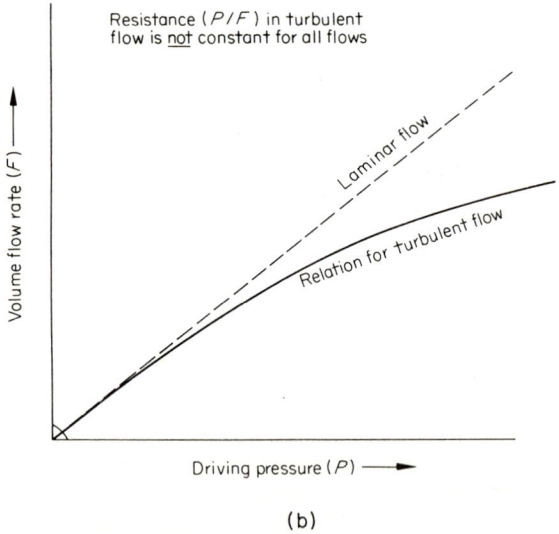

Fig. 2.16. Relation between driving pressure and flow, for (a) laminar and (b) turbulent flow.

force is required to achieve this acceleration. During quiet breathing this force is negligible, but during forced expiration it is not [6].

During forced expiration under sluice conditions the pressure drop from alveolus to EPP (ΔPA–EPP) must be accounted for by pressure drops due to frictional resistance to both laminar (ΔPla) and turbulent (ΔPtu) flow, as well as to convective acceleration (ΔPca).

$$\Delta P_{\text{A–EPP}} = \Delta P\text{la} + \Delta P\text{tu} + \Delta P\text{ca} \tag{2.12}$$

The following equations relate those pressure drops to the major physical variables L, length of tube; D, diameter of tube; DEPP, diameter of tube at equal pressure point; μ, viscosity of gas; ρ, density of gas; and $\dot{V}$, volume flow rate of gas. We find that [5]

$$\Delta P\text{la} \propto \frac{L}{D^4} \cdot \mu \cdot \dot{V}, \quad \text{where} \propto \text{means 'varies with'} \tag{2.13}$$

$$\Delta P\text{tu} \propto \frac{L}{D^{4 \cdot 75}} \cdot \mu^{0 \cdot 25} \cdot \rho^{0 \cdot 75} \cdot \dot{V}^{1 \cdot 75} \tag{2.14}$$

$$\Delta P\text{ca} \propto \frac{L}{(D\text{EPP})^4} \cdot \rho \cdot \dot{V}^2 \tag{2.15}$$

Dividing both sides of the equations by $\dot{V}$, to give resistance on the left-hand side, we have

$$R\text{la} \propto \frac{L}{D^4} \cdot \mu \quad \text{as in Poiseuille's equation} \tag{2.16}$$

$$R\text{tu} \propto \frac{L}{D^{4 \cdot 75}} \cdot \mu^{0 \cdot 25} \cdot \rho^{0 \cdot 75} \cdot \dot{V}^{0 \cdot 75} \tag{2.17}$$

$$R\text{ca} \propto \frac{L}{(D\text{EPP})^4} \cdot \rho \cdot \dot{V} \tag{2.18}$$

and

$$R\text{la} + R\text{tu} + R\text{ca} = R\text{us} \tag{2.19}$$

where Rus is again the total resistance upstream to the EPP under sluice conditions.

In equations 2.16–2.18 it is seen that resistance due to laminar flow is independent of density, while resistance due to turbulent flow and convective acceleration is not. It happens to be very easy to change the density of inspired gas. Oxygen 20% plus helium 80% has a density of only 36% of air, and it is only 12% more viscous. If a MEFV curve is performed first with air, then with helium-oxygen mixture, no great difference should be seen if Rus is mainly due to laminar flow, in fact a small decrease in maximum flows might occur because of the small increase in viscosity. If on the other hand Rus is mainly due to turbulent flow and convective acceleration, then markedly greater maximum flows may be achieved on helium-oxygen mixture: this in fact occurs in normal subjects, for the EPPs are sited in the large bronchi where flow is turbulent and much convective acceleration has occurred. In patients with chronic fixed airways obstruction due to chronic bronchitis, no change in maximum flows on helium-oxygen mixture is found. In them, there is a marked increase in resistance in small airways of less than 2 mm diameter. The EPPs are therefore sited peripherally, in the 'bell of the trumpet', and upstream to those EPPs flow is presumably laminar, with little pressure drop due to convective acceleration.

SURFACE TENSION [7], ALVEOLAR STABILITY [8], AND INTERDEPENDENCE [9]

It is time we made certain definitions.

Force is mass times acceleration (Newton).

$$F = m.a \tag{2.20}$$

The magnitude of a force may be expressed in dynes; or as grammes weight, when it is understood that the relevant acceleration is that due to gravity.

A force may be applied in theory at a point, or in practice over an area. The mean distribution of force over that area is force/cm^2, and is called either pressure or stress. While the units of pressure and stress are identical, the intuitive sense is different. Thus if you take hold of a piece of wood by both ends and push the hands together, you exert pressure; if you pull your hands apart you exert stress. Pressure presses—stress stretches: the units are the same.

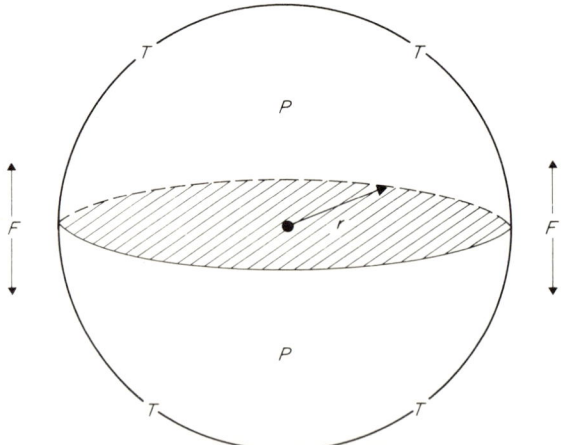

Fig. 2.17. A spherical bubble with radius r. Pressure in the bubble (P) is sustained by surface tension (T) in the wall. F is the force tending to separate the bubble at the equator.

Tension will be used here in the pure sense of surface tension. Since we are dealing with films only a few molecules thick, the area over which the force is applied is less relevant than its length. Thus the units of surface tension are dynes/cm, or force per unit length of film.

It is true that the word tension is widely used as equivalent to pressure or stress, especially in muscle mechanics. This practice can only lead to confusion, and will not be followed here.

Consider a spherical soap bubble of radius r as in Fig. 2.17. Inside it is a pressure P, opposed by the surface tension T in the soap film. The relation between T and P may be obtained by considering the forces tending to separate the bubble into two halves at the equator. This force is P times the area of the section πr^2

$$F_1 = P . \pi . r^2 \tag{2.21}$$

It is opposed by an opposite force, F_2 in the wall of the bubble, namely T times $2\pi r$, the circumference round the equator.

$$F_2 = T . 2 . \pi . r \tag{2.22}$$

In equilibrium

$$F^1 = F^2 \tag{2.23}$$

and

$$P . \pi . r^2 = T . 2 . \pi . r \tag{2.24}$$

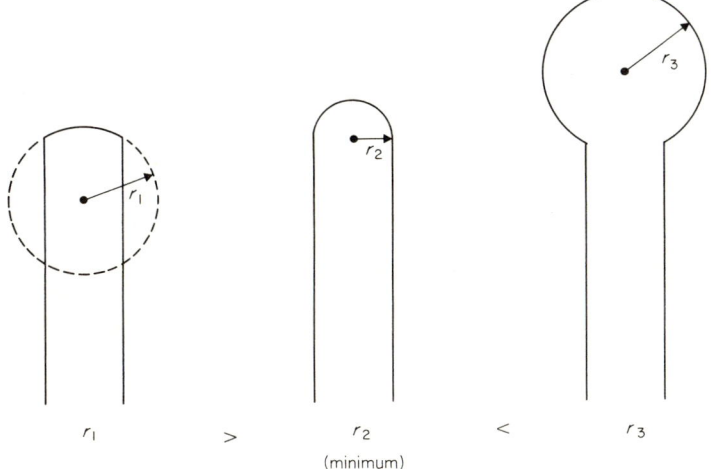

Fig. 2.18. As a bubble is blown on the end of a tube, the radius r starts large, decreases to a minimum when hemispherical, and then increases again.

On simplification,

$$P = 2 \cdot T/r \tag{2.25}$$

which is recognisable as the form of the Laplace relation peculiar to a sphere. Note that this bubble has only one air-liquid interface, i.e. that it is a soap bubble in water. If it were a bubble in air it would have two surfaces, inside and outside, and the tension in the wall would be distributed over twice the circumference or $4\pi r$.

Now consider a bubble on the end of a tube (Fig. 2.18). As the bubble is gradually blown up, the radius starts very large, decreases to a minimum when the bubble is hemispherical, and then increases rapidly again.

Assume a constant surface tension T. What are the pressure-volume characteristics of this bubble?

From equation 2.25, the changes in P as the bubble volume increases will be in the opposite direction to changes in r. Therefore P starts small, gets larger to reach a maximum when the bubble is hemispherical, and then decreases (Fig. 2.19). From the origin of the graph to point P_1, the bubble is stable. A further increase in pressure will burst the bubble, since it does not exist at higher pressures. A further increase in V above V_1 will be accompanied by a decrease in P. The bubble is unstable.

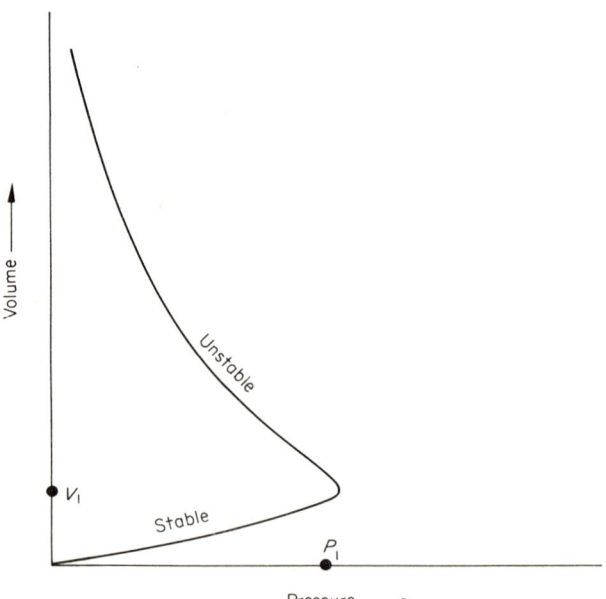

Fig. 2.19. Pressure-volume relation of the bubble shown in Fig. 2.18. ($P = 2T/r$, with T constant.)

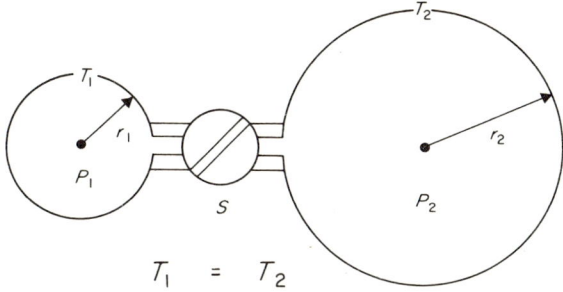

Fig. 2.20. Two bubbles connected by a tube with a stopcock S. Wall tension $T_1 = T_2$, radius r_1 $< r_2$. What happens when the stopcock is opened to allow communication between the bubbles?

Next consider two bubbles connected by a tube which may be opened or closed by a stop-cock, as in Fig. 2.20. Both bubbles have identical surface tension T. What will happen if the stop-cock is opened? Contrary to most people's first thought, the small bubble will empty into the larger one, and collapse. This is because in the bubbles r_1 is less than r_2, T_1 equals T_2, and therefore from equation 2.25 P_1 must be greater than P_2.

It is clearly fortunate that alveoli are not soap bubbles. They are however lined with surfactant substance.

The first difference between bubbles and alveoli is that alveolar walls contain supporting connective tissue with its own pressure-volume characteristics, and the alveoli resemble more an elastic balloon with a soapy lining. Fig. 2.21a shows arbitrary but possible curves for elastic and surface pressures at varying volumes. Since the elastances of lining and balloon are in series, the total pressure may be calculated as the sum of tissue and surface pressures. This is done in Fig. 2.21b, where it is seen that the instability in the surface pressure graph has been ironed out. The elastic balloon is conferring stability over a wider pressure range.

At last, let us come to a real, albeit isolated, lung. If such a lung is alternately expanded with gas and deflated, the pressure-volume relation will show hysteresis, with smaller pressure for a given volume during deflation than during inflation (Fig. 2.22). If the lung is now filled with saline instead of air, and again inflated and deflated, two things happen. First, the whole curve is displaced to the left; second, there is minimal hysteresis. The effect of changing gas for saline is to remove the air-liquid interface and thus to negate the effect of surface forces. We may conclude from the shift to the left that in the air-filled lung about two-thirds of pressure applied during expansion is used to overcome surface forces, and from the change in shape that most of the hysteresis can be accounted for by surface properties.

The surfactant lining the lung has one curious and important property.

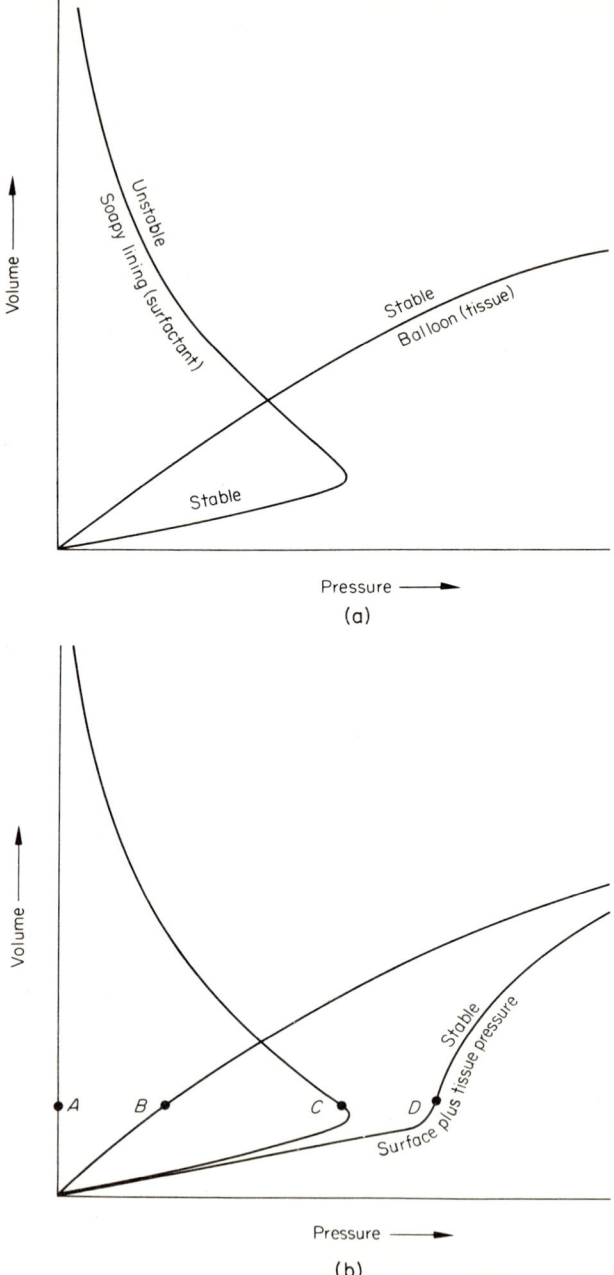

Fig. 2.21. (a) As for Fig. 2.19, with additional curve representing Pressure-volume relation of elastic balloon, or tissue. (b) Surface and tissue pressures are added (e.g. distance AB plus AC gives point D), to give a combined pressure-volume curve. This is stable throughout.

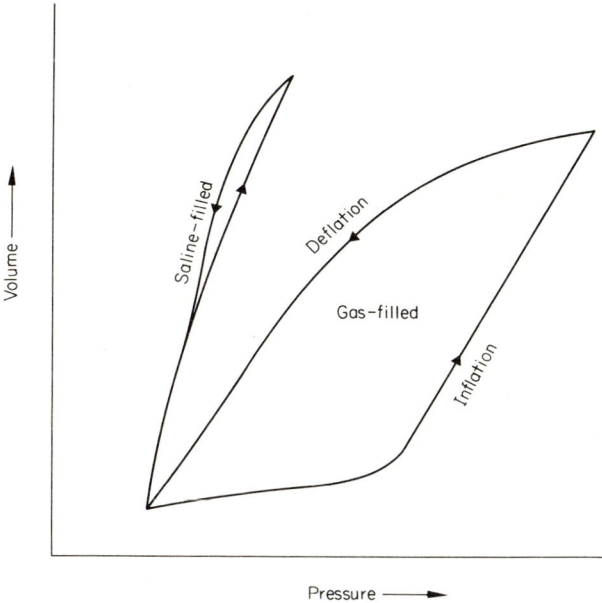

Fig. 2.22. Pressure-volume relation of an isolated lung on inflation and deflation, when filled with gas or with saline.

During inflation and expansion of the film it maintains a constant surface tension of about 40 dynes/cm. During deflation and compression of the film, the surface tension falls to about 2 dynes/cm.

Again from equation 2.25, at a given volume and radius, if T is smaller in deflation, then P will also be smaller than at an identical volume during inflation. This is an important cause of the hysteresis in Fig. 2.22 in the gas-filled lung. Does this matter? It certainly does, for the presence of surfactant accounts for the ability of the lung to remain inflated at the end of the first breath of the neonate. Without surfactant there would be very little human physiology.

Thus, in Fig. 2.23, when the lung is first expanded there is an initial pressure increase with very little change in volume (segment a–b). Here the pressure increase is mainly used to overcome critical opening pressures of collapsed lung units. In the next segment (b–c) the alveoli are filling with air, surface tension remaining constant. During deflation (c–d) the surfactant film is being compressed and surface tension is falling. For a given volume pressure will be less, or, for a given pressure, volume will be more. At zero pressure, air remains in the lung (point d)—the functional residual capacity or FRC. Subsequent breaths (dotted lines) occur using economically small pressure swings, with volumes above FRC. Without the property of the surfactant film to decrease surface tension on compression, at the end of the first breath the lung would not return to point *d*, but collapse completely to point *a*, and for every subsequent breath large pressure changes would be required to overcome the opening pressures of collapsed alveoli.

While these properties of the surfactant are vital for the first breath of the neonate, and deficiency of surfactant in hyaline membrane disease accounts for the tendency to collapse and difficulty of reinflation of the lungs in babies with that condition, the presence of surfactant film is of equal importance in adults as a defence against the natural tendency of airspaces to collapse completely on deflation.

In pulmonary embolism, for example, there is surfactant deficiency in the wedge of tissue beyond the block, accounting in part for the tendency of embolised lung parenchyma to collapse. There is also some evidence that continuous breathing of pure oxygen causes defective surfactant function, which could account in part for pulmonary changes seen in oxygen toxicity.

One further property of the film is that if it is continuously cycled over small volumes, it gradually loses its ability to decrease surface tension on compression, and alveoli tend to collapse completely on deflation. This may be shown to occur progressively during artificial respiration at constant tidal volume, with a gradual fall in arterial oxygen tension due to shunting of blood past collapsed unventilated lung parenchyma. The peculiar properties of the

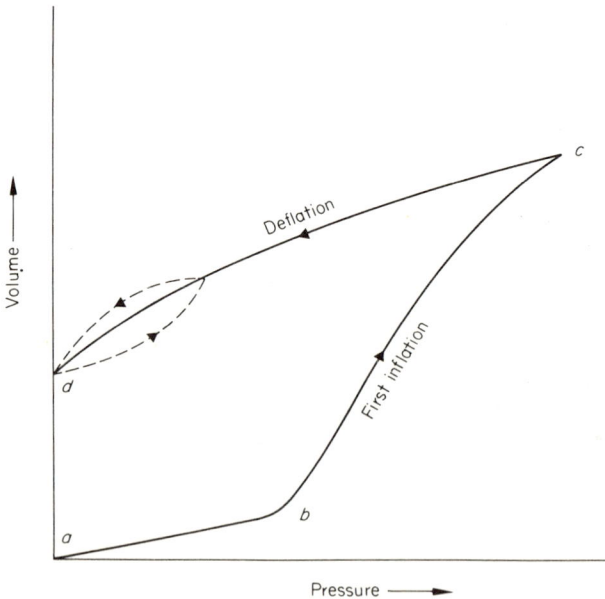

Fig. 2.23. First inflation from the gas-free state in the neonate. See text.

surfactant may be restored by occasional large expansions of the film, during artifical ventilation by periodic hyperinflation, and in real life by occasional sighs.

In summary we have so far considered several reasons whereby alveoli might be unstable and collapse. The first relates purely to geometry and the relation of distending pressure to radius according to Laplace (Fig. 2.19). The elastic properties of the tissue act like splints to iron out unstable regions from the pressure-volume curve (Fig. 2.21). The second relates to the fact that alveoli are connected in parallel, and if they are unequal in size may empty into each other instead of into the airway (Fig. 2.20). Tissue elasticity is again important since it tends to prevent overinflation of one space at the expense of another. The third lies in the tendency (if surface tension were constant) for collapsed alveoli to remain collapsed unless large opening pressures are achieved with every breath (Fig. 2.23). The quality of surfactant to decrease surface tension as lung volume diminishes acts to prevent this.

One further important determinant of alveolar stability remains, and it relates to the fact that alveoli are connected, not only in parallel, but gummed together so that deformation of one alveolus must tend to deform its neighbours in the opposite direction. This property of lung tissue is called interdependence [9, 11] and explains the observation that the specific compliance of the lung, studied within the lung, is smaller than the specific compliance of that segment when separated from the rest of the lung, and of the specific compliance of the whole lung. It is easier to deform a segment of lung in isolation than when it is surrounded by other lung tissue. The relevant mathematics are difficult [10], but the main conclusions relative to alveolar stability are as follows.

1 When the lung is distended at constant pressure, gas pressure in all airspaces is the same. Therefore there are no pressure differences across alveolar walls from space to space. Therefore all distending pressures must arise from tissue attachments.

2 In a perfectly homogeneous and evenly distended lung, the effective distending pressure would be the same everywhere and equal to transpulmonary pressure.

3 In a non-homogeneous lung with local deformations, local distending pressures will differ from transpulmonary pressure in a direction tending to minimise the local deformity.

This is the sort of concept which seems obvious at first sight, but becomes increasingly less so with further consideration. One way of looking at it is this. Since the lung is a highly complex and convoluted meshwork, quite large local deformities can be taken up by tiny compensatory deformities from the vast reserve of mesh.

It is a rather impressive piece of engineering to maintain a sponge with airspaces separated from blood by thin and permeable membranes, and to keep the airspaces dry and open. It seems positively arrogant to arrange to vary the air volume of the sponge by a factor of up to four, sometimes at 30–40 cycles per minute, for many decades. It is perhaps curious that although the effects of splinting by connective tissue, and of variation in surface forces have been studied for many years, only recently has it been realised that the stability of a mesh lies also in the intrinsic mechanical properties of meshes, or their interdependence.

COLLATERAL VENTILATION [12]

It is a surprising fact that if beads of 1–2 mm diameter are inserted down the trachea of a dog so that there is widespread airways occlusion, there is no fall in vital capacity and no fall in dynamic compliance with increasing frequency of breathing. This implies that the tidal ventilation of the parts of the lung subtended by occluded airways is normal and that it must be supplied by collateral routes.

These collateral routes are of two types, alveolar-alveolar (pores of Kohn) and bronchiolar-alveolar.

(a) No collateral ventilation

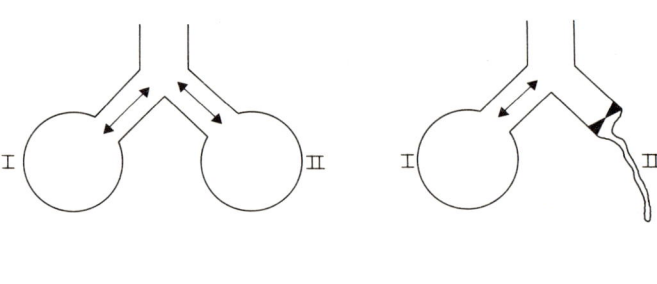

(b) Collateral ventilation

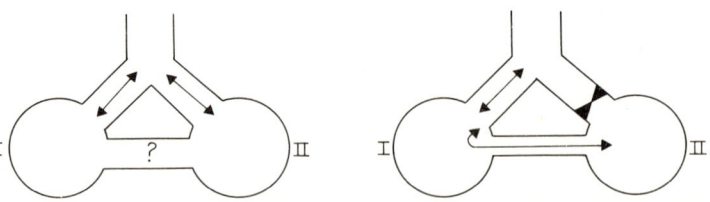

Fig. 2.24. (a) If there is no collateral ventilation, blockage of an airway leads to collapse of the subtended air space. (b) If collateral channels are present, ventilation of both air spaces can continue, but space II is ventilated through space I and therefore its first inspirate will be alveolar gas from space I, followed by further dead space gas from the airway. Contrariwise, all fresh inspired gas to both spaces must pass through space I. Thus the conditions for ventilation of the two spaces are far from normal.

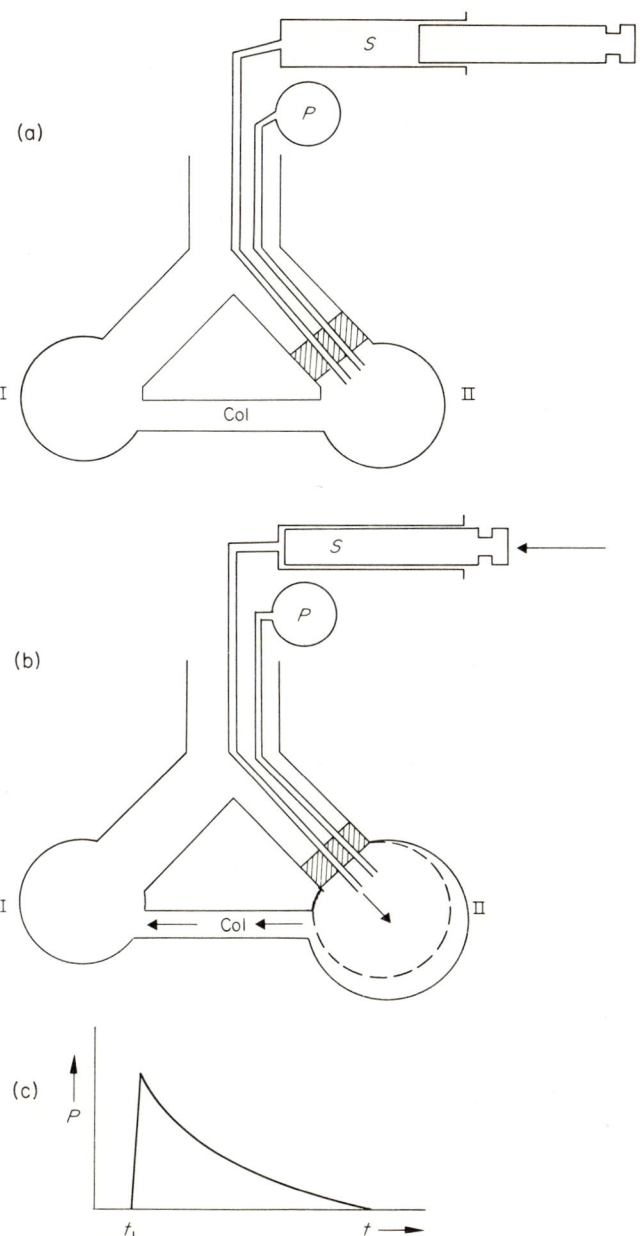

Fig. 2.25. An airway to a segment of lung is blocked by a plug through which pass two catheters (a), one connected to a syringe *S* for inflation the other to a pressure gauge *P*. If the segment is suddenly inflated (b) the pressure in it will rise abruptly (c) and then fall with time. From the exponential decay an approximate time constant for collateral ventilation can be determined.

The degree of collateral ventilation shows marked species variation depending on the development of interlobular septa. Pigs' lungs are highly lobulated, and it is difficult to demonstrate any collateral ventilation at all. The human lung appears to resemble more closely that of the dog in this respect.

The implications of collateral ventilation on the pathological results of obstruction to an airway are important. If a small airway is blocked and the gas distal to it is no longer in continuity with the inspired gas the airspaces will collapse (Fig. 2.24a). If perfusion continues there will be a shunt. If collateral ventilation takes over gas exchange can continue until the airway block is cleared (Fig. 2.24b). This gas exchange will not be normal, for the alveolus through which collateral ventilation occurs will receive more than its normal share of fresh inspired gas while the alveolus into which collateral ventilation occurs receives more than a fair share of dead space.

When an airway is occluded the degree of ventilation of the subtended air spaces depends on the compliance of those spaces and the resistance to gas flow of the collateral passages. This was tested [12] by plugging a catheter into a peripheral airway, suddenly inflating the occluded segment, and watching the time course of decay of pressure within that segment as gas leaked out via collateral channels (Fig. 2.25). From the decay curve estimates of the time constant (resistance times compliance) of the collateral channels were obtained and found to be about the same as the time constant for the whole lung. This does *not* mean that the resistance to gas flow of the collateral channels is no higher than that of normal channels, for the reverse is the case, but reflects the fact that the effective compliance of a lung segment inflated independently of surrounding parenchyma is lower (stiffer) than the compliance of that segment when inflated synchronously with surrounding parenchyma.

This is another aspect of the property of interdependence of the parenchymal mesh, such that when airway obstruction occurs increased forces tend to hold open the obstructed air spaces, and pari passu to draw in ventilation by collateral channels.

REFERENCES

1 MEAD J. (1960) Volume displacement body plethysmograph for measurements on human subjects. *J. Appl. Physiol.* **15**, 736–740.

2 DUBOIS A.B., BOTELHO S.H., BEDELL G.N., MARSHALL R., & COMROE J.H. (1956) A rapid plethysmographic method for measuring thoracic gas volume: a comparison with a nitrogen washout method for measuring functional residual capacity in normal subjects. *J. Clin. Invest.* **35**, 322–326.

3 DUBOIS A.B., BOTELHO S.H. & COMROE J.H. (1956) A new method for measuring airway resistance in man using a body plethysmograph: values in normal subjects and in patients with respiratory disease. *J. Clin. Invest.* **35**, 327–334.

4 PRIDE N.B. (1971) The assessment of airflow obstruction. Role of measurements of airways resistance and of tests of forced expiration. *Brit. J. Dis. Chest* **65**, 135–169.

5 MEAD J., TURNER J.M., MACKLEM P.T. & LITTLE J.B. (1967) Significance of the relationship between lung recoil and maximum expiratory flow. *J. Appl. Physiol.* **27**, 95–108.

6 HYATT R.E. & WILCOX R.E. (1963) The pressure-flow relationships of the intrathoracic airway in man. *J. Clin. Invest.* **42**, 29–39.

7 CLEMENTS J.A. & TIERNEY D.F. (1965) Alveolar instability associated with altered surface tension. *Handbook of Physiology*, Section 3 Volume II, American Physiological Society, Washington D.C.

8 MEAD J. (1973) Mechanical properties of lungs. *Physiol. Rev.* **41**, 281–351.

9 MEAD J., TAKISHIMA T. & LEITH D. (1970) Stress distribution in lungs: a model of pulmonary elasticity. *J. Appl. Physiol.* **28**, 596–608.

10 WILSON T.A. (1972) A continuum analysis of a two-dimensional model of the lung parenchyma. *J. Appl. Physiol.* **33**, 472–478.

11 MEAD J. (1973) Respiration; pulmonary mechanics. *Ann. Rev. Physiol.* **35**, 169–192.

12 WOOLCOCK A.J. & MACKLEM P.T. (1971) Mechanical factors influencing collateral ventilation in human, dog and pig lung. *J. Appl. Physiol.* **30**, 99–115.

Chapter 3. Gas Exchange

The following symbols are used frequently throughout the chapter, and the reader should make himself familiar with them before proceeding.

Relating to gas volumes and flow rates

V, unqualified		lung volume	L
qualified by T, i.e.	V_T	tidal volume	L
A	V_A	alveolar volume	L
D	V_D	dead space volume	L
$\dot{V}$, unqualified		total ventilation rate	L/min
qualified by I, i.e.	$\dot{V}_I$	inspired ventilation rate	L/min
E	$\dot{V}_E$	expired ventilation rate	L/min
A	$\dot{V}_A$	alveolar ventilation rate	L/min
f		respiratory frequency	breaths/min

Relating to gas concentrations

C	blood gas content	L/L
F	fractional concentration of gas	L/L
P	partial pressure of gas, in gas or blood	mmHg (or kPa)

which may be qualified by the following

a	arterial
v	venous
$\bar{v}$	mixed venous
ec	end-capillary
A	alveolar
$\bar{A}$	mixed alveolar
et	end-tidal
I	inspired
E	mixed expired

For example, $P\bar{v},_{CO_2}$ is the partial pressure of CO_2 in mixed venous blood.

Relating to gas exchange

$\dot{V}_{O_2}$	oxygen uptake	L/min
$\dot{V}_{CO_2}$	carbon dioxide uptake	L/min
$R = \dot{V}_{CO_2}/\dot{V}_{O_2}$	the respiratory quotient	

Relating to blood flow

$\dot{Q}$, unqualified   blood flow rate   L/min

qualified by t, i.e. $\dot{Q}t$ total cardiac output   L/min

         s $\dot{Q}s$ blood flow shunted past gas-   L/min

                          exchanging tissues

Other variables will be defined in the text.

SHUNTS, DEAD SPACE, AND ALVEOLAR VENTILATION

Many of the equations concerned with lung gas exchange are based on the principle of conservation of mass and state simply that since mass cannot be destroyed it must be accounted for at the beginning and end of any transport

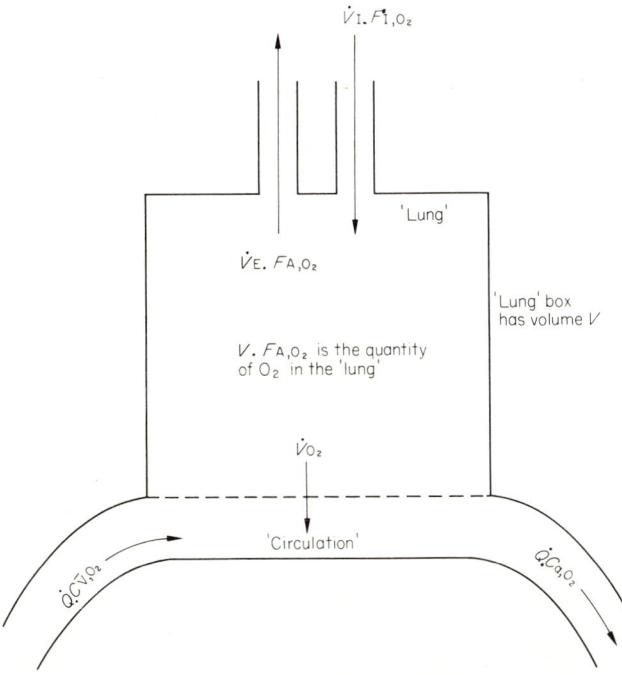

Fig. 3.1. A simple lung-circulation model. O_2 enters in the inspired ventilation $\dot{V}I$ and leaves in the expired ventilation $\dot{V}E$ It passes across to the circulation $(\dot{V}O_2)$, arterialising the mixed venous blood. For other symbols see pp. 42–3 and text.

process. This is not necessarily true on the cosmic scale, but is altogether a sufficient approximation for our purposes.

     In a system where blood flows past a ventilated lung (Fig. 3.1) we may say that the rate of change of quantity of O_2 in the lung, which is the rate of change of fractional concentration $(dF_{A,O_2}/dt)$ times the lung volume V, is equal to the rate of entrance of O_2 to the system in venous blood and inspired gas, minus the rate of exit from the system in expired gas and arterial blood.

$$\frac{V \cdot dF_{A,O_2}}{dt} = \dot{Q} \cdot C_{\bar{v},O_2} - \dot{Q} \cdot C_{a,O_2} + \dot{V}_I \cdot F_{I,O_2} - \dot{V}_E \cdot F_{A,O_2} \tag{3.1}$$

The difference between O_2 ventilatory inflow $\dot{V}_I \cdot F_{I,O_2}$ and outflow $\dot{V}_E . F_{A,O_2}$ is the oxygen uptake $\dot{V}_{O_2}$, and substituting this, we have

$$\frac{V \cdot dF_{A,O_2}}{dt} = \dot{Q} \cdot (C_{\bar{v},O_2} - C_{a,O_2}) + \dot{V}_{O_2} \tag{3.2}$$

If we now suppose a steady state, where F_{A,O_2} is constant, its derivative $dF_{A,O_2}/dt$ becomes zero, and

$$\dot{Q} = \frac{\dot{V}_{O_2}}{(C_{a,O_2} - C_{\bar{v}O_2})} \tag{3.3}$$

which is the steady state form of the Fick equation. The reader should derive the corresponding expression for $\dot{V}_{CO_2}$, C_{a,CO_2}, and $C_{\bar{v},CO_2}$.

Consider now a system (Fig. 3.2) where part $(\dot{Q}s)$ of the total blood flow is

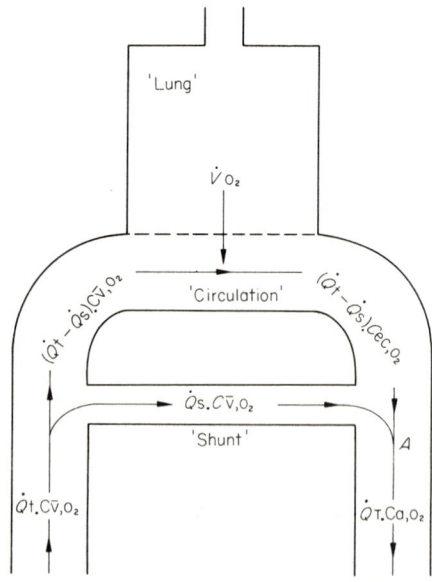

Fig. 3.2. A similar system with a 'shunt' whereby some blood bypasses the lung. For symbols see pp. 42–3 and text.

shunted right to left past the gas-exhanging tissues (an anatomic shunt). Steady-state mass-balance equations around mixing point A in the diagram give

$$(\dot{Q}t - \dot{Q}s) \cdot Cec,o_2 + \dot{Q}s \cdot (C\bar{v},o_2) = \dot{Q}t \cdot (Ca,o_2) \qquad (3.4)$$

and after rearrangement

$$\frac{\dot{Q}s}{\dot{Q}t} = \frac{(Cec,o_2 - Ca,o_2)}{(Cec,o_2 - C\bar{v},o_2)} \qquad (3.5)$$

Thus the ratio between shunted and total blood flow may be determined by measurement of O_2 content of arterial and mixed venous blood, and of end-pulmonary-capillary blood which has undergone gas exchange. (The last, Cec,o_2, is obviously most difficult to sample, and this technical problem is discussed below.) If a separate measurement of total cardiac output, $\dot{Q}t$, is available, the magnitude of $\dot{Q}s$ can be calculated.

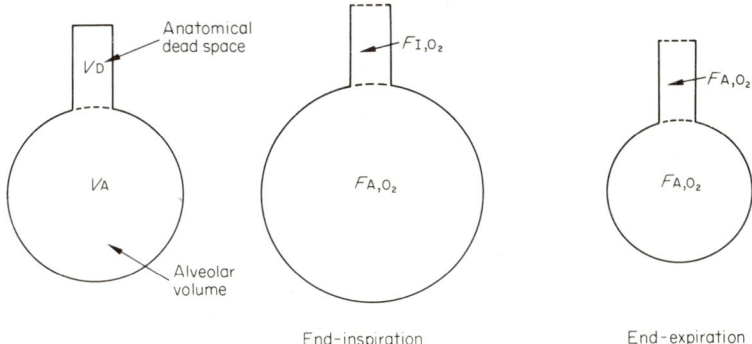

Fig. 3.3. A simple lung model incorporating dead space.

Again in a very simple model (Fig. 3.3) we may consider the lung as made up of gas-exchanging alveolar tissue, of variable volume V_A, and of a fixed volume space in airways where no gas exchange takes place, the anatomic dead space, V_D. After an inspiration the lung contains alveolar gas and the dead-space or airway contains unchanged inspired gas. On expiration, dead-space gas is first driven out, followed by alveolar gas for the remainder of the tidal volume. If the expirate is collected, the amount of CO_2 in it is made up of a portion from the dead space ($V_D \cdot Fi,co_2$) and a portion from the alveolar compartment (($V_T - V_D) \cdot FA,co_2$). Then

$$V_T \cdot FE,co_2 = V_D \cdot Fi,co_2 + (V_T - V_D) \cdot FA,co_2 \qquad (3.6)$$

and on rearrangement

$$\frac{V_D}{V_T} = \frac{(FA,co_2 - FE,co_2)}{(FA,co_2 - Fi,co_2)} \qquad (3.7)$$

Note the close similarity of equations 3.5 and 3.7. They are both 'shunt' equations, the latter also being known as the Bohr equation. In effect dead-space air is 'shunted' in that it is inspired but does not see the alveolus. It is 'wasted' in the sense that it is air which is breathed in – but does no good.

We can now see the concept of alveolar as opposed to total ventilation, in the sense of ventilation of gas-exchanging areas as opposed to wasted dead-space ventilation. Since

$$\dot{V} = V_T . f \tag{3.8}$$

$$\dot{V}_A = (V_T - V_D) . f \tag{3.9}$$

This leads to the 'alveolar ventilation equation', again a mass balance equation, which states that in the steady state the net CO_2 output ($\dot{V}_{CO_2}$) is equal to the difference between the rate at which CO_2 leaves the lung ($\dot{V}_A . F_{A,CO_2}$) and the rate at which it enters ($\dot{V}_A . F_{I,CO_2}$).

$$\dot{V}_{CO_2} = \dot{V}_A . F_{A,CO_2} - \dot{V}_I . F_{I,CO_2} \tag{3.10}$$

and when air is breathed, F_{I,CO_2} is effectively zero, and

$$\dot{V}_A = \dot{V}_{CO_2}/F_{A,CO_2} \tag{3.11}$$

where $\dot{V}_A$ and $\dot{V}_{CO_2}$ are measured in the same units. Since we normally express $\dot{V}_{CO_2}$ as STPD, and $\dot{V}_A$ under BTPS conditions, and remembering that $P_{A,CO_2} = F_{A,CO_2} . (P_B - 47)$, as in equation 3.13b, we have

$$\dot{V}_A \text{ in L/min BTPS} = \frac{(\dot{V}_{CO_2} \text{ in L/min STPD}) . 310/273 . 760/(P_B - 47)}{P_{A,CO_2}/(P_B - 47)}$$

or

$$\dot{V}_A \text{ BTPS} = \frac{\dot{V}_{CO_2} \text{ STPD} . 863}{P_{A,CO_2}} \tag{3.12}$$

There is a hyperbolic relation between alveolar ventilation and alveolar P_{CO_2}—if $\dot{V}_{CO_2}$ is constant. For example, if $\dot{V}_A$ doubles, P_{A,CO_2} halves.

THE OXYGEN-CARBON DIOXIDE DIAGRAM

We will spend considerable time on this concept [1]. It is a highly theoretical approach, and the reader will find that he will frequently ask himself what, if any, its relevance to real life may be. It is justified in the author's view, first because it has given him and others many hours of quiet intellectual amusement, which he hopes some readers may share at a cost of a few pencils and some reams of paper only, and second because its graphical basis allows a visual intuitive grasp of fundamental principles of gas exchange which leavens the underlying mathematical analysis. Since we shall make many simple calculations based on this graph, SI units will not be given in the text, but will be found on the figures.

The total pressure in an air-breathing alveolus, if we ignore the small breath-to-breath fluctuations, is equal to atmospheric pressure P_B, taken as 760 mmHg. At 37°C, 47 mm of this is accounted for by water vapour pressure. The remaining 713 mmHg are taken up by the partial pressures of the resident gases, so that

$$P_{A,O_2} = F_{A,O_2} . 713 \tag{3.13a}$$

$$P_{A,CO_2} = F_{A,CO_2} . 713 \tag{3.13b}$$

$$P_{A,N_2} = F_{A,N_2} . 713 \tag{3.13c}$$

where

$$F_{A,O_2} + F_{A,CO_2} + F_{A,N_2} = 1 \tag{3.14a}$$

and therefore

$$P_{A,O_2} + P_{A,CO_2} + P_{A,N_2} = 713 \tag{3.14b}$$

In the right-angled isosceles triangle of Fig. 3.4, any possible combination of alveolar P_{O_2} and P_{CO_2} may be plotted. The length of the axes (713 mmHg) ensures that neither variable can exceed 713, and the right-hand diagonal bound at 45° ensures that the sum of P_{O_2} and P_{CO_2} cannot be greater than 713. Any point lying on the diagonal bound, such as point Y, has a P_{N_2} of zero. Any point lying within the triangle, such as point X, has a P_{O_2} and P_{CO_2} which can be read off the axes and a P_{N_2} which is equal to the horizontal distance XZ between point X and the diagonal bound. The reader should satisfy himself of these points using equation 3.13 and 3.14 and the properties of similar triangles.

On a part of this diagram (Fig. 3.5a) plot first the inspired air point I (P_{O_2} 150, P_{CO_2} 0 mmHg). Take the respiratory exchange ratio R, which is $\dot{V}_{CO_2}/\dot{V}_{O_2}$, equal to 1·0. Then for any ten molecules of CO_2 coming into the alveolus from the blood, 10 molecules of O_2 will be taken up. For any 10 mm rise in P_{A,CO_2} there will be a 10 mm fall in P_{A,O_2}. All possible alveolar points, for $R = 1·0$, must lie on a line with slope -1, starting at the inspired gas point I.

Taking for example alveolar point A (P_{O_2} 110, P_{CO_2} 40 mmHg), we may easily plot the position of mixed expired gas. If V_D/V_T is 1/3, then the gas expired from the alveoli is diluted by half its volume of gas from the anatomic dead space (P_{O_2} 150, P_{CO_2} 0 mmHg, point I), and the mixed expired point E

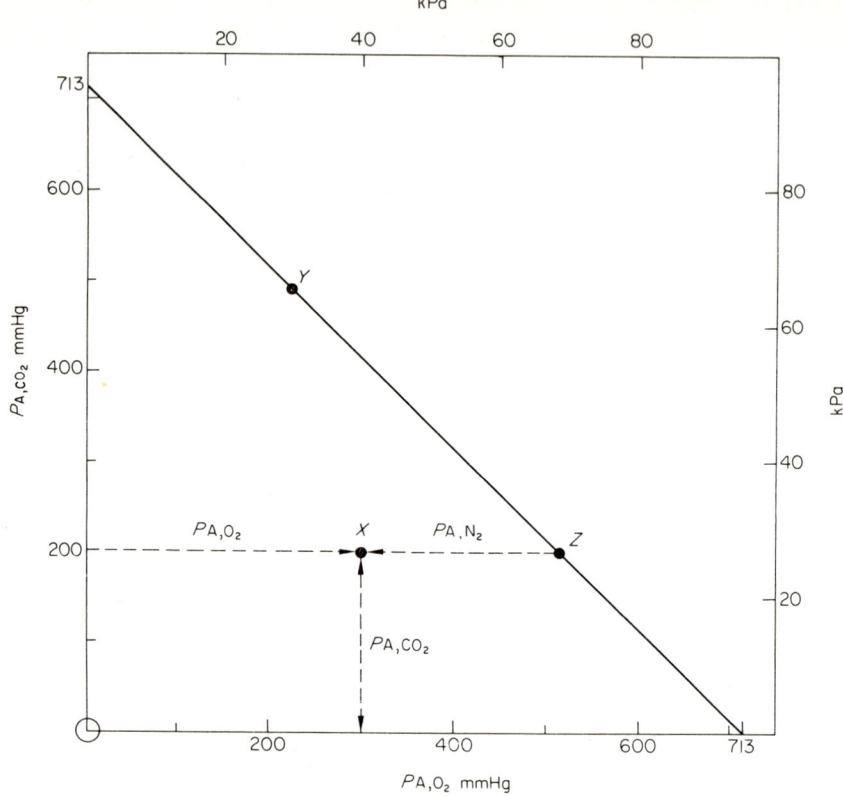

Fig. 3.4. The Oxygen–Carbon dioxide diagram.

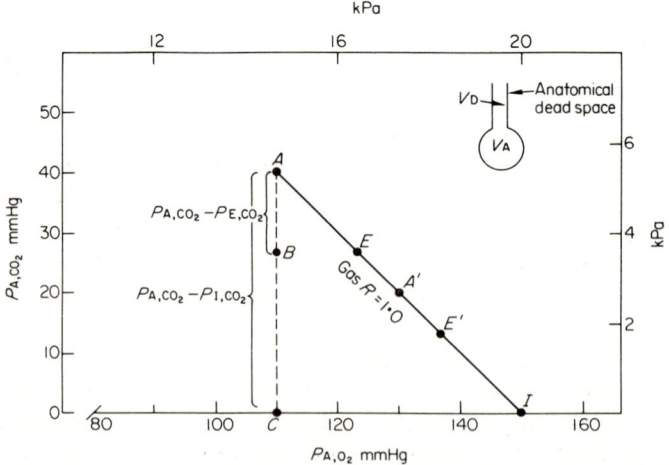

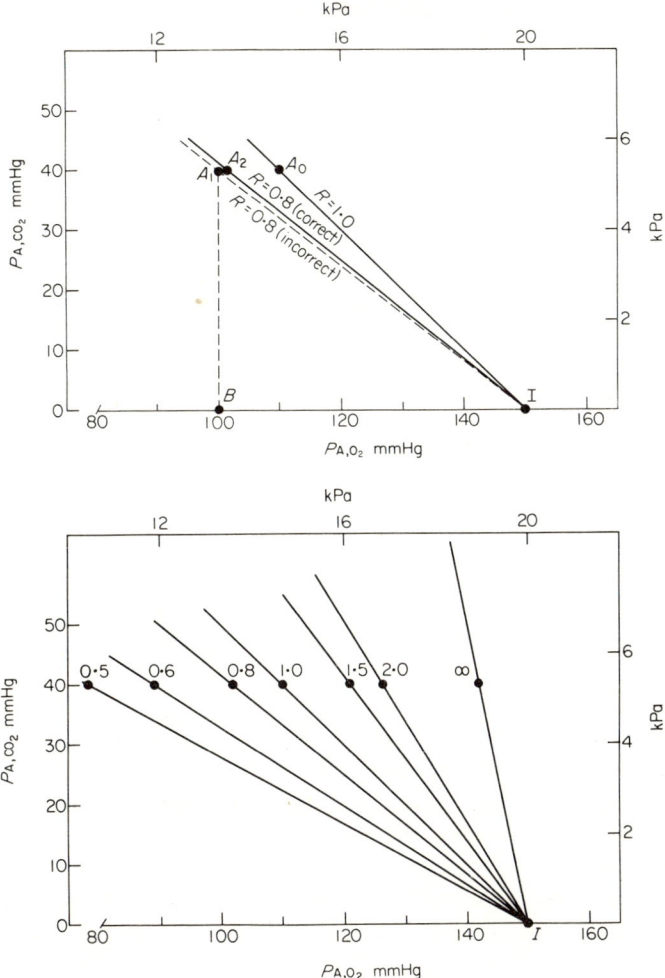

Fig. 3.5. (a) The gas $R = 1 \cdot 0$ line. Effect of added dead space on mixed expired point E, and of change of ventilation on position of alveolar point A. (b) The effect of correction for inspired-expired volume difference (see text) on the gas $R = 0 \cdot 8$ line. (c) A fan of gas R-lines for different values of R.

will be one third of the way down line AI. From the properties of similar triangles,

$$\frac{AE}{AI} = \frac{AB}{AC} = \frac{P_{A,CO_2} - P_{E,CO_2}}{P_{A,CO_2} - P_{I,CO_2}} = \frac{V_D}{V_T}$$

as we have previously shown with equation 3.7 and 3.13b. P_{I,CO_2} is of course effectively zero during air breathing. In general the larger V_D/V_T, the more mixed expired point E approaches the inspired gas point I. If V_D/V_T equals 1, no gas exchange occurs, and E coincides with I. The smaller V_D/V_T, the more point E approaches alveolar point A. If V_D equals 0, V_D/V_T equals 0 and mixed expired point E coincides with point A.

What happens if ventilation is doubled? With $\dot{V}_{CO_2}$ constant, P_{A,CO_2} must halve (equation 3.12) and alveolar point A moves to a new position A' halfway toward I. E must also move to E', one third of the way between A' and I.

Now take R equal to 0·8. Then for every eight molecules of CO_2 put into the alveolus, ten molecules of O_2 are taken out, or if P_{A,CO_2} rises by 8 mm, P_{A,O_2} must fall by 10 mm. Then all alveolar gas points for $R = 0·8$ must lie on a line with a slope of $-0·8$ starting at the inspired gas point I and passing through point A_1, where P_{A,O_2} is 100 and P_{A,CO_2} is 40 mmHg. Apparently if we know P_{A,CO_2} and R, we can calculate P_{A,O_2}. Thus in Fig. 3.5b

$$R = \frac{A_1 B}{BI} = \frac{P_{A,CO_2}}{(P_{I,O_2} - P_{A,O_2})},$$

and rearranging

$$P_{A,O_2} = P_{I,O_2} - (P_{A,CO_2}/R) \tag{3.15}$$

This simple relation is given frequently in the early literature, and unfortunately it is not quite right. The reason for this is that if R is not equal to 1·0, the volume of gas breathed in does not equal the expired volume. Thus over the course of a single breath with inspired tidal volume 0·5 L, and $R = 0·8$, if 16 ml CO_2 were put into the lung, 20 ml of O_2 would be taken out. Then the expired tidal volume is 496 ml. The true form of equation 3.15 can be found by simple but rather tedious algebra [1] and will not be derived here. It is

$$P_{A,O_2} = P_{I,O_2} - \frac{P_{A,CO_2}}{R} + \frac{P_{A,CO_2} \cdot F_{I,O_2} \cdot (1 - R)}{R} \tag{3.16}$$

a form of the 'alveolar gas equation'. The third term on the right corrects for the above problem of volume changes. Note that with physiological values it is rarely more than 2–3 mm, and that when $R = 1·0$, the correction factor is equal to zero, which we would expect since the problem of difference between inspired and expired gas volumes does not arise.

Returning to Fig. 3.5b, calculate from equation 3.16 P_{A,O_2} for P_{A,CO_2} 40 and $R = 0·8$. It is 102 mmHg. The correct R line passes through that point A_2, as shown. By a similar process, starting in each case with $P_{A,CO_2} = 40$, we may build up a table of values of P_{A,O_2} for any R, thus.

P_{A,CO_2}	R	P_{A,O_2}
40	0·5	78
40	0·6	89
40	0·8	102
40	1·0	110
40	1·5	121
40	2·0	126

This enables us to draw a fan of R lines, as in Fig. 3.5c.

In addition look again at equation 3.16 and ask what happens when R approaches infinity, that is when CO_2 is added to alveolar gas without removal of O_2. If you note that $(1 - R)/R = 1/R - 1$, you should be able to see that for $R = \infty$, $P_{A,O_2} = P_{IO_2} - P_{A,CO_2} . F_{I,O_2}$, which enables us to plot the $R = \infty$ line.

If intrigued, try to answer the following questions.
• What is the intersection of the $R = \infty$ line with the CO_2 axis?
• Where is the $R = 0$ line?
• What is the lowest R value possible for an alveolus with P_{CO_2} of 40?

The next step is to plot on the diagram the point corresponding to the P_{CO_2} and P_{O_2} of mixed venous blood (Fig. 3.6), with typical values of, say,

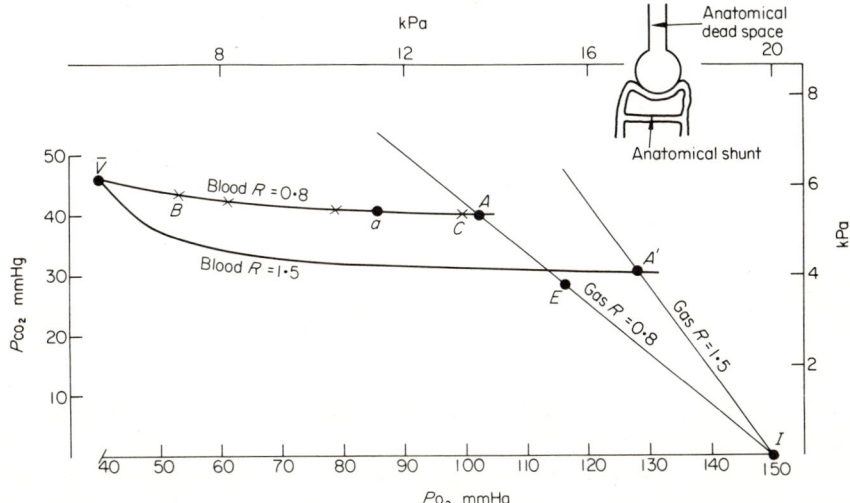

Fig. 3.6. Blood and gas R-lines. Effect of shunt in moving arterial point 'a' along blood R-line, compared with effect of dead space in moving mixed expired point E down gas R-line.

$P_{\bar{v},CO_2} = 46$, $P_{\bar{v},O_2} = 40$ mmHg. The problem is to plot R lines for blood, radiating from the mixed venous point. Whereas for gas this involved merely making one calculation and drawing a line with a ruler, for blood we must calculate a number of points and draw a curve to fit them. This is because in the gas phase the relation between gas partial pressure and quantity of gas is linear, but the relation between blood gas partial pressure and the quantity (content) of gas in the blood is described by the blood gas dissociation curves which are not linear. Therefore in order to derive blood R lines we need some convenient numerical expression of the blood O_2 and CO_2 dissociation curves, such as the Dill nomogram [1] or the Severinghaus blood gas calculator [2]. The precise relative merits of different numerical representations of the dissociation curves are fortunately not particularly important here, for we are far more interested in finding general principles of gas exchange than in an obsessional exactitude in the placement of plotted points.

Then if in mixed venous blood P_{CO_2} is 46 and P_{O_2} is 40 mmHg, $C\bar{v},_{CO_2}$ and $C\bar{v},_{O_2}$ are 0·528 and 0·145 L/L respectively (Fig. 3.7). If this blood

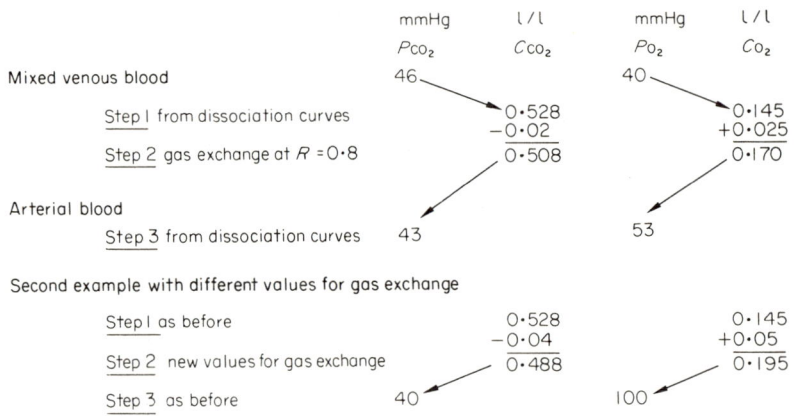

Fig. 3.7. Specimen calculations for plotting blood R-lines.

exchanges at $R=0·8$, 0·02 L/L CO_2 might be lost from the blood and 0·025 L/L O_2 gained, giving by subtraction $C\bar{v},_{CO_2}=0·508$ and $C\bar{v},_{O_2}=0·17$ L/L. From the dissociation curve, P_{CO_2} is 43 and P_{O_2} 53 mmHg, giving us point B in Fig. 3.6 on the blood $R=0·8$ line. A second point C is calculated in Fig. 3.7 and plotted in Fig. 3.6. Others may be also plotted and a line drawn to fit, as shown.

The blood $R=0·8$ line has one, and only one, intersection with the gas $R=0·8$ line at point A, which means that with $P_{I},_{O_2}$ and $P\bar{v},_{O_2}$ fixed, and this particular value for R, in an alveolus exchanging gas in the steady state (where blood $R=$ gas R), there is one and only one possible pair of values for P_{O_2} and P_{CO_2}, 102 and 40 mmHg respectively in this instance. Similar lines may be drawn and intersections found for any other value of R (e.g. $R=1·5$ in Fig. 3.6).

Note now that just as an anatomic dead space (Fig. 3.3) moved the mixed expired point down the gas R line (Fig. 3.5a) according to equation 3.7, so an anatomic right-to-left shunt will move the mixed arterial point to the left along the blood R line according to equation 3.5, say to point 'a' in Fig. 3.6. It must do this because the mixed arterial blood contains red blood which has equilibrated with gas at point A, plus desaturated mixed venous blood from the shunt. Here is a reason why the arterial blood might have a lower P_{O_2} than alveolar gas. Remember anyway that deadspace moves the mixed expired point down the gas R line, and shunt moves the mixed arterial point left along the blood R line.

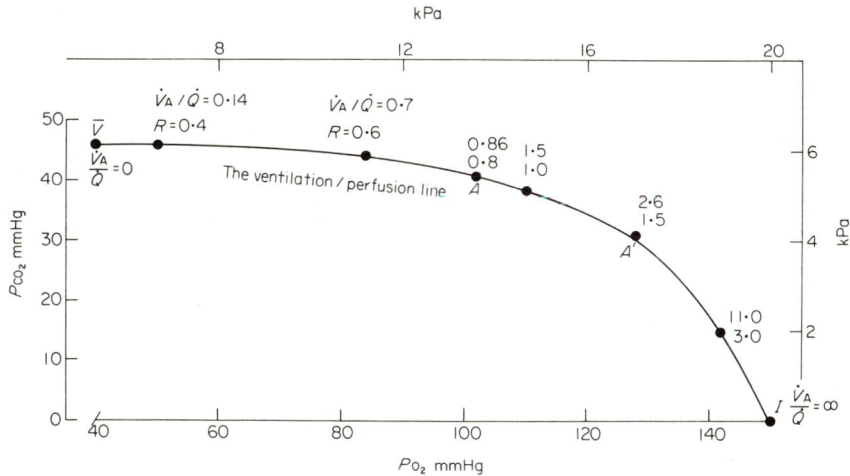

Fig. 3.8. The $\dot{V}_A/\dot{Q}$ line obtained by joining the intersection points of blood and gas R-lines. Any point on the line has a single value for R (lower number) and a single value for $\dot{V}_A/\dot{Q}$ (upper number).

In Fig. 3.8 is a series of intersections between blood R lines and gas R lines. The locus of all such points is a curve joining the mixed venous to the inspired points, and it is called the ventilation-perfusion line. Any point on the line is characterised not only by certain values of R, P_{CO_2} and P_{O_2}, but by a certain value of the ratio of ventilation to perfusion ($\dot{V}_A/\dot{Q}$) for a lung unit exchanging at that R value. The value of $\dot{V}_A/\dot{Q}$ is obtained as follows. We have already seen that

$$\dot{V}_A = \frac{\dot{V}_{CO_2} \cdot 863}{P_{A,CO_2}} \tag{3.12}$$

and that

$$\dot{Q} = \frac{\dot{V}_{O_2}}{(C_{a,O_2} - C_{\bar{v},O_2})} \tag{3.3}$$

Remembering that $R = \dot{V}_{CO_2}/\dot{V}_{O_2}$, we divide equation 3.12 by equation 3.3, and after simplification obtain

$$\frac{\dot{V}_A}{\dot{Q}} = \frac{R \cdot (Ca,_{O_2} - C\bar{v},_{O_2}) \cdot 863}{Pa,_{CO_2}} \tag{3.17}$$

Assume for the moment that the blood leaving a lung unit has the same gas tensions as the alveolar gas, i.e. that $Pa,_{O_2} = Pa,_{O_2}$. Then for each point of intersection on the $\dot{V}_A/\dot{Q}$ line, R is known, $Pa,_{CO_2}$ is known, $Ca,_{O_2}$ is obtained by the dissociation curve from $Pa,_{O_2}$ which we just set equal to the (known) $Pa,_{O_2}$, and $C\bar{v},_{O_2}$ can be obtained by dissociation curve from $P\bar{v},_{O_2}$, which is plotted in Fig. 3.8. The $\dot{V}_A/\dot{Q}$ ratio for each point on the $\dot{V}_A/\dot{Q}$ line is then calculated from equation 3.17, as shown in Fig. 3.8.

Note again the implications of this finding. With inspired and mixed venous gas tensions fixed, for a gas exchanging unit with a given ratio of ventilation to perfusion, that $\dot{V}_A/\dot{Q}$ ratio determines one and only one pair of values for alveolar P_{O_2} and P_{CO_2}, with one and only one value for R. The locus of all these points of differing $\dot{V}_A/\dot{Q}$ is a curve which joins the mixed venous to the inspired gas points. The mixed venous point may be considered to have a $\dot{V}_A/\dot{Q}$ ratio of zero, and the inspired gas point a $\dot{V}_A/\dot{Q}$ ratio of infinity.

The concept of the perfect lung

If the object of a perfect blood-gas exchanger is to move CO_2 from blood to gas and O_2 from gas to blood, in a perfect lung the blood leaving that lung should have exactly the same gas tensions as the gas leaving the lung. Even in normal man, there is in fact a gradient for oxygen between alveolar and arterial blood, and we have already seen one reason for such a gradient, namely a right-to-left anatomic shunt, as shown in Fig. 3.6 where the arterial point is displaced to the left of alveolar point A.

A second and far more important reason is the mixing of blood and gas from parts of the lung with differing $\dot{V}_A/\dot{Q}$ ratios to form mixed arterial blood and mixed alveolar gas respectively. We need only consider mixing from two different lung regions to illustrate the point (Fig. 3.9). Note particularly that there is *no* dead space and *no* shunt, and also that each lung unit is behaving 'perfectly' in that the blood leaving it, here called end-capillary (ec) blood, has the same tensions as alveolar gas. $Pa,_{O_2} = Pec,_{O_2}$, and $Pa,_{CO_2} = Pec,_{CO_2}$. End-capillary blood mixes to form mixed arterial blood: alveolar gas mixes to form mixed alveolar gas.

In the example given, both lung units have been given ventilation of 1 L/min, but the unit on the left has a perfusion of 0·67 L/min giving a $\dot{V}_A/\dot{Q}$ ratio of 1·5, while that on the right has a perfusion of 7·15 L/min, giving a $\dot{V}_A/\dot{Q}$ ratio of 0·14. These two sets of values are chosen not because they are

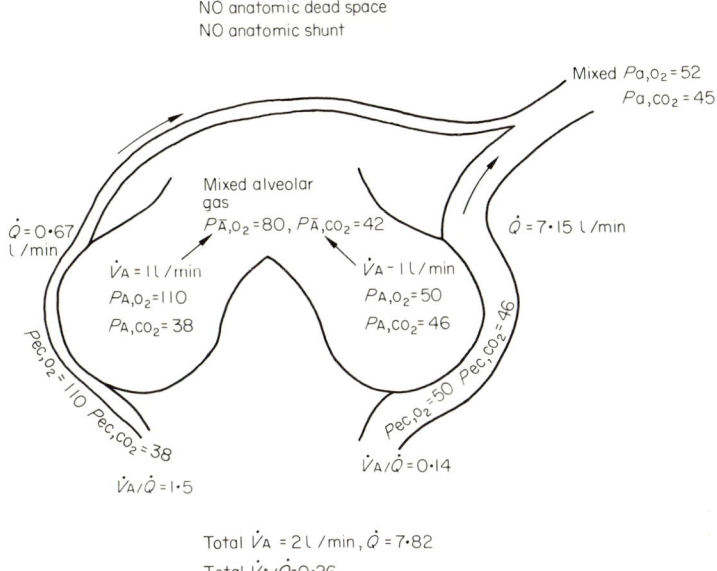

NO anatomic dead space
NO anatomic shunt

Mixed $Pa,O_2 = 52$
$Pa,CO_2 = 45$

Mixed alveolar gas
$P\bar{A},O_2 = 80$, $P\bar{A},CO_2 = 42$

$\dot{Q} = 0.67$ l/min

$\dot{V}A = 1 l/min$
$PA,O_2 = 110$
$PA,CO_2 = 38$

$\dot{V}A - 1 l/min$
$PA,O_2 = 50$
$PA,CO_2 = 46$

$\dot{Q} = 7.15$ l/min

$Pec,O_2 = 110$ $Pec,CO_2 = 38$

$\dot{V}A/\dot{Q} = 1.5$

$Pec,O_2 = 50$ $Pec,CO_2 = 46$

$\dot{V}A/\dot{Q} = 0.14$

Total $\dot{V}A = 2 l/min$, $\dot{Q} = 7.82$
Total $\dot{V}A/\dot{Q} = 0.26$

Fig. 3.9. Effect of mixture of blood and gas from two lung units of different $\dot{V}A/\dot{Q}$. There is no dead space and no shunt in this model.

physiologically particularly likely, but for illustrative reasons, being widely separated on the $\dot{V}A/\dot{Q}$ line. The alveolar gas tensions of these two units are taken from Fig. 3.8 and plotted again in Fig. 3.10a. They are, on the right, Po_2 50 and Pco_2 46 mmHg, and on the left, Po_2 110 and Pco_2 38 mmHg.

The mixed alveolar gas tensions are easily calculated, for since $\dot{V}A$ is equal at 1 L/min for both units, and since partial pressure in the gas phase is proportional to quantity of gas present, the mixed alveolar gas tensions are the mean of the gas tensions in the two units, at $\bar{A}$ (Po_2 80, Pco_2 40 mmHg), halfway along the line joining points L and R in Fig. 3.10a. (If $\dot{V}A$ for one unit were 1 L/min and for the other were 2 L/min the mixed alveolar gas point would be one third of the way along the line.)

Remember the assumption that each of these lung units behaves perfectly in the sense that the blood leaving them has completely equilibrated and has the same gas tensions as alveolar gas. What are the partial pressures of O_2 and CO_2 in the mixed arterial blood from the two units? Once again, because of the alinearity of the blood dissociation curves, we cannot calculate the mixed gas tensions directly on Fig. 3.10a with a ruler and pencil, but must go to the dissociation curve (Fig. 3.10b) on which the points for left (L) and right-hand (R) lung units are plotted.

Point L (Po_2 110) has an O_2 content of 0·198 L/L. Point R (Po_2 50 mmHg) has an O_2 content of 0·164 L/L. Then from Fig. 3.9, every minute

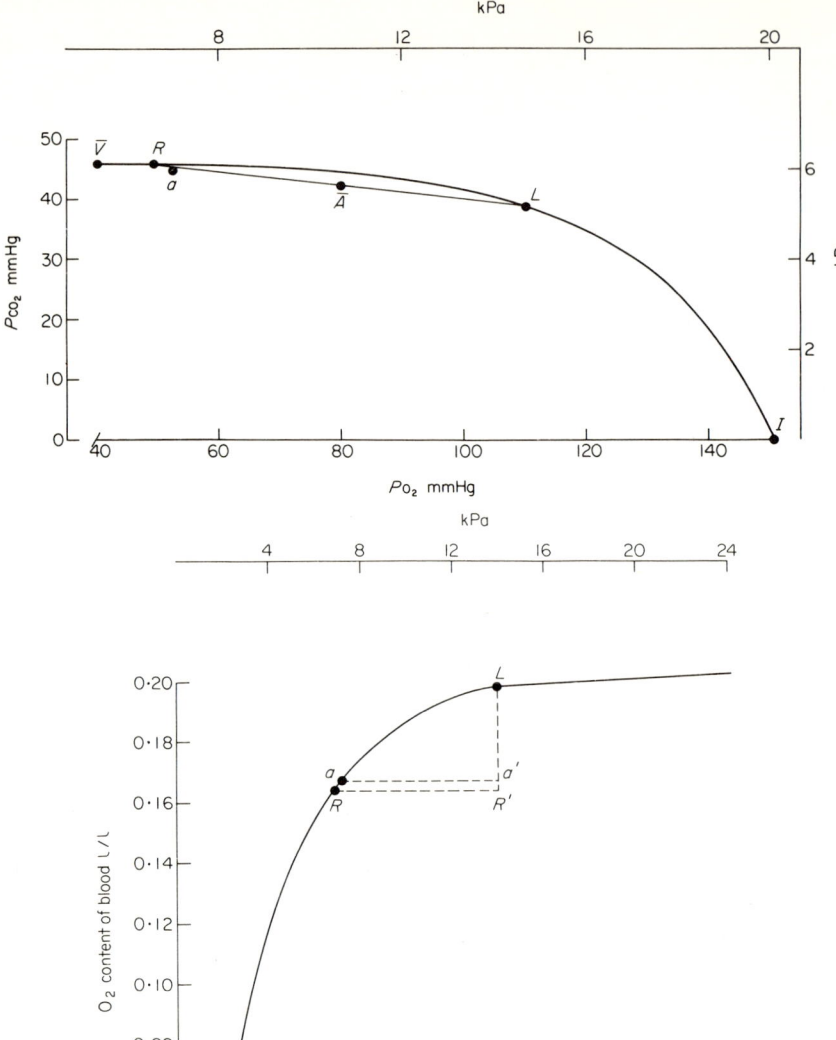

Fig. 3.10. (a) The same two lung units (R and L of Fig. 3.9) plotted on the O_2–CO_2 diagram, with resulting points for mixed alveolar gas ($\bar{A}$) and arterial blood (a). (b) The Po_2 and O_2 content of blood leaving the two lung units (R and L) of Fig. 3.9, plotted on the Hbo_2 dissociation curve.

0·67 L of blood containing 0·198 L of oxygen per L of blood mixes with 7·15 L of blood containing 0·164 L oxygen per L blood. Then the total flow traversing the system in one minute, 7·82 L, contains $(0·67 \times 0·198) + (7·15 \times 0·164)$ L of O_2. Therefore the content of the mixture is

$$\frac{(0·67 \times 0·198) + (7·15 \times 0·164)}{7·82} \text{ L } O_2/\text{L blood}$$

or 0·167 L O_2/L blood

The Po_2 of the blood mixture is read off the dissociation curve as 53 mmHg (Fig. 3.10b, point a). Similar calculations with a CO_2 dissociation curve give a mixed arterial Pco_2 of 45 mmHg. The mixed arterial point is plotted in Fig. 3.10a. But the Po_2 of mixed alveolar gas is 80 mmHg, giving a gradient of 27 mmHg between mixed alveolar gas and mixed arterial blood, even though both lung units were functioning 'perfectly' in the sense that blood and gas leaving each unit had the same gas tensions, and even though there was no dead space and no shunt.

We will now proceed from this physiologically grotesque example to draw general conclusions about the position of the arterial and mixed alveolar points on the O_2–CO_2 diagram.

In Fig. 3.11, 4 lung units with varying $\dot{V}_A/Q$ but with equal $\dot{V}_A$ of 1 L/min

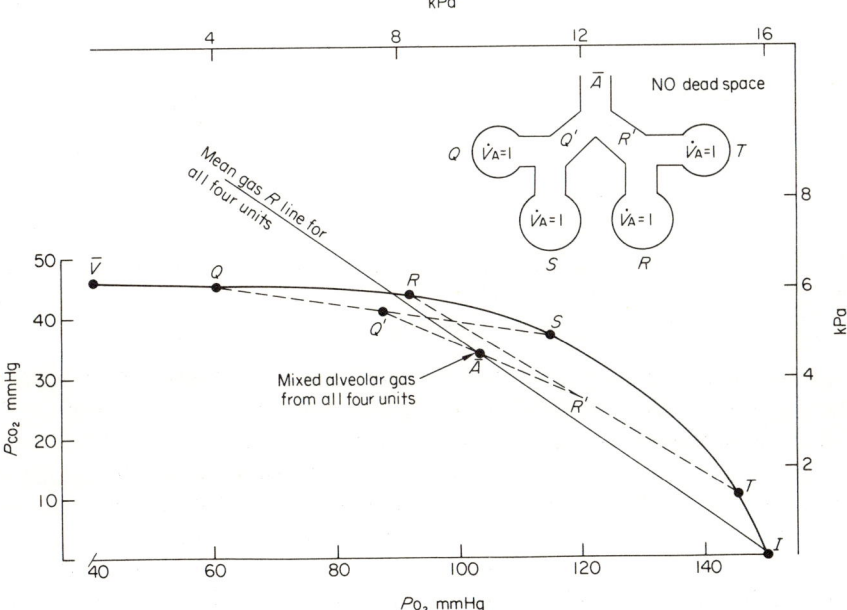

Fig. 3.11. The effect of mixing gas from 4 different lung units, plotted on the O_2–CO_2 diagram. There is *no* dead space in this model.

are shown on the $\dot{V}_A/\dot{Q}$ line. There is no dead space. Alveolar gas from Q mixes with gas from S to give gas of composition Q', with similar mixture of gas from R and T to give R'. The final mixed alveolar gas $\bar{A}$ is half-way between Q' and R', *and must lie on the mean R line for the 4 units functioning together*. Q', R' and $\bar{A}$ are half-way along QS, QT, and $Q'R'$ in each case because the gas contribution from each of the paired sources is the same. The important general point is that mixing gas from lung units of different $\dot{V}_A/\dot{Q}$ values moves the mixed alveolar point down the mean R line away from the $\dot{V}_A/\dot{Q}$ line.

What is more, just as alveolar gas mixture pushed the mixed alveolar point down the mean gas R line, arterial blood mixture from areas of differing $\dot{V}_A/\dot{Q}$ pushes the mixed arterial point to the left along the blood R line, as shown in Fig. 3.12. Compare now Fig. 3.12 with Fig. 3.6. Fig. 3.12 represents a system

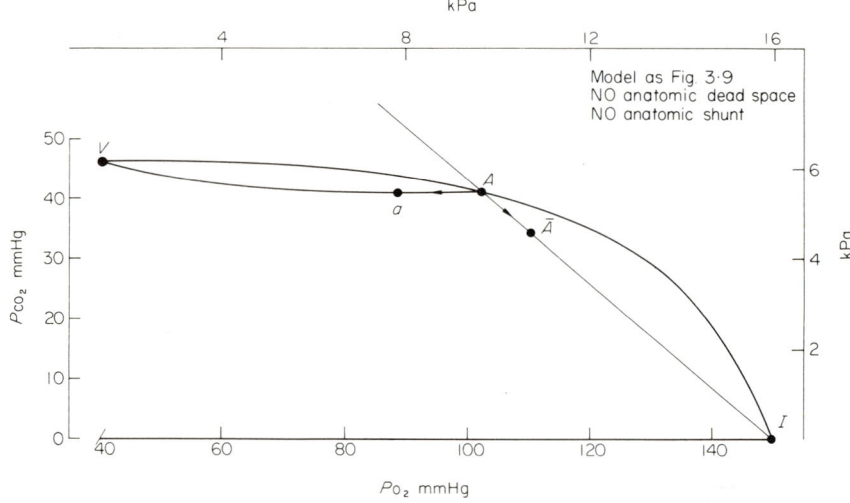

Fig. 3.12. Effect of $\dot{V}_A/\dot{Q}$ mismatch in moving arterial point away from alveolar point along blood R-line, and mixed expired point away from alveolar point down gas R-line, even though no shunt or dead space was present in the model.

with no dead space and no shunt, but admixture of blood from two units of differing $\dot{V}_A/\dot{Q}$ ratios. Yet this system behaves *as if* there were a shunt, in that the arterial point is pushed out along the blood R line, and *as if* there were a dead space, in that a mixed alveolar point is pushed down the gas R line. Indeed, it might be useful to quantitate these $\dot{V}_A/\dot{Q}$ effects in terms of shunt and dead space, and this is what we shall later do.

As a corollary of this argument note that our original definition of a perfect lung as one where the gas and the mixed arterial blood leaving the lung have identical gas tensions demands not only that there be no shunt or dead space, but that $\dot{V}_A/\dot{Q}$ be *everywhere the same*.

At this point we shall define the constitution of 'ideal alveolar gas' as the point A in Fig. 3.12. In a lung of varying $\dot{V}A/\dot{Q}$ units, with shunt and dead space, exchanging in the steady state with a certain identical blood and gas R, with known mixed venous and inspired gas tensions, the ideal alveolar point is defined by the intersection of blood and gas R lines on the $\dot{V}A/\dot{Q}$ line. If there were no shunt or dead space and $\dot{V}A/\dot{Q}$ ratios were the same throughout the lung, the mixed arterial blood and the gas leaving the lung would have the same gas tensions as ideal alveolar gas. The deviations of arterial and mixed alveolar gas from the ideal alveolar point could be taken as a measure of the lung's imperfections.

Two important qualitative effects should now be noted. In Fig. 3.10b look at a normal alveolar point such as P_{O_2} 100 mmHg. If blood from a low $\dot{V}A/\dot{Q}$ area with a low P_{O_2} is mixed with blood at P_{O_2} 100 mmHg, say in equal quantities, there must be an appreciable gradient between ideal alveolar and mixed arterial blood, for the dissociation curve to the left of the P_{O_2} 100 point is markedly concave down. If blood of high P_{O_2}, say 150 mmHg, is mixed with blood at P_{O_2} 100 mmHg, there will be almost no such gradient at all, for the dissociation curve is almost linear to the right of the P_{O_2} 100 point. Thus for purely geometrical reasons, the magnitude of the A–a gradient is much more affected by admixture of blood from low than from high $\dot{V}A/\dot{Q}$ areas.

Look at the shape of the $\dot{V}A/\dot{Q}$ line in Fig. 3.12. The general effect of mixing alveolar gas from different $\dot{V}A/\dot{Q}$ areas is to drive the mixed alveolar point down the gas R line. Taking a normal alveolar point P_{O_2} 100, P_{CO_2} 40 mmHg, note that the admixture of alveolar gas from a high $\dot{V}A/\dot{Q}$ area to the right of the normal point will drive the mixed alveolar point appreciably down the resultant mean gas R line, away from the $\dot{V}A/\dot{Q}$ line, for the latter is markedly concave down to the right of the $P_{O_2} = 100$ point. On the other hand, admixture of gas from points to the left of $P_{O_2} = 100$, from low $\dot{V}A/\dot{Q}$ areas, will have much less effect in pushing the mixed alveolar point down the gas R line away from the $\dot{V}A/\dot{Q}$ line, for the $\dot{V}A/\dot{Q}$ line is much less concave in that area.

Therefore when abnormally low $\dot{V}A/\dot{Q}$ areas are present, the most sensitive measure for detecting them will be a gradient between ideal alveolar and mixed arterial blood (A–a D_{O_2}), which might be expressed in terms of a blood shunt. Contrariwise when abnormally high $\dot{V}A/\dot{Q}$ areas are present, the most sensitive measure for detecting them will be a gradient between ideal and mixed alveolar gas (A–$\bar{A}$ D_{CO_2}), which may be thought of as due to dead space.

This distinction is qualitative only. Since the $\dot{V}A/Q$ curve is *everywhere* concave down, *any* variation in $\dot{V}A/\dot{Q}$ must produce *both* an A–a D_{O_2} *and* an A–$\bar{A}$ D_{CO_2}. The presence of one gradient demands the presence of the other. Nevertheless low $\dot{V}A/\dot{Q}$ shows mainly as A–a D_{O_2} or shunt, and high $\dot{V}A/\dot{Q}$ as A–$\bar{A}$ D_{CO_2} or dead space.

We will now quantitate the effect of $\dot{V}A/\dot{Q}$ variation in terms of shunt and dead-space effects. Having just defined 'ideal alveolar' gas, we now need to know how to calculate its gas tensions. It is relatively easy to collect and analyse mixed expired gas from a subject in the steady state, and to calculate $\dot{V}_{O_2}$, $\dot{V}_{CO_2}$ and hence R. F_{I,O_2} and hence P_{I,O_2} are also known. From the alveolar gas equation (equation 3.16) we could then calculate ideal P_{A,O_2} if ideal P_{A,CO_2} were known, and *vice versa*. Look at the blood R lines in Fig. 3.6, and note how flat they are as they approach the ideal alveolar point. The arterial and ideal alveolar P_{CO_2} are nearly the same, unless the arterial point is pushed very far to the left. It seems reasonable therefore to make the approximation that ideal P_{A,CO_2} is equal to P_{a,CO_2}, and this is what is done. The approximation is excellent unless A–a D_{O_2} is very large. Since P_{a,CO_2} can be measured, ideal alveolar P_{O_2} can be calculated by substituting P_{a,CO_2}, F_{I,O_2}, P_{I,O_2} and R into equation 3.16.

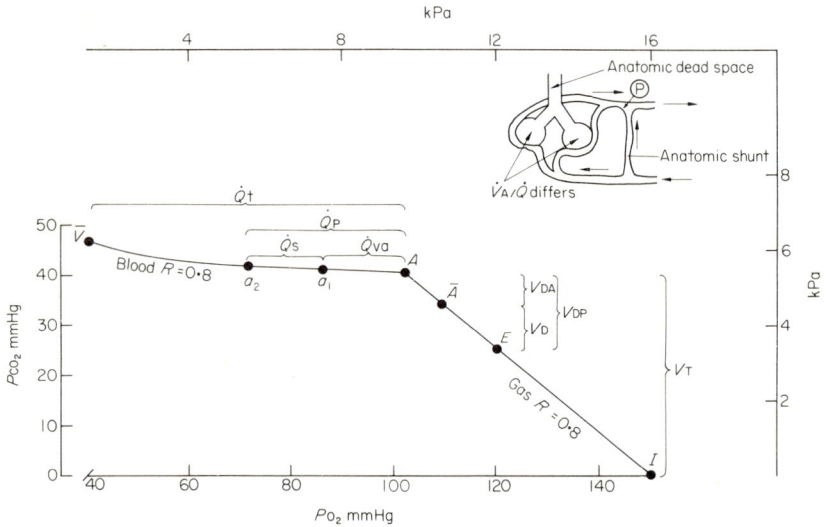

Fig. 3.13. A model with dead space, shunt, and two lung units of differing $\dot{V}_A/\dot{Q}$. Gradients used for calculation of various 'shunts' and 'dead spaces'. See text.

Let us finally examine a model which has dead space, shunt and $\dot{V}_A/\dot{Q}$ variation (Fig. 3.13). The mixed alveolar point $\bar{A}$ is pushed down the gas R line because of $\dot{V}_A/\dot{Q}$ variation, and the mixed expired point E is further down because of dead space. Then by analogy with equation 3.7, or by the graphical method of Fig. 3.5a, and remembering our approximation that P_{A,CO_2} = P_{a,CO_2}, we may define a theoretical 'alveolar dead space', V_{DA}, such that

$$\frac{V_{DA}}{V_T} = \frac{P_{a,CO_2} - P_{\bar{A},CO_2}}{P_{a,CO_2} - P_{I,CO_2}} \tag{3.18}$$

Because of $\dot{V}_A/\dot{Q}$ variation the lung behaves 'as if' there were additional dead space in alveolar tissue.

The anatomic dead space in airways, V_D, is now defined by the following relation, as seen in Fig. 3.13

$$\frac{V_D}{V_T} = \frac{P\bar{A},CO_2 - P_E,CO_2}{P_a,CO_2 - P_I,CO_2} \tag{3.19}$$

The sum of these two spaces, one theoretical, one real, is the badly-named 'physiologic dead space', V_{DP},

$$V_{DP} = V_D + V_{DA} \tag{3.20}$$

$$\frac{V_{DP}}{V_T} = \frac{P_a,CO_2 - P_E,CO_2}{P_a,CO_2 - P_I,CO_2} \tag{3.21}$$

P_a,CO_2 and P_E,CO_2 are easily measured. At first sight $P\bar{A},CO_2$ should be obtainable by measuring the plateau of end-tidal CO_2 on a continuous recording of CO_2 concentration in a single expirate. Actually there are important reasons, which we come to later, why this is unsatisfactory, especially with abnormal lungs.

Therefore by far the commonest measure of dead space in the literature is the physiologic dead space V_{DP} (usually referred to in other texts as simply V_D). Since anatomic dead space does not vary greatly in disease, if physiologic dead space is abnormally high it may reasonably be assumed that this is due to an increase in alveolar dead space, and therefore to the presence of an abnormal proportion of high $\dot{V}_A/\dot{Q}$ areas.

In the same model (Fig. 3.13) the arterial point is pushed to the left by $\dot{V}_A/\dot{Q}$ variation to point a_1, and then further to the left by right-to-left shunting to a_2. By analogy with equation 3.5, we may calculate the total shunt-like effect, which is sometimes called the physiologic shunt, $\dot{Q}p$. Here we take the ideal alveolar P_A,O_2 equal to P_{ec},O_2, and derive the relevant O_2 contents from the dissociation curve. Then (cf. equation 3.5)

$$\frac{\dot{Q}p}{\dot{Q}t} = \frac{C_{ec},O_2 - C_a,O_2}{C_{ec},O_2 - C\bar{v},O_2} \tag{3.22}$$

$\dot{Q}p/\dot{Q}t$ is analogous to V_{DP}/V_T. The implication is that the lung behaves 'as if' a certain proportion of the cardiac output were shunted past it. Part of this shunt is real, the anatomic shunt $\dot{Q}s$. The remainder is theoretical, occurs because of admixture of blood from low $\dot{V}_A/\dot{Q}$ areas, and is often called the 'venous admixture effect', $\dot{Q}va$. If we could calculate $\dot{Q}s$ we could obtain $\dot{Q}va$ by subtraction from a known $\dot{Q}t$. From Fig. 3.13, to do this we need apparently to sample blood at point a_1 (equivalent to point $\bar{A}$ in the previous dead space calculations) which is a theoretical point where blood from alveoli of differing $\dot{V}_A/\dot{Q}$ ratios has mixed, before the entry of the pure venous blood from the true shunt $\dot{Q}s$. This point P is shown diagrammatically in Fig. 3.13, but since in the vast majority of lung disease the true shunt occurs inside the lung, it is quite impossible to sample such blood in real life.

One way round the problem is to give the subject 100% O_2 to breathe. After about 20 minutes, all nitrogen should have been washed out of the lungs and the alveolar gas tensions of all alveoli, whatever the $\dot{V}A/\dot{Q}$, must lie on the diagonal bound of Fig. 3.4 where $Po_2 + Pco_2 = 713$. Since the Pco_2 cannot be higher than that in the mixed venous blood, say 50 mmHg, the Po_2 cannot be lower than 713–50 or 663 mmHg. Then blood coming from *all* alveoli of whatever $\dot{V}A/\dot{Q}$, must be fully saturated. The only unsaturated blood will be that from a true shunt.

Again assuming ideal alveolar equals arterial Pco_2, ideal alveolar Po_2

$$P_{A,O_2} = 713 - P_{a,CO_2} \tag{3.23}$$

Then

$$\frac{\dot{Q}s}{\dot{Q}t} = \frac{Cec,o_2 - Ca,o_2}{Cec,o_2 - C\bar{v},o_2} \tag{3.24}$$

where Cec,o_2 is derived by dissociation curve from Pec,o_2, taken equal to P_{A,O_2} (equation 3.23).

At this stage the symmetry in the various shunt and dead-space equations should be obvious. We may make a table to set the relevant terms in parallel (Table 3.1).

Table 3.1. 'Shunts' and 'Dead-spaces'

Real or anatomic shunt	$\dot{Q}s$	V_D	Real or anatomic dead space
	+	+	
Theoretical shunt due to $\dot{V}A/\dot{Q}$ variation 'venous admixture effect'	$\dot{Q}va$	V_{DA}	Theoretical dead space due to $\dot{V}A/\dot{Q}$ variation 'alveolar dead space'
Total shunt-like effect 'physiologic shunt'	$=\dot{Q}p$	$=V_{DP}$	Total dead-space-like effect 'physiologic dead space'

We shall now leave the O_2–CO_2 diagram, but will return to it in discussion of the practical assessment of defects of gas exchange. (The reader may prefer to proceed directly to p. 72 while the concepts of shunt and dead-space are fresh in his mind, and return later to the intervening material.)

Here are some final problems for keen players of the O_2–CO_2 diagram game.

1   Draw the $\dot{V}A/\dot{Q}$ line with pure oxygen as the inspired gas.

2 Draw the $\dot{V}_A/\dot{Q}$ line with pure CO_2 as the inspired gas. The organism is not allowed to die.

3 (Very difficult) What would be the implications for gas exchange if the O_2 or CO_2 dissociation curves were concave up?

DIFFUSION

Throughout the previous section we have made the invariable assumption that in each lung unit alveolar gas and capillary blood completely equilibrate so that individual alveolar and end-capillary gas tensions are identical. This implies that there is no effective impediment to gas exchange due to diffusion across the membrane, an assumption which at first sight appears poor.

The diffusing capacity D for a gas across the alveolar-capillary membrane is defined in terms of gas volume transported per minute, per mmHg gradient of partial pressure across the membrane.

Thus if the diffusing capacity of a gas-membrane-blood system were 20 ml/mmHg/min, and the partial pressure of the gas was 15 mmHg in the gas phase and 10 mmHg in the blood phase, the rate of gas transfer $\dot{V}$gas from alveolus to blood is $(15-10).20$ or 100 ml/min.

Rearranged,

$$D = \dot{V}gas/(P_A,gas - P_c,gas) \tag{3.25}$$

where P_A and P_c are the alveolar and capillary partial pressures of the gas in question. Both these, and the overall gas transfer rate must be known if the diffusing capacity is to be calculated.

It is the pulmonary capillary pressure which presents the problem, for in the capillary the partial pressure of a gas which is being taken up by the blood is low at the venous end and rises progressively along the capillary as gas transfer occurs. The rate of transfer is highest at the venous end where the alveolar-capillary gradient is maximal, and lowest at the arterial end of the capillary. (Our previous assumption for O_2 and CO_2 is in fact that complete equilibration has occurred in end-capillary blood and that the transfer rate at this point is zero.) In the lung then, the total gas transfer rate is the sum of an infinitely large number of transfer rates deriving from different points with different alveolar-capillary gradients along the course of different capillaries. The relevant gradient to use with the overall gas transfer rate would be the *mean* alveolar-capillary gradient, if one could only calculate it.

Although the difficulties are enormous, methods for obtaining the diffusing capacity of the lung (D_L) for oxygen have been devised. The procedures are tedious, the calculations onerous, and the necessary assumptions more than usually worrying, with the result that this measurement finds no common clinical application and will not be further considered.

A better approach is to use a gas with physical properties which simplify the problem. Such a gas is carbon monoxide, and its special property is that its affinity for haemoglobin is so great that, when breathed in low concentrations, its partial pressure in pulmonary capillary blood is negligibly low and can (with certain precautions) be ignored. Then DL for carbon monoxide is simply the transfer rate divided by the mean alveolar concentration (equation 3.25) of that gas. Mean alveolar concentration is obtained from an end-tidal sample. Transfer rate can be measured in a number of ways, during steady-state CO breathing, during rebreathing or during breath-holding. The single-breath or breath-holding technique is quick to perform, and while the necessary circuitry is complicated the procedure has now been largely automated and is finding increasing popularity in lung function laboratories. The theory behind the calculation is however rather more difficult than that which applies to steady-state and rebreathing techniques, with the result that increasing numbers of respiratory workers are pressing buttons on apparatus which they do not understand and plugging the resulting numbers into an equation which they cannot derive. This seems a pity, and the following section is intended to help such people.

The single-breath test for pulmonary diffusing capacity for CO (DL,CO)

A subject takes a breath of air containing a very little CO and holds it. As CO passes into the blood the alveolar concentration FA,CO falls with time. Starting from the beginning with the mass balance equation, we have

$$VA \cdot \frac{dFA,CO}{dt} = DL,CO \cdot (PA,CO - Pc,CO) \tag{3.26}$$

which states that the rate of change of quantity of CO in the alveolar compartment of the lung is equal to the diffusing capacity times the gradient across the membrane between alveolus and capillary (Pc) blood. Fortunately we may take Pc, CO as equal to zero, and expressing PA,CO as FA,CO $\cdot$ ($PB - 47$) as in equation 3.13, we then have

$$VA \cdot \frac{dFA,CO}{dt} = DL,CO \cdot FA,CO \cdot (PB - 47) \tag{3.27}$$

This equation takes the form of

$$\frac{dy}{dt} - k \cdot y = 0 \tag{3.28}$$

where y is equivalent to FA,CO, and k to

$$\frac{DL,CO \cdot (PB - 47)}{VA}$$

Equation 3.28 is a simple and basic differential equation, applying not only to the transfer of CO from alveolus to blood as here, but also to processes as disparate as the time-course of radio-active decay and the emptying of leaky buckets. The method of solution is given early in any book treating differential equations and will not be repeated here. The solution is [3]

$$y = y_0 . e^{-kt} \quad \text{or} \quad y = y_0 . \exp(-kt) \tag{3.29}$$

where y_0 is a constant, the value of y at time zero, and e is the transcendental number, the base of natural logarithms ($\log_e$), approximately $2 \cdot 718$. Equation 3.29 has the form seen in Fig. 3.14a. Returning to our original variables, we obtain as solution to equation 3.27,

$$F_{A,CO} = F_{A,CO_0} . \exp \left(- \left[\frac{D_{L,CO} . (P_B - 47)}{V_A} \right] . t \right) \tag{3.30}$$

which takes the form of the graph plotted in Fig. 3.14b. The initial concentration of CO, F_{A,CO_0}, occurring immediately after inhalation, falls off 'exponentially' with time as the breath is held.

The problem now is how to make measurements so that we can solve for $D_{L,CO}$ in equation 3.30.

At the next step it is important to realise that the logarithmic ($y = \log_e x$) and exponential ($y = e^x$) functions are inversely related, like the functions $y = x^2$ and $y = \sqrt{x}$. Note that $\sqrt{(x^2)} = x$, and that $(\sqrt{x})^2 = x$ also. Similarly since $y = e^x$ and $y = \log_e x$ are inverse functions, $e^{(\log_e x)} = x$, and $\log_e (e^x) = x$. Many people find this difficult or mysterious, so we will put it into words.

The square of the square root of a number is that very number; the square root of the square of a number is also, equally obviously, that number. We say that these two functions, square and square root, are inversely related. The logarithmic and exponential functions are also inversely related. Thus the logarithm of the exponential function of a number is that number, and the exponential of the logarithm of a number is—that number.

Now take the logarithm of both sides of equation 3.30.

$$\log_e F_{A,CO} = \log_e \left[F_{A,CO_0} . \exp \left(- \left[\frac{D_{L,CO} . (P_B - 47)}{V_A} \right] . t \right) \right] \tag{3.31}$$

and from the properties of logarithms whereby $\log ab = \log a + \log b$,

$$\log_e F_{A,CO} = \log_e F_{A,CO_0} + \log_e \exp \left(- \left[\frac{D_{L,CO} . (P_B - 47)}{V_A} \right] . t \right)$$

$$= \log_e F_{A,CO_0} - \frac{D_{L,CO} . (P_B - 47)}{V_A} . t \tag{3.32}$$

$\log_e F_{A,CO_0}$ and $\dfrac{D_{L,CO}(P_B - 47)}{V_A}$

are both constants.

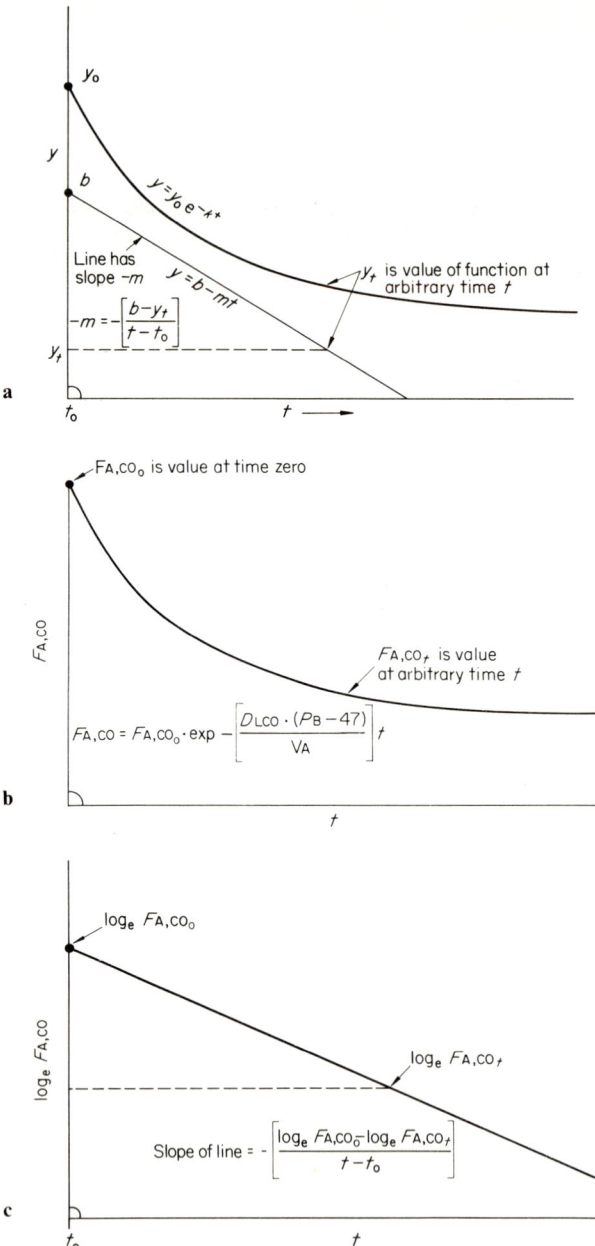

Fig. 3.14. (a) Schematic graphs of $y = y_0\,e^{-kt}$ and $y = b - mt$. (b) Schematic graph of $F_{A,CO}$ $= F_{A,CO_0}\cdot\exp\left(-\left[D_{L,CO}\cdot(P_B - 47)/V_A\right]\cdot t\right)$. (c) Schematic graph of same function as in Fig. 3.14b, having taken logarithms of both sides. This result may be obtained by plotting the function on semi-logarithmic graph paper.

Equation 3.32 has the form of

$$y = b - mt \qquad (3.33)$$

which is a straight line with intercept b on the y axis, as in Fig. 3.14a and slope $-m$. In equation 3.32, b corresponds to $\log_e FA,CO_0$ and $-m$ to $-DL,CO \cdot (PB - 47)/VA$. Thus if we plot FA,CO on a logarithmic scale we shall obtain a straight line with intercept FA,CO_0 on the y axis and slope $-DL,CO \cdot (PB - 47)/VA$, as in Fig. 3.14c. But the slope of this line is also

$$-\left[\frac{\log_e FA,CO_0 - \log_e FA,CO_t}{(t - t_0)} \right]$$

where FA,CO_t is the value of the function FA,CO at some time t, say at the end of the breath-holding manoeuvre. If we take these last two expressions for the slope of the line, equate them and simplify, we obtain

$$DL,CO = \frac{(\log_e FA,CO_0 - \log_e FA,CO_t)}{(t - t_0)} \cdot \frac{VA}{(PB - 47)} \qquad (3.34)$$

FA,CO_t is obtained by asking the subject to breathe out at some time t and sampling the alveolar (end-tidal) concentration, while $(t - t_0)$ is the breath-holding time. What we now need is the alveolar volume in which the CO is diluted (VA) and the initial concentration of CO at time zero (FA,CO_0).

These are obtained by including some helium in the inspired gas and measuring the end-tidal helium concentration (FA,He_t) after breathholding at the same time as the CO concentration (FA,CO_t). Then since helium is not absorbed from the lung into the bloodstream, the amount of helium in the lung at the end of breathholding is the same as the amount which went in with the tidal breath,

$$VA \cdot FA,He_t = (VI - VD) \cdot FI,He \qquad (3.35)$$

where VD is here the apparatus dead space (known) plus anatomic dead space (assumed with little error) and VI is the inspired volume of the breath. Rearrangement of equation 3.35 gives

$$VA = \frac{FI,He}{FA,He_t} \cdot (VI - VD) \qquad (3.36)$$

We now have VA for equation 3.34. Assume next that CO is distributed and diluted as the helium is. Then the ratio of alveolar to inspired helium (which does not exchange with the blood), at time t, is the same as the ratio of *initial* alveolar to inspired CO.

$$\frac{FA,CO_0}{FI,CO} = \frac{FA,He_0}{FI,He} = \frac{FA,He_t}{FI,He} \qquad (3.37)$$

or

$$FA,CO_0 = \frac{FA,He_t \cdot FI,CO}{FI,He} \tag{3.38}$$

We now have FA,CO_0 for equation 3.34. Substitute therefore equations 3.36 and 3.38 into equation 3.34, remembering that a property of logarithms is that $\log a - \log b = \log (a/b)$, and obtain

$$DL,CO = \frac{\log_e \left[\dfrac{FA,He_t \cdot FI,CO}{FI,He \cdot FA,CO_t} \right] \cdot (VI - VD) \cdot \left[\dfrac{FI,He}{FA,He_t} \right]}{(t - t_0) \cdot (PB - 47)} \tag{3.39}$$

This equation may look intimidating, but FI,CO and FI,He are known, FA,CO_t and FA,He_t are measured from the end-tidal sample, VI and $(t - t_0)$ are easily measured, and VD is assumed. All is not yet quite over for the units of measurement do not match, and it is convenient to work in logarithms to base 10, rather than to base e. On the left hand side of equation 3.39, DL,CO is measured in ml STPD/min/mmHg.

$(VI - VD)$ is measured in BTPS,
            therefore multiply the right hand side by $(273 \cdot 713)/(310 \cdot 760)$.
$(VI - VD)$ is measured in litres,
            therefore multiply the right hand side by 1000.
$(t - t_0)$ is measured in seconds,
            therefore multiply the right hand side by 60.

Note that $PB - 47$ occurs in the divisor, and take PB equal to 760. To convert natural logarithms to logarithms to base 10, multiply the right hand side by $2 \cdot 3026$ [4].

Combining all these constants, we finally obtain

$$DL,CO = 160 \cdot \log_{10} \left[\frac{FI,CO \cdot FA,He_t}{FI,He \cdot FA,CO_t} \right] \cdot \frac{(VT - VD)}{(t - t_0)} \cdot \left[\frac{FI,He}{FA,He_t} \right] \tag{3.40}$$

Many people use this equation. A little quiet amusement may usually be otained by asking them what the number 160 is there for. The keen European will doubtless wish to repeat the calculations using SI units.

While the demonstration of the mathematics behind the calculation of single-breath DL,CO is satisfying, the underlying principles of the measurement may have disappeared in the welter of algebra. We may restate them as follows.

1   A known quantity of CO is inhaled into the lung and the breath is held.
2   The initial concentration of CO is determined from a simultaneous measure of VA by helium dilution.

3   The resulting decay of alveolar CO concentration is sampled by exhaling and measuring the CO in the end tidal sample.

4   Provided that the decay has the single exponential form of equation 3.29, the two points F_{A,CO_0} and F_{A,CO_t} characterise that exponential completely (Fig. 3.14b). The exponent $(D_{L,CO} . (P_B - 47))/V_A$ is then defined and $D_{L,CO}$ may be calculated.

Put this way three questions are immediately apparent. First, is the decay, in real life, a single exponential function? The answer is that multiple alveolar sampling experiments show that it is a very reasonable approximation to such a function.

Second, what is this alveolar volume V_A? If we were trying to measure lung volumes by helium dilution, we would ask the subject to rebreathe the helium mixture until equilibration between lung and spirometer had occurred. Here we use a single breath and surely complete equilibration cannot have occurred during the breath-hold. The answer is that it would be better to refer to it as an 'effective' alveolar volume V_A,eff. The helium behaves 'as if' it were distributed in such a volume. Since the CO is 'effectively' distributed in the same volume, the procedure is reasonable and practical.

Third, does not CO transfer continue to occur during inspiration and expiration as well as during the breath-hold? Certainly it does, and correction factors to $(t - t_0)$ may be applied. Cotes gives a full discussion of the technique, these and other assumptions, and correction factors [5].

The interpretation of the diffusing capacity of the lung for CO ($D_{L,CO}$)

Certain diseases are characterised by thickening of the alveolar-capillary membrane, for example fibrosing alveolitis and pulmonary oedema. These conditions are usually associated with a low arterial P_{O_2} and a normal or low P_{CO_2}. Since CO_2 is about 40 times more diffusible than O_2, it was once thought that the arterial hypoxia in such conditions was due to diffusion block to oxygen, CO_2 being relatively unimpeded.

This mechanism is easy to comprehend, and was called alveolar-capillary block, a phrase with an excellent and apparently scientific ring to it. As we will show, it is rare or non-existent.

$D_{L,CO}$ is a *capacitance*-type measurement expressed as flow per unit driving pressure. Its reciprocal $1/D_L$ (driving pressure required to produce unit flow) reflects the *resistance* to diffusion between alveolus and blood. We have so far considered that all the resistance is in the membrane, but in fact part of that resistance is to the passage of CO from the capillary side of the membrane through the plasma and across the membrane of the red cell. The total resistance $1/D_L$ may then be subdivided into two parts; $1/D_M$ which is the resistance across the alveolar-capillary membrane, and $1/(\theta . v_c)$ which is the resistance through the plasma and across the red cell membrane to the haemoglobin. θ is the reaction rate of carbon monoxide with haemoglobin, and vc is the pulmonary capillary blood volume.

Since resistances in series may be added

$$\frac{1}{D_L} = \frac{1}{D_M} + \frac{1}{\theta \cdot vc} \tag{3.41}$$

The reaction rate θ is not a constant. It varies with the oxygen tension in the blood, and the relation between θ and P_{O_2} has been determined in vitro. If $D_L,_{CO}$ is measured at two levels of oxygenation, with the subject breathing air and then a hypoxic gas mixture, and two values of θ are taken from the in vitro data, two equations of the form of equation 3.41 are obtained, with two unknowns, D_M and vc, the values of which may then be calculated. This would seem to be an excellent manoeuvre, since it gives an important variable, the pulmonary capillary blood volume, and separates out the alveolary-capillary membrane component of the lung diffusing capacity. There are however technical and theoretical difficulties which include

1   the calculation of the relevant P_{O_2} from which to obtain θ;

2   the fact that θ is derived from *in vitro* experiments and then applied to an *in vivo* measurement; and

3   the fact that breathing a hypoxic gas mixture will itself cause changes in the pulmonary microcirculation. The equations are simultaneous but the measurements are not.

For these and other reasons the separate measurement of the membrane component of the diffusing capacity and of the pulmonary capillary blood volume has not found a place in standard pulmonary function testing.

We may now usefully make a list of physiologic and pathologic variables which may affect the overall diffusing capacity of the lung D_L.

1   The membrane component D_M. Certainly if the membrane is thicker than normal there will be an increased resistance to diffusion, though not necessarily enough to prevent equilibration between alveolar and end-capillary gas tensions.

Far more importantly, if the area of the alveolar capillary membrane is diminished, the overall transfer rate of CO, and $D_L,_{CO}$ must be diminished also.

2   The pulmonary capillary volume, vc, changes with posture, exercise, certain types of respiratory acrobatics such as the Valsalva manoeuvre, and with disease. An increase in capillary volume tends to accompany a rise in pulmonary venous pressure (mitral stenosis) or an increase in pulmonary blood flow (left-to-right intracardiac shunt). A fall in capillary volume accompanies the loss of capillary bed in severe destructive chronic lung disease. Note that this destruction of capillary bed will decrease D_L by two theoretically separate mechanisms, first by diminishing vc, second by diminishing D_M due to loss of membrane area.

3 The reaction rate with haemoglobin, θ, is proportional to the amount of haemoglobin present. Anaemia decreases D_L,CO, other things being equal. The reaction rate is inversely related to capillary Po_2. The higher the Po_2 in the capillary, the lower D_L,CO.

Plainly there are many other reasons for a decreased D_L,CO than a thick alveolar-capillary membrane. Partly for this reason, many workers in Europe refer to 'transfer capacity' T_L,CO rather than diffusing capacity of the lung. Unfortunately there has been a recent counterbid for the use of the phrase transfer factor by immunologists. While that discipline is certainly invasive, little confusion has yet occurred in context.

Can a thick membrane *ever* cause an alveolar-end capillary gradient for Po_2? It was once widely assumed that in patients with severe diffuse fibrosing alveolitis this did occur. In 1962 Finley, Swenson and Comroe [6] published a study on a series of such patients. They used nitrogen wash-out methods to characterise the ventilation-perfusion abnormalities present and then calculated the arterial Po_2 which should result from the measured $\dot{V}_A/\dot{Q}$ abnormalities. They found that the arterial hypoxia in the patients could be entirely accounted for by the demonstrated $\dot{V}_A/\dot{Q}$ mismatch. This really underlines the importance of the dependence of D_L on the area of membrane between blood and gas. In the limit, if in an experimental animal the left main pulmonary artery and the right main bronchus were tied, the pulmonary diffusing capacity would be zero, although the membrane would be normal.

Thus, coincidentally, those very patients who would be expected to have hypoxia due to 'alveolar-capillary block' by a thick membrane also had severe $\dot{V}_A/\dot{Q}$ disturbances sufficient to account for the arterial hypoxia. A recent paper using different techniques in similar patients did find a few cases where diffusion block might be partly responsible for hypoxia [7].

Can the excess fluid of pulmonary oedema, which may increase diffusion distance from gas to blood, cause alveolar-capillary block? Staub's [8] calculations suggest that if the alveolar Po_2 is high, the alveolar wall thickness sufficient to cause an appreciable gradient between alveolus and end capillary would be so great that the alveolus would be unstable and collapse (thus causing a $\dot{V}_A/\dot{Q}$ mismatch if perfusion continued). In pulmonary oedema the ideal alveolar Po_2 is indeed almost always high since the Pco_2 is normal or low. (Take representative values and calculate P_{A,O_2} from the alveolar gas equation.)

Thus in man, breathing air, at rest, at sea level, even with grossly thickened membranes, the thick membranes are rarely if ever responsible for arterial hypoxia. Yet if one asks a medical student what the causes of arterial hypoxia are, he will more often than not mention first alveolar-capillary block. It would do no harm if this phrase were forgotten.

The reader may at this stage wonder what, if anything, is the point of measuring D_L,CO, since it is affected by a large number of variables which he does not wish to concern himself with, and does not detect the pathological abnormality which he thought was the main object of the exercise. A further problem is the wide range of normal values. Thus, from Cotes [5], if a predicted normal value for DL,CO were 25 ml/min/mmHg, and two standard deviations are ± 10, the DL,CO would have to be less than 15 before we could say with any confidence that it was abnormally low.

Yet, properly regarded and used, it is a very useful test. Regard it, first, as a sensitive test of overall efficiency of gas exchange, admittedly influenced by several variables. Use it, second, in serial estimations in the same patient to assess disease progression or response to treatment, rather than as a single estimation to try and support a diagnosis. The single-breath test is admirably suited to this, for it is rapid, non-invasive, and well-tolerated by the patient.

Thus, one of the commonest uses of the DL,CO is to assess the progress of patients with pulmonary sarcoid and the response to steroid therapy. In sarcoid the alveolar-capillary membrane may be thickened. It is ironic that this is *not* the reason why measurements of DL,CO are used to assess these cases.

CAUSES OF ARTERIAL HYPOXIA

We can now list in reasonable order of importance the possible mechanisms which produce arterial hypoxia, namely

> Ventilation-perfusion mismatch,
> Anatomic (right-to-left) shunt,
> Hypoventilation,
> Diffusion block.

Of these the last we may for practical purposes forget.

In a young normal subject, Pa,O_2 is about 100 mmHg (13·3 kPa) and Pa,CO_2 about 40 mmHg (5·3 kPa). If blood gas tensions and respiratory quotient are measured and ideal alveolar PO_2 calculated (equation 3.6), a small gradient (A–a DO_2) of about 5 mmHg (0·7 kPa) will be found, caused by the small normal right-to-left shunt of about 1% of the cardiac output, and some normal variation in ventilation-perfusion ratios.

The alveolar-arterial gradient for oxygen (A–a DO_2) increases with age, a $Pa O_2$ of 80 mmHg (10·7 kPa) and A–a DO_2 of 20 mmHg (2·7 kPa) being quite normal in an elderly person [9].

Anatomic shunt. If it is required to quantitate the anatomic shunt, this may be done by giving pure oxygen to breathe (p. 62), and sampling arterial and mixed venous blood, the latter by float catheter. It might be thought that in severe emphysema where much lung parenchyma has been destroyed the anatomic shunt would be very large, but surprisingly this is not so [10]. A large shunt may be seen in pulmonary oedema, especially after myocardial infarction [11], and may be partially reversed by a few vital capacity breaths suggesting that alveolar or airways closure may partly account for its presence [12]. Patients with pneumonia or heart failure who require intermittent positive pressure respiration often need also a very high concentration of oxygen in the inspired gas to maintain a Po_2 of more than 50 mmHg (6·7 kPa), and here again large shunts may be demonstrated. Practically, it is rarely necessary for clinical reasons to quantitate $\dot{Q}s/\dot{Q}t$. An abnormal shunt is present when arterial Po_2 is surprisingly low even with high concentrations of O_2 in the inspired gas. Thus with pure oxygen inspired, in normal lungs, Pa,o_2 should be more than 600 mmHg (80kPa); with 60% oxygen (nasal catheter or M–C Mask) the Pa,o_2 should be more than 350 mmHg (47 kPa). An arterial Po_2 of less than 150 and 100 mmHg respectively (20 and 13·3 kPa) suggests an important degree of true shunting.

Hypoventilation. By this we mean that *alveolar ventilation* $\dot{V}A$ (equation 3.9) is too low to maintain a normal Pa,co_2, which must therefore rise. (We do not refer to total ventilation $\dot{V}$ (equation 3.8) which is related to alveolar ventilation by the size of the dead space (equation 3.9), in this case the physiologic dead space since we are referring to arterial Pco_2 (equation 3.21)).

If Pa,co_2 rises, Pa,o_2 must fall. The question is, when interpreting blood gas measurements which show high Pa,co_2 and low Pa,o_2, is all of the hypoxia due to the hypoventilation, or is some of it due to other factors?

While the effect of changing ventilation is to move the alveolar point up or down the gas R-line (Fig. 3.5a) it should not change the magnitude of A–a Do_2 much. Therefore in a patient with high Pa,co_2 and low Po_2, if the A–a Do_2 is normal, it is reasonable to assume that the hypoxia is entirely accounted for by hypoventilation. In clinical practice it is rarely possible to make a rigorous measurement of A–a Do_2, either because the apparatus or personnel is unavailable or because the patient is too ill for the collection of expired gas. It turns out that a reasonable estimate of A–a Do_2 may be made by adding Pa,co_2 and Po_2 together and subtracting the sum from 140 mmHg (18·7 kPa). Then as a simple rule of thumb if that estimate of A–a Do_2 is greater than 20 mmHg (2·7 kPa), suspect an important cause of arterial hypoxia other than known hypoventilation.

Ventilation-perfusion mismatch. This is the most important cause in more than 90% of cases with arterial hypoxia in clinical practice. It is possible to assess the magnitude of importance of the mismatch in producing hypoxia by collecting and analysing expired gas, arterial and mixed venous blood, and calculating the physiologic shunt $\dot{Q}p/\dot{Q}t$, then giving pure O_2 to breathe and from similar collections and analyses calculating $\dot{Q}s/\dot{Q}t$ (pp. 61–2). The difference is $\dot{Q}va/\dot{Q}t$, the venous admixture effect of ventilation-perfusion mismatch. This is rarely done in clinical practice. A simpler approach is to regard ventilation-perfusion mismatch as the cause of arterial hypoxia in the absence of evidence for hypoventilation or anatomic shunt.

Then a logical approach to blood gas results which show hypoxia would be as follows.

1   Disregard diffusion block as a possibility.

2   Is Pa,co_2 high?

   (a) If so, alveolar hypoventilation accounts for at least part of the hypoxia.

   (b) Is hypoventilation the only cause of the hypoxia? Add Pa,o_2 to Pa,co_2 and subtract the sum from 140 mmHg (18·7 kPa). If the answer is less than 20 mmHg (2·7 kPa), hypoventilation is probably the only important cause of hypoxia, and some measure of improving ventilation alone may bring Pao_2 to a satisfactory level. If the answer is more than 20 mmHg (2·7 kPa) some other important abnormality is present other than hypoventilation; it must be either shunt or $\dot{V}A/\dot{Q}$ mismatch.

   (c) Be cautious with oxygen administration (p. 236).

3   Is Pa,co_2 normal or low?

   (a) If so, the cause of hypoxia is anatomic shunt and/or $\dot{V}A/\dot{Q}$ mismatch.

   (b) Give oxygen in high concentration. If Pa,o_2 remains below 150 mmHg (20 kPa) on 100% O_2 or below 100 mmHg (13·3 kPa) on 60% O_2, suspect an important increase in anatomic shunt. If Pa,o_2 rises above those levels, ventilation-perfusion mismatch is the *only* important cause of the hypoxia.

DISTRIBUTION OF VENTILATION AND PERFUSION WITHIN THE LUNG [13]

Distribution of blood flow

Effect of gravity on flow through alveolar capillaries

Most of the work describing distribution of blood flow is based on techniques of radio-active gas measurement. If a solution of xenon-133 is injected into a peripheral vein it will be carried to the lung capillaries and since it is highly insoluble will pass immediately into the alveolar gas. The more the blood flow to a given part of the lung, the more xenon will arrive in the alveoli there. After the injection the lungs are scanned from top to bottom with moving pairs of counters. The counts obtained at each level in the lung are proportional to the blood flow to that level. Then the subject rebreathes into a spirometer until the xenon has equilibrated, when its concentration is the same throughout the lung-spirometer system. Again the lungs are scanned. Since the concentration of xenon in all alveoli is the same, the counts obtained at each level in the lung are now proportional to the volume of alveoli at that level. Further calculations using both sets of counts will then give blood flow per unit alveolar volume. Such measurements made on erect normal man show that the pulmonary blood flow per unit lung volume is very small or zero at the apices of the lungs, gradually increasing down the lung towards the bases.

The reasons for this distribution of pulmonary arterial flow within the lung were elucidated in a series of papers by West and colleagues [13] using an isolated dog lung preparation which could be ventilated or held at known alveolar pressures and perfused with control of flow rate, and of arterial and venous pressures (Fig. 3.15a). The lungs may be scanned after injection of xenon on the venous side, with the respirator temporarily stopped. Alveolar pressure is then everywhere zero in reference to atmospheric pressure. It is then instructive to divide the lung into three zones (Fig. 3.15b).

In zone I alveolar pressure is greater than pulmonary artery pressure, which is greater than pulmonary venous pressure ($PA > Pa > Pv$). In essence, the pulmonary artery pressure is in this zone insufficiently high to pump blood to the top of the lung, and there is no blood flow to zone I, the pulmonary capillaries being collapsed.

In zone II alveolar pressure is lower than pulmonary artery pressure, but still higher than pulmonary venous pressure ($Pa > PA > Pv$). Here the lung capillaries behave like a floppy tube in a Starling resistor. The equilibrium position of a floppy tube is that where the pressure inside the tube equals the pressure outside. Therefore it will narrow at the downstream end until the alveolar pressure outside the capillary equals the pressure inside, and during flow the pressure within the downstream end of the capillary will always be equal to PA. Therefore the driving pressure during flow in this zone will always be ($Pa - PA$). Alterations in Pv do not affect flow, provided Pv is kept less than PA. Blood flow increases down zone II, since PA is everywhere zero under these conditions and Pa increases down the lung.

In zone III $Pa > Pv > PA$. Here driving pressure is ($Pa - Pv$). It might be expected that blood flow would be constant down zone III since the difference between Pa and Pv is constant at any level within the zone. Blood flow does tend to increase down the zone despite this, for while the driving pressure is constant the values of Pa and Pv individually increase down the lung and the capillary transmural pressure increases similarly since alveolar pressure is everywhere zero. Hence the capillaries are progressively distended with lower resistance down the zone, and flow progressively increases towards the bottom of the lung.

Effect of lung volume on extra-alveolar vessels

While the alveolar capillaries may be considered to be exposed to alveolar pressure, the extra-alveolar vessels, in particular the larger veins, are exposed to pleural pressure. At high lung volumes they are held open by the negative intrapleural pressure; at FRC and lower lung volumes they are relatively narrow and contribute an important resistance. This effect will be more important at the base then the apex, for there is a pleural pressure gradient (again due to gravity) such that the pleural pressure is less negative, hence less distensive, at base than apex.

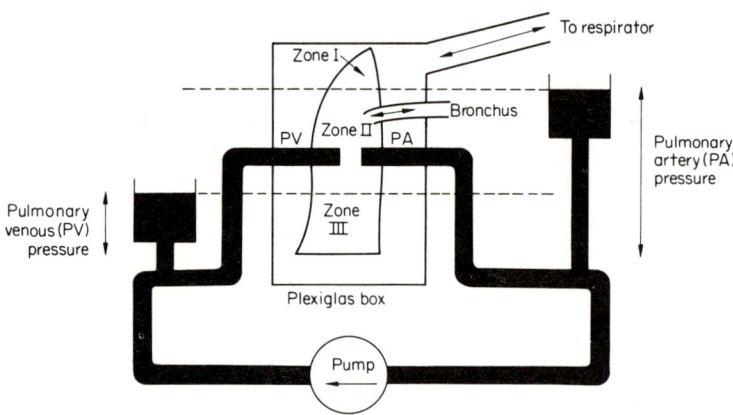

Fig. 3.15. (a) The isolated perfused lung is enclosed in a plexiglass box and may be ventilated by negative pressure by connecting a respirator to that box. Pulmonary arterial, Pa, and pulmonary venous, Pv, pressures may by be set by altering the height of blood reservoirs, and blood flow may be altered by changing the pump speed. Reference point for Pa and Pv pressures is the bottom of the lung. For Zones I–III see text and Fig. 3.15b.

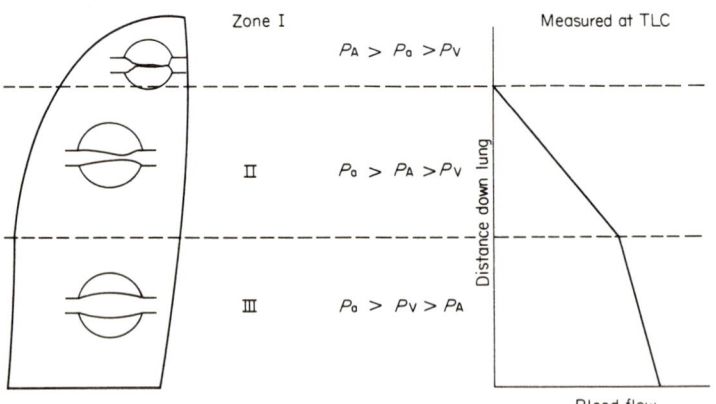

Fig. 3.15. (b) Zone I. Vessels collapsed, no flow. $P_A > Pa > Pv$. Zone II. Starling resistor. Driving pressure is $(Pa - P_A)$. $Pa > P_A > Pv$. Zone III. Driving pressure is $(Pa - Pv)$ which is constant. But transmural pressure is $(Pa - P_A)$ at the arterial end and $(Pv - P_A)$ at the venous end of the capillary, and increases down Zone III. Hence there is progressive dilatation and increased flow down Zone III.

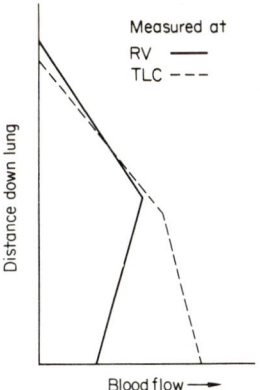

Fig. 3.15. (c) Effect of lung volume on blood flow distribution.

The combined result is that at high lung volumes approaching TLC, alveolar-capillary resistance is dominant, and flow distribution resembles that shown in Fig. 3.15b. At low lung volumes, particularly below FRC, the influence of extra-alveolar vessel resistance becomes dominant in zone III, with the result that flow decreases down that zone, as in Fig. 3.15c.

Although much of the experimental work was done on dog lungs with non-pulsatile flow of blood, the results correspond well with those from normal human subjects with two minor exceptions. First, pulsatile blood flow blurs the well-differentiated distinctions between zones in the steady-flow preparation, but the general conclusions remain intact. Second, in human lungs, the pulmonary artery pressure is sufficient to perfuse the apices in the erect position in many subjects, so that a well defined zone I is rarely found.

In a diseased lung the normal distribution of flow may be markedly altered, either because of altered perfusion pressures, or because of change in vessel calibre due to chemical changes (hypoxia for example) or to intrinsic structural alteration of the vessel wall. These three factors are frequently so intricately combined that it is difficult to separate them. Thus in mitral stenosis or in left ventricular failure the lung apices are well perfused since pulmonary artery pressure is high and there is no zone I. The bases are under-perfused, due partly to perivascular oedema, partly to structural narrowing of the vessel lumen, and partly to hypoxic vasoconstriction. The result may be that the normal perfusion gradient is reversed, flow per unit lung volume being higher at the apex than at the base. It is in such cases that the upper lobe veins appear dilated on the chest X-ray film.

Finally it should be recalled that while the airways down to the terminal bronchioles are supplied by the bronchial arteries, the more peripheral airways and pulmonary parenchyma are dependent on the pulmonary blood flow for their metabolism. It is tempting to relate the apical distribution of some lung disorders (e.g. post-primary pulmonary tuberculosis) to the possibly disadvantageous nutrition of the apical lung regions.

Distribution of ventilation

The pleural pressure gradient [14]

The pleural pressure is more negative at the apex of the lung than at the base. Therefore the force distending the alveoli at the apex is greater than that distending those at the base and in the resting position at FRC apical alveoli are larger than basal ones.

The reason for this pleural pressure gradient has proved quite hard to determine. In the following discussion it is assumed that if the lung were removed from the chest cavity and freed from the stress of gravity, there would be no systematic regional variation in size or mechanical properties of alveoli.

Initially it was felt that since the pleural cavity contained some fluid, there must be a simple hydrostatic pressure gradient down the pleural cavity so that if a fine catheter were to be passed progressively downwards in that cavity a pressure gradient of 1 cmH$_2$O/cm down the lung would be observed. This was wrong for two reasons. First the pleural space is a virtual not an actual space, and second pleural pressure is a surface not a hydrostatic pressure. If two glass microscope slides are wetted and placed surface-to-surface, quite a large force is required to separate them (as opposed to sliding them apart which is relatively easy). This force is used to overcome surface pressure between the two wet slides and is analogous to the force needed to separate parietal from visceral pleura. It is this type of pressure which is measured as pleural pressure by the oesophageal balloon technique. Unfortunately, if a catheter is placed in the pleural space, the virtual space will be opened up, fluid may accumulate around the catheter (however fine) and a hydrostatic pressure gradient of 1 cmH$_2$O/cm may be observed. This gradient is an artefact of the investigative technique. In any case the pleural pressure gradient measured by methods which do not involve opening the pleural space was found to be not 1 cmH$_2$O/cm but about 0·3 cmH$_2$O/cm.

A better proposition relates to the possibility that chest wall or lung are of different unstressed, or natural, shapes, by which we mean the theoretical shapes which would obtain if the lung or chest wall were separated from each other and freed from the stress of gravity.

Assume that the lung and chest cavity do *not* have the same natural shapes (Fig. 3.16) and that in the lung of natural shape all alveoli are the same size. If the lung is then placed in the chest cavity and sealed by surface pressure to the chest wall, some parts of the lung will be relatively compressed and some will be relatively expanded. Contrariwise some parts of the chest wall will be drawn in and some will be pushed out. If the chest wall were relatively non-

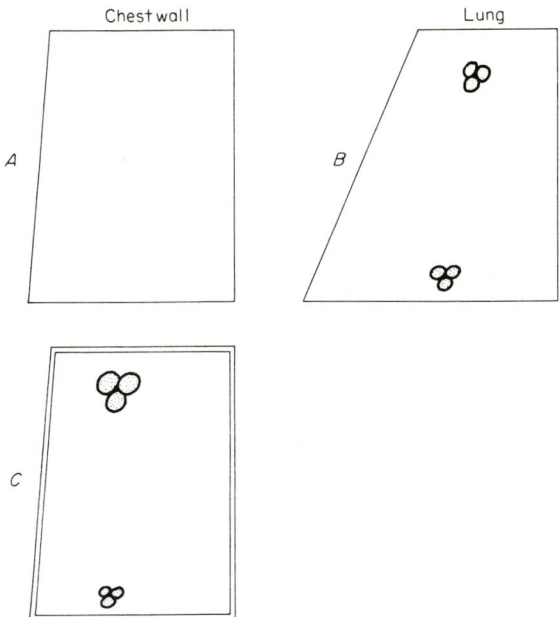

Fig. 3.16. Suppose the natural shapes of the chest wall (A) and lung (B) were different, and that alveoli in (B) were all the same size. If the lung were now placed within and sealed to the relatively stiff chest wall, upper alveoli would be distended and lower ones compressed (C).

distortable there would be quite marked variation in lung compression and expansion relative to the lung's natural shape (Fig. 3.16) and some alveoli would be smaller than others. The important corollary is that for the smaller alveoli the distending pressure under static conditions would be less than for the more expanded alveoli. Therefore pleural pressure is less over the smaller alveoli than over the larger and a pleural pressure gradient must exist.

The main difficulty in accepting this proposition will be in the fact that we normally think of pleural pressure as a force which determines alveolar size. This is the basis for example of the measurement of static compliance. We now encounter the idea that a pleural pressure change is essentially the *result* of a deformation of alveoli imposed by the inclusion of the lung within and sealed to a relatively rigid chest wall. This reversal of causative role for pleural pressure and alveolar volume is logical, but initially difficult to accept intuitively.

The lung of course is never unstressed, but always subjected to gravity. A second proposition is that the pleural pressure gradient is due to the simple effect of gravity on lung mass. If a spring is hung free in space (Fig. 3.17) the upper coils will be further apart than the lower ones since they support more weight and will be stretched more. This is an appealing analogy to the fact that apical alveoli at FRC are bigger than basal ones. However the lung is not supported free in space. Indeed if one were to design a method for supporting the mesh-work of a spherical sponge against gravity, one might support the sponge evenly around the periphery and place within its substance a support structure radiating from a central core. This is not too far from the position of the lung, supported peripherally by surface forces and centrally by airways and blood vessels radiating from an admittedly eccentric hilum.

While the direct effect of gravity on lung mass must produce some variation in alveolar size it need not account entirely for its observed distribution and in the argument so far it is emphasised that there are two reasons why the shapes of chest cavity and lung might differ:

1   their unstressed shapes are different (Fig. 3.16); and

2   the effect of gravity distorts lung parenchyma more than the chest wall (Fig. 3.17).

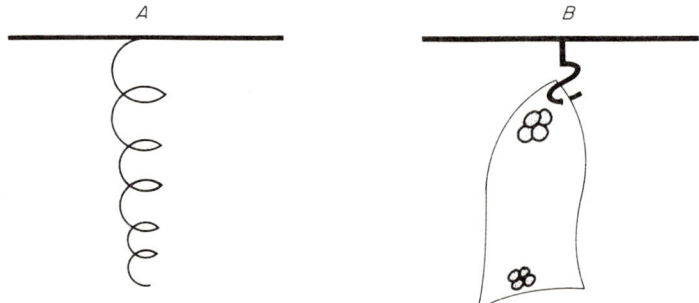

Fig. 3.17. Analogy between a suspended spring (A) where the upper coils support more weight and are therefore more stretched, and a lung similarly suspended (B) where the upper air spaces will be more distended than the lower because of gravity.

It is not clear from the present evidence which of these two effects is the more important.

When the lung and chest wall are considered in the intact animal a third reason for differing shape is apparent, namely that in the erect position the chest wall may be distorted by the weight of abdominal contents which are to some extent supported by or hung from the diaphragm via its attachments to the lower border of the rib cage. This might distort the chest wall in the fashion shown in Fig. 3.18, expanding apical and compressing basal alveoli, to produce a pleural pressure more negative at the top of the lung. It has been shown however that regional variations in alveolar size are not altered when the subject is immersed in water to the level of the xiphisternum [15], a manoeuvre which takes the weight of abdominal contents off the chest wall.

Although the chest wall distortion appears permanent to that extent, it

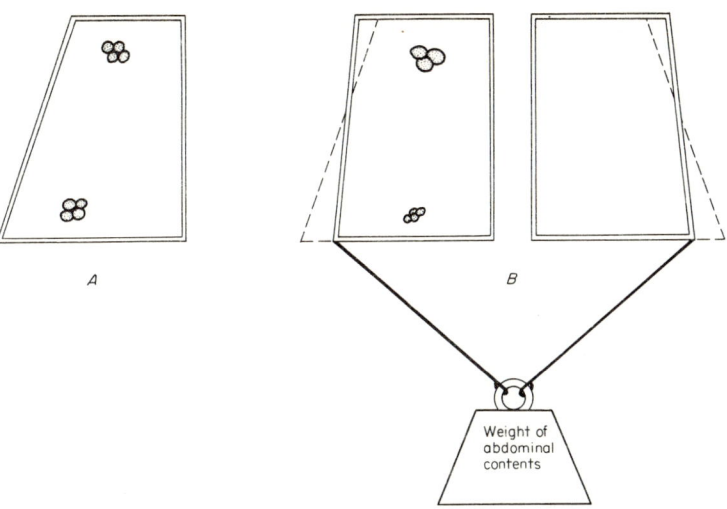

Fig. 3.18. If the chest wall is distorted from its original shape (A, and dotted lines in B), upper alveoli will be distorted and lower alveoli compressed.

may well be even so that it was originally produced by gravitational force on abdominal contents during transition from the horizontal to the erect posture during childhood, and only becomes permanent after long-term adoption of the erect posture. It would be important though ethically difficult to repeat the investigation of Greene and colleagues [15] with small children instead of adult subjects. A further implication is that experiments done on this problem involving change to erect posture in animals whose thorax is normally horizontal may not give comparable results to those from habitually erect man.

We have already met the word interdependence in considering the intrinsic property of the lung parenchymal network to resist distortion. A second type of interdependence may now be shown between lung and chest wall. Suppose (Fig. 3.19) that an airway becomes blocked and a segment of lung undergoes absorption atelectasis. The volume of that segment will shrink, and the area of pleural surface which it subtends will tend to be pulled towards the hilum. If that surface does move inwards, the chest wall must be similarly deformed. In order to deform the relatively non-distortable chest wall the pleural pressure over the distorted area must become more negative. Thus the distending pressure on the alveoli which are collapsing will increase with increasing deformation, a mechanism which tends to prevent collapse and enhance alveolar stability. The relatively stiff chest wall is in effect splinting the lung parenchyma against local distortion.

Consider now the possible effect of varying alveolar size on the distribution of ventilation. The pressure-volume relation of the lung is curvilinear

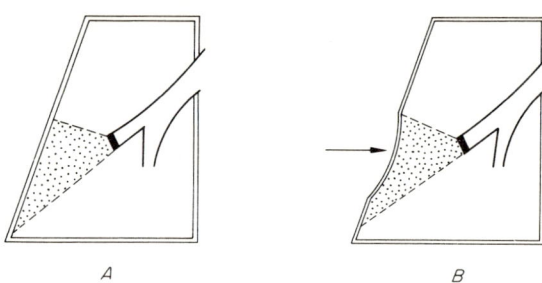

Fig. 3.19. If an airway is blocked (A), the lung it supplies (stippled area) will collapse. As it shrinks it tends to draw the chest wall inwards (B). Since the chest wall is not easily distorted, the pleural pressure over the subtended segment will become more negative.

(Fig. 3.20). Small alveoli at the base of the lung lie on a steep part of the curve where a small increase in distending pressure will produce a large increase in volume. Large alveoli at the apex lie on a relatively flat part of the curve where the same increase in pressure will produce a much smaller increment in volume. If an equal change of distending pressure is applied at apex and base in Fig. 3.20, the basal alveolus of volume 2 units would be increased to $3\frac{1}{2}$

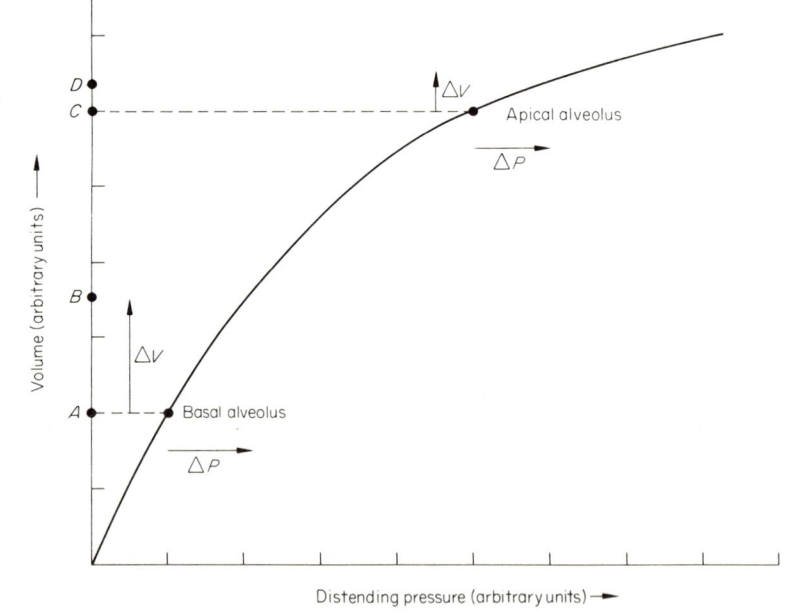

Fig. 3.20. The smaller basal alveolus (volume A) lies on a steeper part of the compliance curve than the larger apical alveolus (volume B). Identical changes in distending pressure applied to both (ΔP) will produce a volume change (ΔV) of $1\frac{1}{2}$ units (distance AB) for the basal, but only $\frac{1}{3}$ unit (distance CD) for the apical alveolus.

units, a ventilation per unit volume of $\frac{3}{4}$, but the apical alveolus of volume 6 units would only increase to 6·3, a ventilation per unit volume of 1/20, giving a steep gradient of ventilation per unit volume down the lung. This gradient would be diminished if the apical swings in pleural pressure were greater than at the base, and by the principle of chest wall-lung interdependence one would expect this to be the case if the apical chest wall were deformed from natural shape by being pushed out and the basal chest wall deformed by being pushed in (Fig. 3.18).

Actually basal pressure swings are probably greater than apical, the reverse of what one would prefer and expect on the above argument, and all this goes to show is that prediction of events when gas is flowing by reference to static compliance properties alone will predictably mislead.

Distribution of resistance

It is very difficult to measure local resistance of a small section of lung, for this requires measurement of the pleural pressure over the relevant subtended pleural area, of the relevant elastic recoil of the segment (taking into account the presence of parenchymal interdependence and of collateral flow), and of flow from the isolated segment.

The distribution of resistance may however be inferred by following the distribution of inspired gas at varying flow rates. At very low flow rates, it is assumed that most of the work is done against the elastic properties of the lung, and hence flow is distributed according to compliance, most of the flow going to more easily distensible areas of high compliance. On the other hand at high flow rates, it is expected that most of the work is done against resistive properties, most of the flow going by routes of low resistance.

Distribution of boluses inhaled from FRC

These proposals have been tested [16, 17] by injecting a bolus of radioactive gas into the inspirate and then scanning the chest to see to which region the labelled portion of the inspirate has been distributed.

The bolus may be injected into the trachea, labelling dead space gas; at the mouth at the beginning of inspiration; or at the end of a 500 ml added dead space, labelling the terminal part of tidal volume. The inspiration may be done very slowly (0·1 L/sec), quite slowly (0·4 L/sec), or fast (more than 2 L/sec). The results are shown in a qualitative manner in Fig. 3.21.

1 During the slow inspirations (0·1 L/sec, Fig. 3.21, top line) one would expect the label to be distributed mainly to the more compliant basal areas (see Fig. 3.20), and this occurs.

2 When inspiratory flow is faster (Fig. 3.21, look down the columns), the faster the flow the more the labelled gas tend to go to the apical lung areas. We

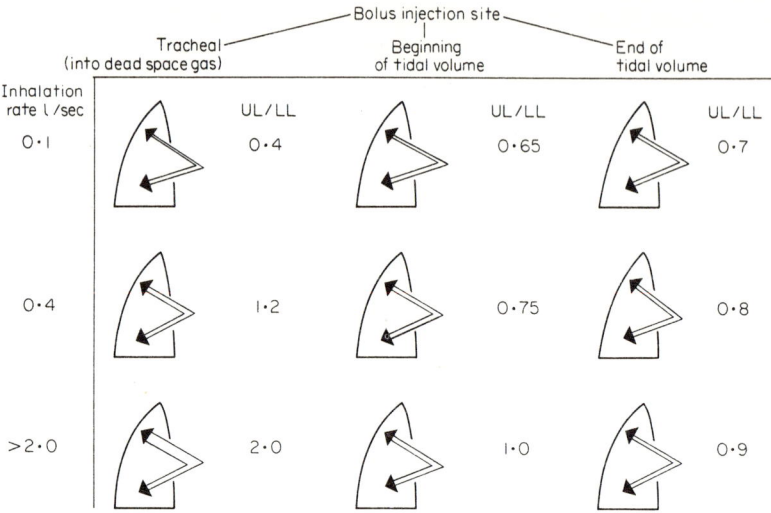

Fig. 3.21. The distribution of a bolus of tracer gas between upper and lower lung regions depends on a) the rate of inhalation (left hand column) and (b) the injection site within the tidal volume (top row). The ratio of the quantity of the bolus going to upper regions divided by that going to the lower lobes (UL/LL) is given for each condition and is represented roughly by the thickness of the respective arrows. The numbers for UL/LL are *not* experimental but obtained by combining and idealising the data of Bake *et al.* [16] and Grant *et al.* [17].

know from morphological measurements on frozen dog lungs that basal small airways are narrower than apical airways at FRC, for the same reason that basal alveoli are smaller than apical. We would therefore expect resistance in the lower parts of the lung to be higher than in the upper parts, and that therefore at high flow rates the labelled gas would be preferentially distributed to apical regions, with a distribution ratio (Fig. 3.21) greater than 1·0. Surprisingly this has not invariably been found, and the data of Bake and colleagues [16] and Grant and colleagues [17] differ on this point. One possibility for which there is some supporting evidence is that although small airway resistance does vary up the lung, being higher at the base, the pleural pressure swings are greater at the base than at the apex, diverting more flow to the bases than would be expected if flow distribution were governed only by the distribution of resistance.

3 The later the bolus is inserted during inspiration, the more even the distribution (Fig. 3.21, look along the rows). While this is in part due to the greater spread of the bolus when inserted at the end of a 500 ml dead space, it also suggests that the distribution of both compliance and resistance becomes more even with progressive inflation, which is intuitively reasonable and supported by the observation that (in dog lung at least) at TLC alveoli and small airways show no systematic regional variation in size.

4 Note that at high flow rates, dead space gas is distributed preferentially to the apices. It is interesting that dead space gas may thus be diverted to high $\dot{V}_A/\dot{Q}$ areas best able to deal with it.

Distribution of boluses inhaled from RV: closing volume

In the previous section the studies were all based on the injection of a bolus of tracer gas while the subject inspired from FRC.

If instead the subject breathes out to *RV* and the bolus is injected at the mouth at the onset of the next inspiration, an entirely different distribution pattern is found. The bolus of tracer gas now goes almost entirely to the apices. This is because at *RV* small airways at the bases are closed and do not open until a certain amount of gas has been inspired: the initial part of the inspirate therefore goes entirely to the upper lung regions.

The lung volume at which airway closure begins to occur may be detected by continuous measurement of the concentration of marker gas in the expirate. Suppose a bolus of helium is given at the beginning of inspiration from *RV* and diverted thereby mainly to upper lung regions. Then during subsequent slow expiration to *RV* (Fig. 3.22) the helium concentration in the expired air is continuously recorded, and plotted against change in lung volumes.

A typical record shows:

Phase I: Zero concentration as the dead space gas is expelled.

Phase II: A sharply rising concentration due to a mixture of dead space and alveolar gas.

Phase III: A plateau, with cardiogenic oscillations, composed of a mixture of alveolar gas from all regions.

Phase IV: A sudden rise in concentration as basal airways begin to close and the expirate comes mainly from upper lung regions with relatively high helium concentrations. The lung volume at which the helium concentration suddenly rises is called the closing capacity. The difference between that volume and residual volume is called the closing volume (Fig. 3.22).

A second method of obtaining this measurement is sufficiently similar to be confusing. After expiring to *RV*, the subject takes a full vital capacity breath of pure oxygen. During subsequent full slow expiration the nitrogen concentration in the expirate is measured and plotted against volume. The resulting trace looks very like that in Fig. 3.22. The important point to realise is that this is not a bolus of oxygen but a full inspiration. At *RV*, basal alveoli are smaller than apical alveoli: at TLC they are about the same size. Therefore during full inspiration of pure oxygen, more oxygen goes to the base than the apex, and nitrogen concentration is higher at the apex than at the base. During the subsequent expiration the onset of basal airway closure is signalled by a rise in nitrogen concentration of predominantly apical origin.

Several immediate questions arise.

1   Do the basal airways actually close, or is it just that the relevant lung units are for some reason not ventilated? The answer is that closure probably occurs.

2   Is the measurement reproducible? The answer is yes, if the phase IV onset is sharply marked. Unfortunately it sometimes is not, and the presence of cardiogenic oscillations also makes it hard to select the take-off point accurately.

3   Is the measurement flow-dependent? The answer is no, at expiratory flows of less than 0·5 L/sec.

4   Do helium bolus and oxygen methods agree? Answer, yes on the average.

When the point at which airway closure occurs is below FRC, as it is in normal young subjects, all lung units must be ventilated during tidal breathing (Fig. 3.22). If closing volume is higher than FRC, basal lung units will close

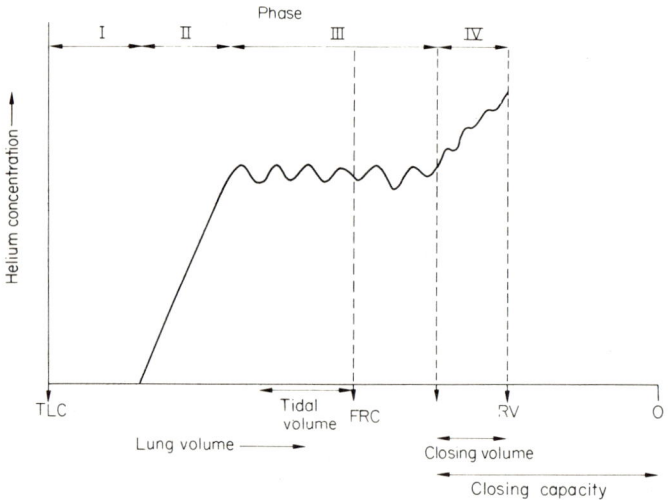

Fig. 3.22. A test for closing volume. A bolus of helium is inspired at *RV* and the inspiration continued to TLC (left). During a subsequent slow expiration to *RV* (right) a record is made of helium concentration in the expired gas plotted against the change in lung volume measured simultaneously at the mouth by spirometer or pneumotachygraph. Note that during normal breathing at rest all tidal ventilation is above closing volume, provided that FRC is greater than closing volume.

during tidal ventilation. Closing volume occupies such a position within the vital capacity in some elderly subjects, with the result that basal ventilation is expected to be inadequate with low $\dot{V}_A/\dot{Q}$ areas. This is believed to be a cause of arterial hypoxia in such subjects, and one reason for the progressive fall in arterial P_{O_2} and rise in $_A$–$_a$ D_{O_2} which occur with increasing age.

It would seem reasonable that in patients with narrowed airways (bronchitis, pulmonary oedema), airways with damaged and more easily collapsible walls (bronchitis), or airways poorly supported by decreased elastic recoil (early emphysema), closing volume would be increased, and this indeed appears to be the case. At present the measurement has become fashionable in the attempt to detect patients with early bronchitis (p. 228), since it is technically relatively simple and suitable for survey work.

Distribution of ventilation/perfusion ratios

Whereas the distribution of perfusion may be summarised relatively simply with some dependence on lung volume (Fig. 3.15c), it is clear that distribution of ventilation is far more complex (Fig. 3.21), being related to the distribution of pleural pressure, of pleural pressure changes with tidal breathing, of resistance, of compliance, and of airway closure. All these factors are dependent on lung volume in a highly interactive way. Nevertheless a general statement may be made that ventilation per unit lung volume tends to increase down the lung at volumes greater than FRC, but that the rate of increase is less than the rate of increase of blood flow down the lung. Thus the overall $\dot{V}_A/\dot{Q}$ ratios tend to decrease down the lung from a value of about 3 at the apex to about 0·6 at the base (Fig. 3.23).

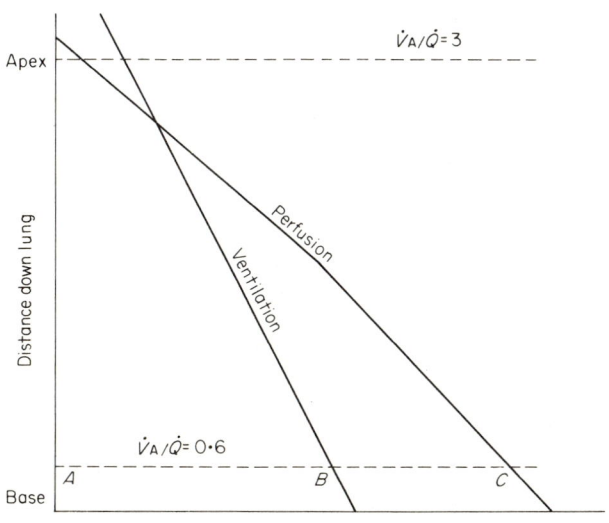

Fig. 3.23. Perfusion per unit lung volume increases from apex to base (cf. Fig. 3.15b). Ventilation also increases but not so much. Thus basal $\dot{V}_A/\dot{Q}$ may be about 0·6, measured as AB/AC, while apical $\dot{V}_A/\dot{Q}$ may be as high as 3·0.

Regional inhomogeneity of ventilation

In the previous sections we have noted a number of reasons relating to the spatial distribution of resistance, compliance and airway closure, whereby ventilation is unevenly distributed within the lung. This type of unevenness is called regional inhomogeneity and refers to distribution of gas between units ventilated in parallel.

The original concept of Otis and colleagues that air spaces of high compliance tended to be supplied by airways of low resistance, resulting in a small variation in regional time constants and therefore small variation in ventilation per unit volume, remains a useful way to begin to think about the problem. We have subsequently seen that regional compliance varies with lung volume, and that regional resistance varies with both lung volume and gas flow rate and may even be infinite when basal airways are closed.

Yet another important factor in the distribution of ventilation refers to the depth to which a tidal inspiration penetrates down conducting airways of differing shape and volume. We are now considering gas passing through structures in series, whereas our previous considerations have been of structures ventilated in parallel. Clearly ventilation may vary in different areas in the sense that the tidal air may penetrate to a different extent down different pathways. This series-type variation in ventilation is called stratified inhomogeneity.

Stratified inhomogeneity of ventilation

As the airways progressively branch, the size of the individual airways becomes progressively smaller, but the total cross-section of airways of a given branching generation becomes progressively larger (Fig. 3.24). The details of

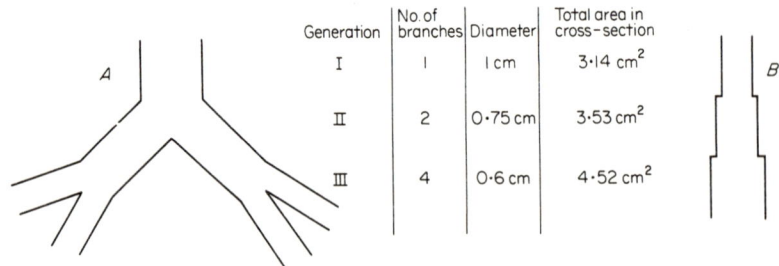

Generation	No. of branches	Diameter	Total area in cross-section
I	1	1 cm	3·14 cm²
II	2	0·75 cm	3·53 cm²
III	4	0·6 cm	4·52 cm²

Fig. 3.24. In the lungs successive branches are smaller (A) but the cross-sectional area of all branches of the generation becomes progressively larger (B).

the branching geometry have been described by Horsfield [19]. The following account ignores the implications of assymetrical branching patterns, as opposed to the symmetrical arrangement of Fig. 3.24, but the general conclusions drawn should still apply.

The most important feature to note is the rapid increase in total cross-sectional area which occurs at the terminal bronchioles (Fig. 3.25; total cross-sectional area 80 cm²), through the transitional zone of respiratory bronchioles (total cross-section 280 cm²), down to the respiratory zone of alveolar ducts and sacs (total cross-section about 7×10^5 cm²).

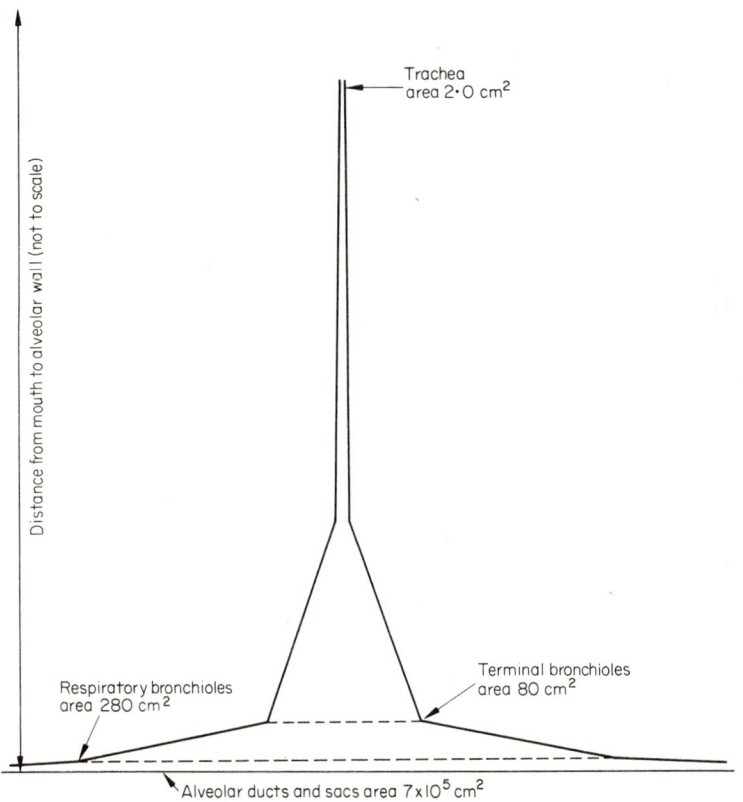

Fig. 3.25. The total cross-sectional area of airways of a given generation increases (Fig. 3.24b) at first slowly, then very rapidly at the level of the terminal bronchioles. The shape of the diagram has been well compared to a tintack (La Force).

One corollary of this anatomical arrangement is that the velocity of gas flow will be very low in the peripheral airways. Thus in the trachea which has a cross-sectional area of say 2·0 cm², the velocity for a volume flow rate of 100 ml/sec is 50 cm/sec. At the same volume flow rate in the respiratory bronchioles (cross-sectional area 280 cm²) the linear velocity is only 100/280 or 0·36 cm/sec.

The important question relates to the depth of penetration of a tidal volume down the conducting pathways. Assume for the moment that the inspired gas has a square-wave front, and that an inspirate of 0·6 L will take the gas front down to the junction between respiratory bronchioles and alveolar ducts in the model shown in Fig. 3.25. This leaves about 2 mm distance between the gas front and the far end of the alveoli, and gas mixing beyond this point must occur by diffusion only. The basic question is, will diffusion equilibration be complete within the time course of a single breath, or will the composition of gas near the alveolar wall differ from that near the mouth of the alveolus? If the latter case were true, there would be a gradient of

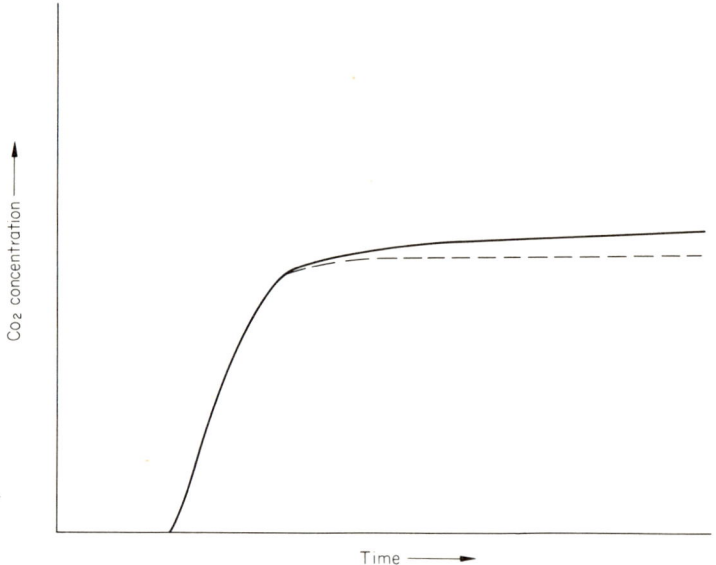

Fig. 3.26. If the CO_2 concentration in a single expirate is instantaneously recorded, the alveolar 'plateau' slopes upward (solid line). The slope of this plateau is diminished after a thirty second breath-hold (dotted line). Cardiogenic oscillations (Fig. 3.22) have been omitted for clarity.

gas tensions from the alveolar wall towards the airways: for example, CO_2 tension would be highest at the wall and lowest at the alveolar mouth. It is this type of variation in gas tension within a single lung unit which would be described as 'stratified inhomogeneity' of ventilation.

It is certainly true that if the concentration of CO_2 is instantaneously recorded at the mouth during expiration, the so-called alveolar plateau is not horizontal, but rises gradually (Fig. 3.26). (A similar phenomenon is seen if nitrogen concentration is measured after a single breath of oxygen. The nitrogen concentration then gradually rises, reflecting a progressive fall in oxygen concentration in the expirate. Thus early portions of the expirate contain, during a normal expiration, relatively low CO_2 concentrations, and following a breath of O_2, relatively high O_2 concentrations. Much published work has been done by the O_2 method but for simplicity the argument will be continued here on the basis of the CO_2 technique).

Two possible explanations for the rise in CO_2 (Fig. 3.26) are

1   That there is a stratified gradient for CO_2, because there has been insufficient time for diffusion equilibrium to occur. Naturally then gas with lower CO_2 concentration from more central regions of the lung unit would precede more peripheral gas with higher CO_2 concentration from near the alveolar wall, and the alveolar plateau would slope upwards, due to stratified inhomogeneity.

2   That there is a variation in time constants in the pathways to different lung units such that areas with smaller time constants will, in a given time, receive a greater proportion of the inspired ventilation per unit volume. These regions will therefore have a lower CO_2 concentration, will fill quicker, and empty earlier, than regions with longer time constants. Hence the early part of the expirate will contain gas predominantly from areas of fast time constants, with the lower CO_2 concentrations—and the alveolar plateau will slope upwards due to regional inhomogeneity.

Historically, Krogh was the first to enquire the reason for the rise in concentration of CO_2 during a single expirate. He concluded on theoretical grounds that this was due to a diffusion gradient—stratified inhomogeneity. This explanation was accepted until 1946 when Rauwerda calculated from the available anatomical data that the diffusion equilibration was so rapid that it could not account for a gradient in CO_2. He gave no explanation for the rise in CO_2 concentration during expiration but this was provided by the time constant approach of Otis and colleagues in 1956, and the theory of regional inhomogeneity was then accepted.

In 1966 Cumming and colleagues [20] re-examined the model used by Rauwerda and made it more realistic. They assumed a square wave front to the tidal gas and lumped the terminal airways together to form a cone. Their calculations suggested that a significant gradient due to diffusion disequilibrium did in fact exist over the time taken for a single expirate. Since that time various different models have been explored, usually of increasing sophistication, but not necessarily the more realistic for that. Each model produces a different conclusion. La Force and Lewis [21], for example, used a symmetrically branching model of the terminal airways, as opposed to a lumped cone, and concluded that stratified inhomogeneity was unimportant.

It can be seen from Fig. 3.25 that because the cross-sectional area peripherally is so large, a very small error in assessing the true dimensions may produce a very large error in estimating the terminal distance across which gas exchange must occur by diffusion alone. It should also be remembered that airway branching is assymetrical [19] and that pathway lengths differ, as opposed to the implicit assumption in Fig. 3.25 that all pathways have the same length.

One is left with the uneasy feeling that the purely theoretical modelling approach is unlikely to determine the relative importance of stratified as opposed to regional inhomogeneity because of the anatomical complexities of the peripheral airways, and turns therefore with relief to the experimental evidence.

Much of this evidence is based on the effect on the slope of the alveolar plateau of (a) breath-holding or (b) inspiring gas of different densities.

If the breath is held for thirty seconds before expiring, the upward slope of the alveolar plateau is diminished (Fig. 3.26). Since no gas is flowing during the breath-hold, this must be due to the evening-out of gas concentration gradients by diffusion. Unfortunately this does not tell us if the diffusion equilibration is occurring between different lung units (regional) or within the same lung units (stratified). It was originally thought that the pathways for diffusion between different lung units would be too long, for gas would have to diffuse up one airway and down another, but the existence of collateral ventilation means that such inter-unit diffusion pathways may be in fact very short.

Since the rapidity of diffusion of a given gas is inversely proportional to the square root of its molecular weight, one would expect large diffusion gradients and a more steeply sloping alveolar plateau for heavy gases such as SF_6 and smaller gradients and less steeply sloping gradients for light gases such as neon [22].

When a volume of one of these foreign gases is inspired, if a diffusion gradient exists, the first portion of the expirate will contain a higher proportion of the foreign gas, and the alveolar plateau should slope downwards. This indeed occurs [22] and the slope is steeper for the heavier gas SF_6 and the difference between SF_6 and neon slopes diminishes with breath-holding. While this strongly supports the presence of stratified inhomogeneity for SF_6, by its comparison with neon, it does not tell us that such inhomogeneity exists for the normal relatively light respiratory gases O_2 and CO_2. In theory the alveolar plateau slope for neon (molecular weight 20, cf molecular weight for O_2 of 32 and for CO_2 of 40) might be due to regional inhomogeneity, and the difference in slopes for neon and SF_6 might be due to stratified inhomogeneity which relates only to the pharmacology of breathing SF_6. A comparison between a gas of molecular weight 32–40 and, say, helium would be more appropriate.

Because of the difficulties in interpretation of the theoretical models of diffusion in the gas phase, and of the experimental results on single expirates with or without breath-holding, combined with the known evidence for regional inhomogeneity of ventilation recounted in the previous section, it is fasionable at present to place more importance on regional than stratified inhomogeneity. The question is however far from settled, and in particular it should be noted first that most experimental work on the regional distribution of ventilation has been done on inspiration, not expiration, and second that calculations on the presence of a diffusion gradient have all assumed a square-wave front. The actual mechanisms of gas transport in the airways will now be examined.

Transport of gas molecules down the conducting system

There are three different transport mechanisms, namely
1   Convective flow, also called bulk or volume flow, referring to the movement of molecules resulting from the application of external force.
2   Diffusion.
3   Mechanical mixing due to the churning action of the heart-beat.
    In the largest airways, flow velocity is very high. Flow is turbulent around the larynx, tending to become more laminar as branching proceeds, but disturbed by eddy currents at the branching points. Diffusion is unimportant here, for it is very slow compared with the high velocities of convective flow in these airways.
    In the smallest airways, flow velocity is very low and axial diffusion is the important transport mechanism, since molecular velocity due to diffusion is much faster than convective flow velocity. Since these airways are individually very narrow, radial diffusion will rapidly even out any concentration gradient across the stream, and the gas front should indeed be square. Thus the assumption of a square front in most gas diffusion models is in fact reasonable.
    In intervening generations of airways, flow is still disturbed by eddies and is certainly not laminar in the strict sense, but a definite flow profile exists with a faster central stream. In these airways transport is by convective flow modified by radial diffusion. This combination of processes is known as Taylor diffusion and means that molecules may diffuse into or out of the fast stream. Interesting results are obtained by varying the carrier gas for O_2. This is normally N_2 during air-breathing but helium may be substituted [23].
    It is then found that if N_2 in the alveoli is washed out by helium, the efficiency of O_2 transport increases since O_2 diffuses more rapidly through helium than through N_2. However if the alveoli contain N_2 as normally and a breath of He–O_2 mixture is taken, O_2 transport is less efficient, than for a normal breath of N_2–O_2, for O_2 diffuses out of the central fast streams of inspired gas more easily if the carrier gas is He (Taylor diffusion) and so penetrate less far into the lung for the He–O_2 than the N_2–O_2 inspirate.

Conclusions

We may conclude that both stratified and regional inhomogeneity of ventilation exist in the normal human lung. Their relative importance is obscure and even more so in diseased lungs. It is attractive to think that in diseases where the gas diffusion pathway in the airways may be lengthened, (e.g. centrilobular or panacinar emphysema), gas exchange may be disturbed by increased stratified inhomogeneity. Yet in these diseases increased regional inhomogeneity is also certainly present, and we have as yet no test for distinguishing the two mechanisms in disease.

REFERENCES

1 RAHN H. & FENN W.O. (1955) *A Graphical Analysis of the Respiratory Gas Exchange.* The American Physiological Society, Washington, D.C.

2 SEVERINGHAUS J.W. (1966) Blood gas calculator. *J. Appl. Physiol.* **21**, 1108–1116.

3 DEFARES J.G. & SNEDDON I.N. (1960) *An Introduction to the Mathematics of Medicine and Biology.* p. 253. North-Holland Publishing Co.

4 Ibid., p. 252, Eqn. 1.

5 COTES J.E. (1968) *Lung Function.* 2nd Edn. pp. 384–385. Blackwell Scientific Publications.

6 FINLEY T.N., SWENSON E.W. & COMROE J.H. (1962) The cause of arterial hypoxia at rest in patients with 'alveolar-capillary block syndrome'. *J. Clin. Invest.* **41**, 618–622.

7 ARNDT H., KING T.K.C. & BRISCOE W.A. (1970) Diffusing capacities and ventilation-perfusion ratios in patients with the clinical syndrome of alveolar-capillary block. *J. Clin. Invest.* **49**, 408–422.

8 STAUB N.C. (1963) Alveolar-arterial oxygen gradient due to diffusion. *J. Appl. Physiol.* **18**, 673–680.

9 RAINE J.M. & BISHOP J.M. (1963) a–a difference in O_2 tension and physiological dead space in normal man. *J. Appl. Physiol.* **18**, 284–288.

10 FRITTS H.W., HARDEWIG A., ROCHESTER D.F., DURAND J. & COURNAND A. (1960) Estimation of pulmonary arterio-venous shunt flow, using intravenous injection of T-1824 dye and Kr^{85}. *J. Clin. Invest.* **39**, 1841–1850.

11 MacKENZIE G.J., TAYLOR S.H., FLENLEY D.C., McDONALD A.H., STAUNTON H.P. & DONALD K.W. (1964) Circulatory and respiratory studies in myocardial infarction and cardiogenic shock. *Lancet* **2**, 825–832.

12 SAUNDERS K.B. (1965) Alveolar-arterial gradient for oxygen in heart-failure. *Lancet* **2**, 160–162.

13 WEST J.B. (1970) *Ventilation/Blood Flow and Gas Exchange.* 2nd Edn. Blackwell Scientific Publications, Oxford.

14 MACKLEM P.T. & MURPHY B. (1974) The forces applied to the lung in health and disease. *Am. J. Med.* **57**, 371–377.

15 GREENE R., HUGHES J.M.B., SUDLOW M.F. & MILIC-EMILI J. (1974) Regional lung volumes during water immersion to the xiphoid in seated man. *J. Appl. Physiol.* **36**, 734–736.

16 BAKE B., WOOD L., MURPHY B., MACKLEM P.T. & MILIC-EMILI J. (1974) Effects of inspiratory flow rate on distribution of inspired gas. *J. Appl. Physiol.* **37**, 8–17.

17 GRANT B.J.B., JONES H.A. & HUGHES J.M.B. (1974) Sequence of regional filling during a tidal breath in man. *J. Appl. Physiol.* **37**, 158–165.

18 TRAVIS D.M., GREEN M. & DON H.F. (1973) Simultaneous comparison of helium and nitrogen 'closing volumes'. *J. Appl. Physiol.* **34**, 304–308. Expiratory flow rate and closing volumes. *J. Appl. Physiol.* **35**, 626–630.

19 HORSFIELD K. (1974) The relation between structure and function in the airways of the lung. *Brit. J. Dis. Chest.* **68**, 145–160.

20 CUMMING G., CRANK J., HORSFIELD K. & PARKER I. (1966) Gaseous diffusion in the airways of the human lung. *Respir. Physiol.* **1**, 58–74.

21 LA FORCE R.C. & LEWIS B.M. (1970) Diffusional transport in the human lung. *J. Appl. Physiol.* **28**, 291–298.

22 CUMMING G., HORSFIELD K., JONES J.G. & MUIR D.C.F. (1967) The influence of gaseous diffusion on the alveolar plateau at different lung volumes. *Respir. Physiol.* **2**, 386–398.

23 JOHNSON L.R. & VAN LIEW H.D. (1974) Use of arterial PO_2 to study convective and diffusive gas mixing in the lungs. *J. Appl. Physiol.* **36**, 91–97.

Chapter 4. Acid-Base Chemistry

This subject provides for many students their greatest intellectual difficulties in clinical medicine. This is hardly surprising, for we are concerned with production and disposal of acid metabolites, and the role of both bicarbonate and protein buffering systems. We consider also the disposal of CO_2, its hydration, the subsequent liberation of hydrogen ions, the dependence of this process on the presence of buffering proteins, the dependence in turn of the buffering powers on the degree of oxygenation of haemoglobin, and the fact that this whole process takes place, not in a test-tube or tonometer, but in a space (the blood volume) which communicates with entirely different systems (extra and intra-cellular fluid). Into these compartments may pour a variety of products of metabolism which tend to disturb the apparently desired acid-base status of the organism. These disturbances are controlled with success in healthy man by elimination of CO_2 gas from the lungs, and by excretion of ions by the kidneys.

The system is complex and multidimensional. To demonstrate its properties we use two-dimensional graphs. Clearly, we may plot a number of combinations of the relevant variables. We may also feel that a logarithmic scale may be helpful on one or other axis, or both. For example hydrogen ion concentration may be plotted as such, $[H^+]$ in mEq/L, or as its negative logarithm, pH. Of the large number of possible diagrams, most have at one time or another been proposed as the most useful way of expressing acid-base relations. Inevitably the subject may be confusing.

The following approach, which is far from original, is designed to help clinicians faced with disturbances of acid-base status in patients, using measurements of pH and P_{CO_2} in arterial blood.

TRANSPORT OF CO_2 IN WATER AND HAEMOGLOBIN SOLUTIONS

Consider first the hydration of CO_2 and the dissociation of carbonic acid.

$$CO_2 + H_2O \underset{}{\overset{(a)}{\rightleftharpoons}} H_2CO_3 \underset{}{\overset{(b)}{\rightleftharpoons}} H^+ + HCO_3^- \tag{4.1}$$

Reaction (a) proceeds slowly unless the enzyme carbonic anhydrase is present. Reaction (b) proceeds rapidly. Although this equation is the start of acid base physiology, it can mislead, for it does not include any term for the protein buffers, which are mainly haemoglobin molecules. Thus in pure water (Fig. 4.1), CO_2 dissolves accordingly to its solubility coefficient (0·03

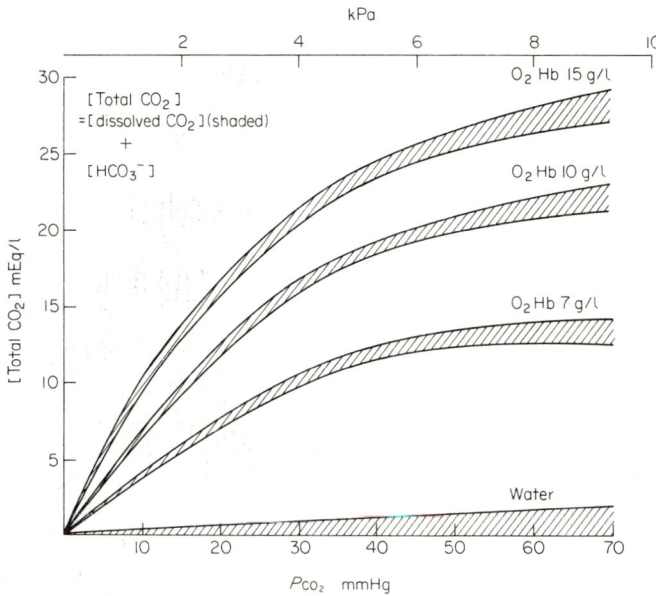

Fig. 4.1. Carriage of CO_2 in water, as dissolved CO_2; and in oxyhaemoglobin (HbO_2) solutions of varying strength, as dissolved CO_2 plus bicarbonate.

mEq/L/mmHg P_{CO_2}, or 0·225 mEq/L/kPa P_{CO_2}). The ratio between CO_2 as dissolved gas and as H_2CO_3 is roughly 1000 to 1, and the ratio between the H_2CO_3 and the product of the H^+ and HCO_3^- ions formed by its ionisation is again roughly 1000 to 1. For all practical purposes the quantity of CO_2 carried as H_2CO_3 and HCO_3^- in pure water can be ignored. In a protein solution of oxyhaemoglobin at 7G/L, a great deal more CO_2 is carried than in pure water, for the presence of H^+ acceptors on the protein enables the reaction of equation 4.1 to proceed to the right with the formation of bicarbonate. Note, from Fig. 4.1, that

1 at a P_{CO_2} of zero there is no bicarbonate whatever the solution:
2 without protein, the bicarbonate concentration is negligible at any P_{CO_2}:
3 the more protein, the more bicarbonate at a given P_{CO_2}.

In Fig. 4.2 is shown a protein molecule with hydrogen ion acceptors which will take up H^+ ions in exchange for sodium. We need an adaptation of equation 4.1 which includes protein buffering.

$$CO_2 + H_2O \rightleftharpoons H_2CO_3 \rightleftharpoons H^+ + HCO_3^-$$
$$+$$
$$PrNa \qquad\qquad (4.2)$$
$$\Updownarrow$$
$$PrH + Na^+$$

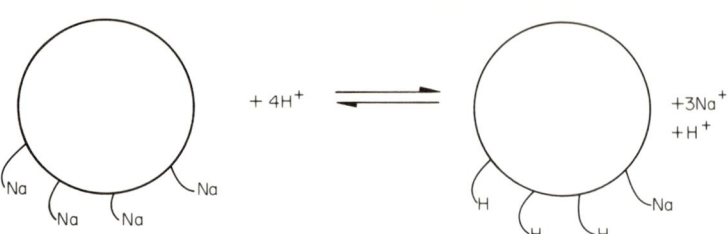

Fig. 4.2. A protein molecule accepting hydrogen ions in exchange for sodium.

In general, the more hydrogen acceptors available on protein molecules, the further the reaction will proceed to the right, and the more sodium bicarbonate will appear. Thus the presence of bicarbonate in this system merely reflects how much hydrogen ion has been buffered, and depends on the number of free hydrogen ion acceptors available. The number available may be increased either by making more free acceptors per protein molecule, or by increasing the number, or concentration, of molecules. The reaction is not linear, for when all the hydrogen ion acceptors are full (saturated), the reaction will stop proceeding to the right due to the build-up of unbuffered free hydrogen ions. At this point the addition of further CO_2 produces no further significant increase in bicarbonate.

These principles, applied to a solution of oxyhaemoglobin in water, may now be applied to a liquid where the haemoglobin is separated off into cells in suspension, namely whole blood.

TRANSPORT OF CO_2 IN WHOLE BLOOD

Carbon dioxide enters the plasma and dissolves therein (Fig. 4.3). A very little CO_2 is hydrated, and buffered by plasma proteins, but this reaction is slow, since there is no carbonic anhydrase, and also clinically unimportant. Dissolved CO_2 also diffuses into the red cell, where it is rapidly hydrated in the presence of carbonic anhydrase, and buffered by hydrogen ion acceptors on the haemoglobin. Bicarbonate accumulates inside the cell, its concentration tending to rise above that in the plasma, and hence bicarbonate ions diffuse out of the cell into the plasma. To maintain electrical neutrality, chloride ions diffuse back from the plasma into the cell. Note that

1 addition of CO_2 to whole blood causes a rise in bicarbonate concentration in the plasma. This reflects the fact that hydrogen ions have been buffered within the cell.

2 Therefore although most of the CO_2 is hydrated and buffered *in the cell*, most of the CO_2 is carried, as bicarbonate, *in the plasma.*

3 The contribution of carbamino compounds is not mentioned. While it would complicate the issue, this would not lead to clearer understanding of applied clinical problems, and it is therefore omitted here, although men-

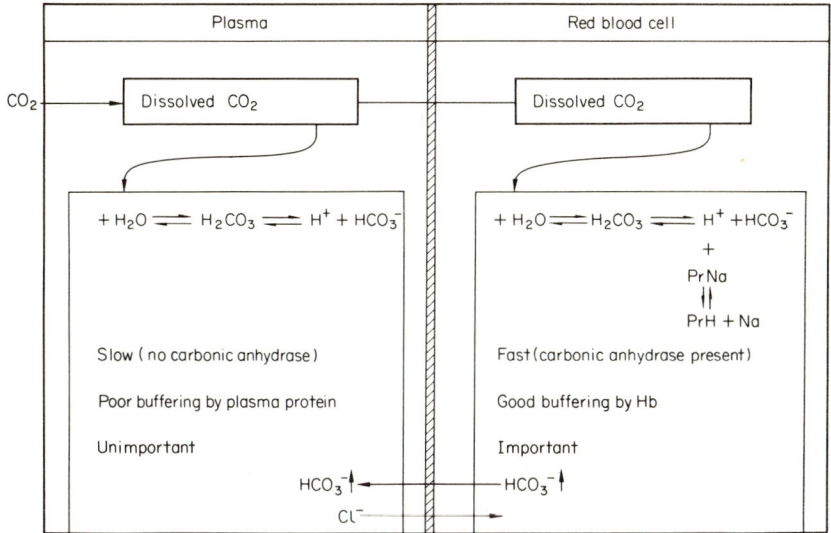

Fig. 4.3. Buffering of CO_2 in plasma and red blood cell.

tioned below in the context of the Haldane effect. A good account of carbamino compounds is given by Davenport [1].

BUFFERING IN *VIVO* AND *VITRO*

Thus far we have considered the addition of CO_2 to whole blood in a test-tube. In the body, the extracellular fluid contains little protein, and little bicarbonate is formed there. Bicarbonate may diffuse from the powerfully-buffered blood to the extravascular, extracellular, fluid. Thus the powerful buffers of the blood are in effect diluted, and the whole body does not buffer CO_2 as well as blood in vitro.

If then in an animal breathing CO_2 the arterial P_{CO_2} were to rise from 40 to 60 mm Hg (5·3 to 8 kPa) the accompanying pH fall would be greater than if that animals blood were equilibrated from 40 to 60 mmHg (5·3 to 8 kPa) in a tonometer.

CHRISTIANSEN–DOUGLAS–HALDANE (C–D–H) AND BOHR EFFECTS

Bohr effect

An increased acidity in the blood, produced, for example, by addition of CO_2, decreases the affinity for O_2 of haemoglobin and shifts the O_2 dissociation curve to the right (Fig. 4.4). Thus at a given tissue P_{O_2} (say 40 mmHg or 5·3 kPa), more O_2 is released, and O_2 uptake thus facilitated.

C–D–H effect

The reduction of oxyhaemoglobin makes available a further supply of hydrogen ion acceptors. Reduced haemoglobin is thus a better buffer than oxyhaemoglobin, and more CO_2 is hydrated and more bicarbonate formed

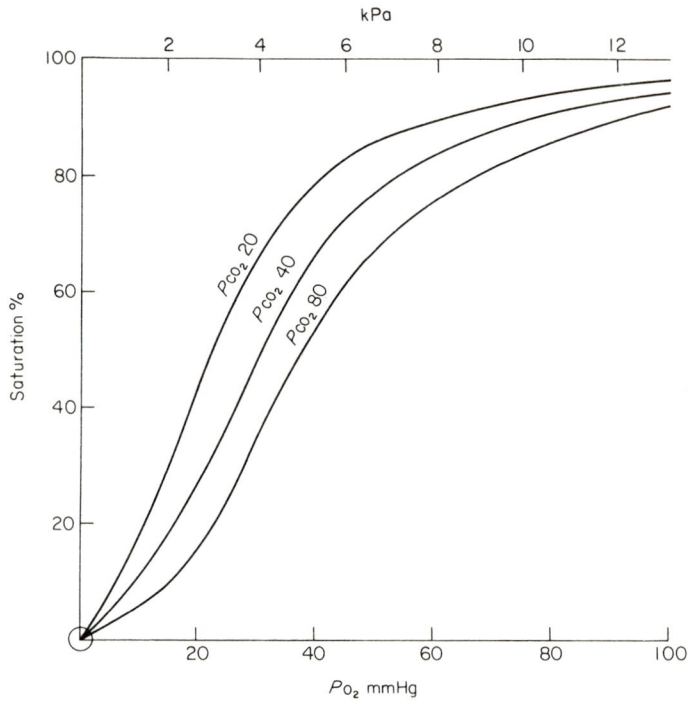

Fig. 4.4. The oxygen dissociation curve and the Bohr effect.

when oxyhaemoglobin is reduced. Moreover reduced blood can carry more CO_2 as carbamino compounds than oxygenated blood.

    If we look at both effects together, when CO_2 is added to the blood in the tissues, the blood becomes more acid: the O_2 dissociation curve shifts to the right (Bohr) which results in increased O_2 release to the tissues. The reduction of haemoglobin is accompanied by an improvement in buffering powers (C–D–H) and hence more CO_2 is hydrated and transported as bicarbonate. More CO_2 is also carried as carbamino compounds.

    In the lungs, CO_2 is removed and the blood becomes less acid: the O_2

dissociation curve shifts to the left (Bohr) which aids O_2 uptake. The oxygenation of haemoglobin is accompanied by a decrease in buffering power (C–D–H): the CO_2 reaction (equation 4.2) is driven to the left with release of CO_2 gas. CO_2 is also released, with oxygenation of haemoglobin, from carbamino compounds.

THE GREAT pH VERSUS [H⁺] ARGUMENT

Many people prefer to express hydrogen ion concentration as such, instead of as pH

$$pH = -\log_{10} [H^+] \tag{4.3}$$

The main reasons for this are that

1   we denote the presence of most other ions as concentration in mEq/L—why not hydrogen ions as well? This is certainly tidy-minded.
2   Students, it is said, find the concept of pH difficult to understand. It is not intuitively obvious why the negative logarithm of $[H^+]$ should be useful.

Against this,

1   In aqueous solutions it is not possible to measure the hydrogen ion concentration by direct methods, e.g. weighing or flame photometry. The glass electrode is used. This electrode produces a voltage which is related to the tendency for the hydrogen ions to escape from the solution. The concentration calculated from this voltage is strictly, therefore, the effective concentration or activity. It is equal to the actual concentration only in 'ideal solutions' which in practice means in very dilute solutions where interactions between the various ions are negligible. In blood, which is far from being an 'ideal solution' it is thought that the actual concentration may be about 25% higher than the activity seen by the electrode.

By sticking to the simple pH notation we avoid problems of this sort.

2   The measurements are made in millivolts on a meter. The millivolts produced by the glass electrode are directly proportional to pH. Practically, adjustments for drift and electrode scale length are easily made on this linear scale (and could not be so on a logarithmic $[H^+]$ scale). pH is what is measured—why not stick to it?
3   The normal pH may be taken as 7·35–7·45. Numbers smaller than this indicate relative acidity, numbers greater—alkalinity. Is this so difficult?
4   A student may, if he wishes, examine the derivation of the Henderson-Hasselbalch equation (given below). The relation of pH and $[H^+]$ should then be clear. If not, no great harm will occur provided he recognises 3 above. He may go further and consider the implications of the Nernst relation, and should then see that it is the logarithm of $[H^+]$ which is the biologically appropriate number. $[H^+]$ acts biologically in a logarithmic way.

Conclusion

We measure pH. It is a scientifically appropriate scale to use both in the practical measurement, and in its biological implications.

THE HENDERSON–HASSELBALCH EQUATION

The following derivation is given by Davenport [1].

The concentration of gas dissolved in a liquid is proportional to the partial pressure of the gas. Thus, in plasma

$$[\text{Dissolved CO}_2]_p = \alpha^1 P_{\text{CO}_2} \tag{4.4}$$

where subscript p denotes plasma concentration, and α^1 is a solubility coefficient.

Dissolved CO_2 is in equilibrium with carbonic acid,

$$CO_2 + H_2O \rightleftharpoons H_2CO_3 \tag{4.5}$$

and the concentration of H_2CO_3, which is very small, is proportional to the concentration of dissolved CO_2, and therefore also to P_{CO_2}, by equation 4.4. Since both [dissolved CO_2] and [H_2CO_3] are proportional to P_{CO_2}, so is their sum.

$$[\text{Dissolved CO}_2 + H_2CO_3]_p = \alpha P_{\text{CO}_2} \tag{4.6}$$

where α is another solubility constant. In the left-hand term, the concentration of H_2CO_3 is less than one-thousandth of the concentration of dissolved CO_2, and it is convenient to denote the combination as [CO_2]. Thus,

$$[CO_2]_p = \alpha P_{\text{CO}_2} \tag{4.7}$$

Carbonic acid dissociates as follows

$$H_2CO_3 \rightleftharpoons H^+ + HCO_3^- \tag{4.8}$$

By the law of mass action

$$\frac{[H^+][HCO_3^-]}{[H_2CO_3]} = K^1 \tag{4.9}$$

where K^1 is a constant

Carbonic acid concentration is proportional to [CO_2]$_p$, and thus also to αP_{CO_2} by equation 4.7. Then

$$\frac{[H^+][HCO_3^-]}{\alpha P_{\text{CO}_2}} = K \tag{4.10}$$

where K is another constant.

Taking logarithms

$$\log[H^+] + \log\frac{[HCO_3^-]}{\alpha P\text{CO}_2} = \log K \tag{4.11}$$

$$\text{or } -\log[H^+] = -\log K + \log\frac{[HCO_3^-]}{\alpha P\text{CO}_2} \tag{4.12}$$

$-\text{Log}[H^+]$ is called pH: $-\log K$ is called pK. Then

$$pH = pK + \log\frac{[HCO_3^-]}{\alpha P\text{CO}_2} \tag{4.13}$$

a form of the Henderson–Hasselbalch equation.

Of these variables, pH and $P\text{CO}_2$ may be measured; $[HCO_3^-]$ may not, but may be calculated if pK is assumed.

Alternatively, since

$$[HCO_3^-] = [\text{Total CO}_2] - \alpha P\text{CO}_2 \tag{4.14}$$

where $[\text{Total CO}_2]$ is the concentration of CO_2 in all its forms, (dissolved, H_2CO_3 and HCO_3^-),

$$pH = pK + \log\frac{[\text{Total CO}_2] - \alpha P\text{CO}_2}{\alpha P\text{CO}_2} \tag{4.15}$$

Total CO_2 concentration may be measured by the method of Van Slyke. The measurement of any two of the variables in equation 4.15 allows the calculation of the third variable if pK is assumed. When measurements are made on plasma at body temperature,

$$pH = 6\cdot10 + \log\frac{[\text{Total CO}_2]_p - 0\cdot0301 P\text{CO}_2}{0\cdot0301 P\text{CO}_2} \tag{4.16}$$

RENAL EXCRETION OF ACID

Before the kidney can effectively secrete hydrogen ions, it must manufacture them in the tubular cell. This is done by the hydration of CO_2 in the presence of carbonic anhydrase. The bicarbonate formed passes into the plasma. The hydrogen ion passes into the tubule in exchange for sodium.

The hydrogen ion in the tubule may either

(a) combine with HCO_3^-, $H^+ + HCO_3^- \rightarrow H_2CO_3 \rightarrow CO_2 + H_2O$
(b) combine with HPO_4^{--}, $H^+ + HPO_4^{--} \rightarrow H_2PO_4^-$; or
(c) combine with ammonia, $H^+ + NH_3 \rightarrow NH_4^+$

Note that with process (a), one bicarbonate ion has appeared in the plasma (when CO_2 was hydrated in the tubular cell), and one bicarbonate ion has disappeared from the urine. It is 'as if' a bicarbonate ion has been reabsorbed: but the ion appearing in the plasma is not the same ion which disappears from the tubule.

WHICH DIAGRAM?

In modern hospital practice, treatment of acid-base disturbances is controlled by measurement of the relevant variables, namely arterial P_{CO_2} and pH. Total CO_2 and bicarbonate may be calculated by graphical methods or by slide rule. This calculation assumes a normal pK of 6·1, which is not always a fair assumption, and it is in those patients who have the severest disturbances of acid-base status that the assumption is worst.

The Davenport [1] pH-bicarbonate diagram, which has many advantages, has the major disadvantage of having calculated $[HCO_3^-]$ as the dependent variable. The CO_2 dissociation curve [2] $(P_{CO_2}-$ Total CO_2 diagram) again has advantages, but total CO_2 must either be calculated from P_{CO_2} and pH, or rather inaccurately measured. (Autoanalyser techniques do not allow the blood sample to be kept at the original body P_{CO_2}, leading to errors in measured total CO_2. These errors are admittedly usually rather small, about 1–2 mEq/L). More importantly, in the practical treatment of acid-base problems, one is usually trying to correct pH, which is not on the diagram. The $[H^+]-P_{CO_2}$ diagram [3] we exclude since for reasons given above we wish to use pH rather than hydrogen ion concentration.

We shall use the $pH - \log P_{CO_2}$ diagram (Fig. 4.5).

THE pH LOG P_{CO_2} DIAGRAM

If samples of blood are placed in tonometers and equilibrated with gases of varying CO_2 tensions, and the pH of the resulting samples measured, it will be found that the plot of P_{CO_2} against pH will be a straight line if the scale on the P_{CO_2} axis is logarithmic (Fig. 4.5). This is the only reason for using a log scale. There is no need to panic. The slope of this buffer line will vary with the haemoglobin concentration, for the more hydrogen acceptors available, the further the reaction in equation 5.2 will proceed to the right, the more HCO_3^- will be formed, and the smaller will be the pH change for a given P_{CO_2} change. The better the buffering power, therefore, the steeper will be the line.

To try and interpret changes in man, as opposed to tonometer, we need knowledge of the *in vivo* response to CO_2 breathing, for the buffer slope *in vivo* will be less steep than *in vitro* (p. 99). The relevant information is plotted in Fig. 4.6, using the data of Schwartz and his colleagues [4], as modified by

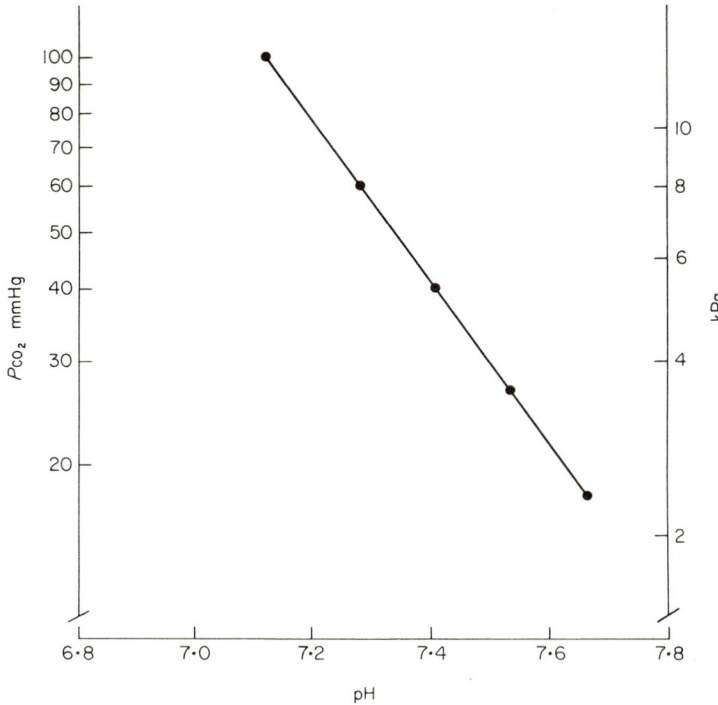

Fig. 4.5. pH–Log P_{CO_2} diagram, showing a normal buffer-line obtained *in vitro*.

Semple [2]. A diagonal shaded area shows the 95% confidence limits for the acute *in vivo* CO_2 dissociation curve in man. Fig. 4.7 shows, in addition, a horizontal stippled band denoting the normal P_{CO_2} (35–45 mmHg or 4·7–6 kPa), and a vertical stippled band for the normal pH range (7·35–7·45). With this diagram we can start to interpret acid-base disturbances by separating them into metabolic and respiratory components.

1 If, in a measurement on arterial blood from a patient, the plotted point lies within the horizontal stippled band, there is *no* respiratory disturbance of acid-base balance, for P_{CO_2} is normal. If the point lies above that area there is a respiratory acidosis (P_{CO_2} high); if it lies below, there is a respiratory alkalosis (P_{CO_2} low).

2 If the point lies within the diagonal shaded area, there is no metabolic disturbance of acid-base balance, for pH is appropriate to the P_{CO_2}. The point lies on the normal *in vivo* CO_2 dissociation curve; therefore the pH change can be totally accounted for by the change in P_{CO_2}. If the point lies to the left of this area, there is a metabolic acidosis; if to the right, a metabolic alkalosis.

3 If the point lies within the rhomboidal transection of horizontal and diagonal bands, clearly acid-base status is normal, for P_{CO_2} is within normal

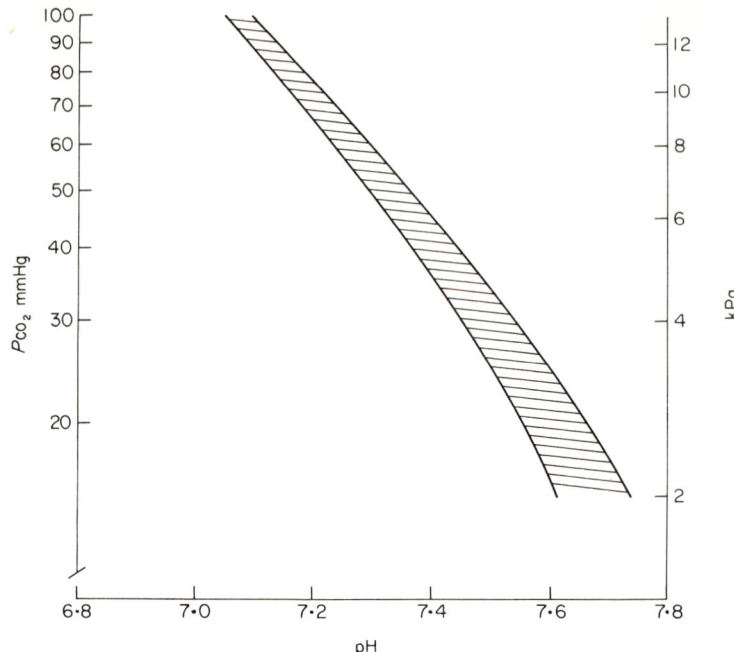

Fig. 4.6. pH–Log P_{CO_2} diagram, with 95% confidence limits for the *in vivo* dissociation curve found by Brackett et al [4].

limits and pH is appropriate to it. If the point lies within the square area bounded by normal pH and P_{CO_2} values, acid-base status is normal by definition, as opposed to by experiment for the rhomboidal area. These two areas coincide sufficiently to cause no clinical confusion, for a point which lies in one but not the other is obviously so nearly normal that it would not cause particular clinical interest, nor would the patient require any therapeutic correction.

To examine now particular points on the diagram:

Point *A*—is indubitably normal.

Point *B*—shows a pure metabolic acidosis, for P_{CO_2} is normal, while pH is reduced, and the point lies to the left of the diagonal shaded area. Such values might be found in a patient with a myocardial infarct and resulting severe hypoxia causing metabolic acidosis.

Point *C*—shows a pure metabolic alkalosis, for P_{CO_2} is normal, while pH is increased, and to the right of the CO_2 dissociation curve.

Point *D*—shows a respiratory alkalosis (P_{CO_2} less than normal) plus a metabolic acidosis (point to left of dissociation curve). This could be caused by severe salicylate overdose, where the respiratory alkalosis is outweighed by metabolic acidosis.

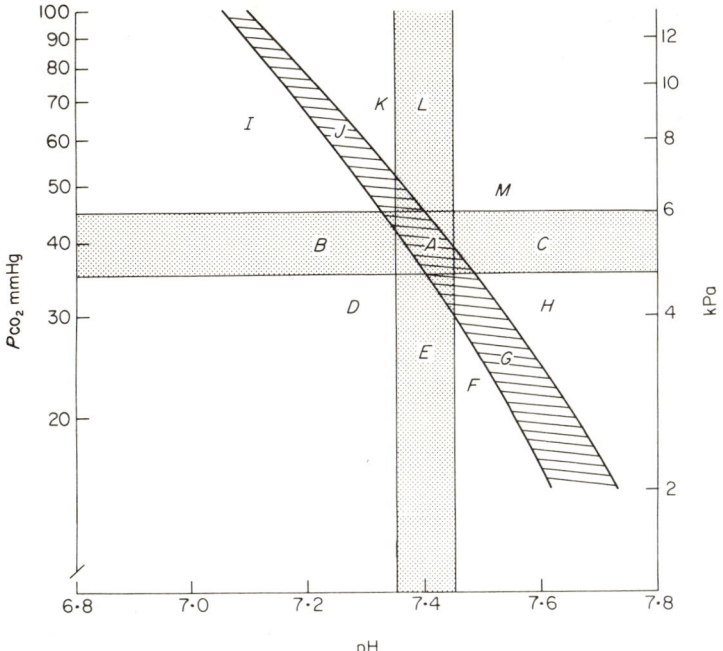

Fig. 4.7. pH–Log P_{CO_2} diagram, with *in vivo* dissociation curve and normal limits for pH and P_{CO_2}. For interpretation of points A to M, see text.

Point *E*—shows a respiratory alkalosis (P_{CO_2} less than normal) plus a metabolic acidosis (point to left of dissociation curve) balanced or perhaps 'compensated', so that pH is normal.

Point *F*—shows a respiratory alkalosis plus a metabolic acidosis (point to right of dissociation curve), where the respiratory alkalosis outweighs the metabolic acidosis, and pH is high. This is the more usual position in salicylate overdose.

Point *G*—shows a pure respiratory alkalosis, as occurs in hysterical hyperventilation.

Point *H*—shows a respiratory plus metabolic alkalosis. This is clinically uncommon, but might be explained by salicylate overdose with loss of acid by vomiting.

Point *I*—shows a respiratory plus metabolic acidosis, most commonly found during resuscitation after cardio-respiratory arrest.

Point *J*—shows a pure respiratory acidosis. While this in physiology laboratories is usually due to CO_2 breathing, in the ward it is invariably due to hypoventilation.

Point *K*—shows a respiratory acidosis plus metabolic alkalosis with pH a little low. This is the classical position in chronic respiratory acidosis (e.g. in

respiratory failure in bronchitis), where the metabolic alkalosis is compensatory, and due to renal retention of bicarbonate. Sometimes the
compensation is complete, and pH is normal—Point *L*.

Point *M*—shows a metabolic alkalosis with respiratory acidosis. The
metabolic alkalosis is the more important, and pH is high. This is seen in
pyloric stenosis, where the metabolic alkalosis is due to prolonged loss of acid
by vomiting, and the respiratory acidosis is compensatory.

THE 'NON-RESPIRATORY pH'

R.J. Linden's group [5] have obtained the *in vivo* CO_2 dissociation curves in
man in varying degrees of metabolic acidosis, as shown in Fig. 4.8. This

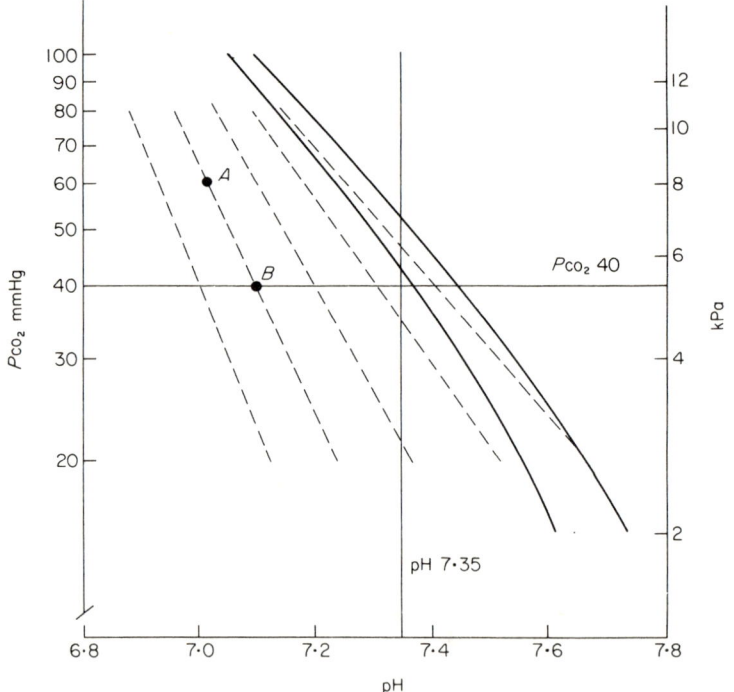

Fig. 4.8. pH–Log P_{CO_2} diagram, with in vivo dissociation curve of Brackett et al [4], and
further *in vivo* curves obtained in metabolic acidosis by Stoker et al [5].

enables us, in acute acidosis, to predict what the pH would be if ventilation
altered to return P_{CO_2} to normal. This 'non-respiratory pH', if less than the
normal lower limit of 7·35, indicates a metabolic acidosis

Thus, a P_{CO_2} of 60 mmHg (8 kPa) and pH of 7·02 gives us point A on Fig. 4.8. Following the diagonal titration line to P_{CO_2} 40 mmHg (5·3 kPa) gives a 'non-respiratory pH' at point B of 7·10, indicating a severe metabolic acidosis in addition to the obvious respiratory acidosis. This is a useful and practical approach.

COMPENSATION

The acid-base system in the body appears to be arranged so that arterial pH and P_{CO_2} (and presumptively cellular pH and P_{CO_2}) are controlled within narrow limits. There are three main defences against excess accumulation or loss of acid, namely

1   the chemical buffers. Blood buffers act immediately. The effect of tissue, or intracellular, buffering is delayed.
2   the lungs. A CO_2 load may be eliminated, or retained, within minutes.
3   the kidneys. Renal excretion, or retention, of acid is the most powerful mechanism for the maintenance of acid-base balance in the sense that it can compensate, in the end, for very large disturbances. It is also the slowest, working on a time-scale of hours, days and weeks, compared with minutes, for the lungs, and seconds, for the chemical buffers.

Thus, in chronic respiratory acidosis due to cor pulmonale, the fall in pH which would be expected from the high level of P_{CO_2} is lessened by the excretion of hydrogen ions and retention of bicarbonate by the kidney. This seems a useful and purposeful action of the body, and the word 'compensation' may be reasonably applied.

This word has been increasingly used wherever the effect of a respiratory disturbance on pH is lessened by a metabolic disturbance, or *vice versa*, regardless of whether this opposition is brought about by the attempt of body control mechanisms to neutralise a single pathological disturbance, as above, or whether the metabolic and respiratory components are both pathological, but happen to have opposing effects on pH. This leads to important misapplications of acid-base measurements to clinical problems.

CLINICAL ACID-BASE PROBLEMS—HOW TO DO THEM

There are only two absolute rules.

Rule 1: Go and see the patient.

A major source of clinical error in these problems is advice based on calculations made on slide rules in the residents' mess.

In the course of history-taking, from a relative if necessary, and a complete physical examination, pay particular attention to:
1   The airway;
2   evidence of hypoxia or CO_2 retention;
3   the pulse, blood pressure, venous pressure and cardiac signs;
4   the state of hydration, and the skin circulation;
5   the state of consciousness and general cerebral function; and
6   the urinary output.
    Then assemble the relevant laboratory data, which should always include:
1   haemoglobin concentration;
2   plasma electrolytes and urea;
3   chest X-ray film;
4   electrocardiogram; besides
5   the blood gas data, which you are only now in a position to interpret.
    During these procedures, try and answer the following questions.
1   How urgent is the problem? How sick is the patient? Obviously extreme urgency, as in resuscitation after cardiac arrest, or transfusion for massive haemorrhage, demands action before full information is at hand. Apart from such obvious exceptions, acid-base disturbances either do not need active correction at all, or need correction much less urgently than most house physicians think.
2   If there is an acid-base disturbance, how long has it been going on for, at what rate has it occurred? In general, a useful approach is to correct an acid-base disturbance at about the same rate as it occurred. Any disturbance which came on over a course of hours or days is usually accompanied by secondary changes in relatively slowly exchanging compartments (e.g. intracellular fluid and especially, brain behind the blood-brain barrier). An attempt at sudden correction based on arterial blood-gas measurements by intravenous infusion may lead to paradoxical and undesired changes in compartments other than the blood volume. For example, infusion of alkali may cause the brain ECF to become more acid (p. 145). The above advice must again be considered against the overall needs of the patient. A patient with a metabolic alkalosis due to pyloric stenosis may have been vomiting for six weeks. Clearly it should not take six weeks to prepare him for surgery, but it should not take six hours either. Two or three days should suffice.

Rule 2: Treat the patient, not the numbers.
The fact that an acid-base disturbance is present does not mean necessarily that it needs correction. Treat it if it endangers the patient's health.
    Always treat the cause of the disturbance rather than the pH. Infuse bicarbonate only if pH needs urgent correction, or the circumstances leading to acidosis cannot easily be controlled. Three examples will illustrate these principles.

1 A man aged 55 has had a myocardial infarct 48 hours previously. He is tachypnoeic and cyanosed, with a raised venous pressure, tachycardia and summation gallop. His blood pressure is 120/80. There are profuse basal crepitations.

Arterial blood gases are P_{CO_2} 30 mmHg (4 kPa)

$\qquad$ P_{O_2} 42 mmHg (5·7 kPa)

$\qquad$ pH 7·27

He therefore, from Fig. 4.7, has a mild respiratory alkalosis with predominant metabolic acidosis (Non-respiratory pH is 7·20, Fig. 4.8).

Question. Does he need bicarbonate?

Answer. No he does not. He needs oxygen, and he needs it in high concentration and he needs it now. Give it and repeat the measurements in about one hour. His metabolic acidosis is probably due to hypoxia.

Question. But while the hypoxia and metabolic acidosis are being corrected, the patient is at risk, for it is well known that lethal arrhythmias are more likely, and their treatment more difficult, in acidosis. Should we not rapidly correct the pH by an infusion of, say, 100 mEq bicarbonate over the next 15 minutes?

Answer. No. That bottle contains, not 'bicarbonate', but sodium bicarbonate. The risk of lethal arrhythmia is putative, but the signs of severe left heart failure are definite. The last thing this patient needs is the rapid infusion of a sodium load. It would be very advisable to treat the heart failure however, since it is his pulmonary oedema which is the cause of his hypoxia, which is the cause of his metabolic acidosis.

Question. Why does he have a respiratory alkalosis?

Answer. Partly because his low P_{O_2} and pH are stimulating respiration via central and peripheral chemoreceptors. This is 'compensatory'. The main reason is that he has high left atrial, pulmonary venous and capillary pressures with pulmonary oedema, which stimulate lung receptors and cause tachypnoea by impulses travelling up the vagus to the brain stem (p. 171). His P_{CO_2} will probably remain a little low until the heart failure resolves.

2 A man aged 66 is admitted. He is stuporose and can give little account of himself. His relatives say that he has been vomiting rather frequently for perhaps a month, and that he has had a productive cough for many years. He is dehydrated, with a tachycardia but normal blood pressure. He has a splash and visible peristalsis. Pyloric stenosis is diagnosed and later demonstrated by barium meal. Initial investigations include:

Plasma Na 135, K 2·3, Cl 96, Total CO_2 35 mEq/L,

Urea 150 mg/100 ml.

Arterial P_{CO_2} 49 mmHg (6·5 kPa), P_{O_2} 60 mmHg (8 kPa), pH 7·49

From Fig. 4.7 he has a predominant metabolic alkalosis, with a respiratory acidosis. Clearly the metabolic alkalosis is due to persistent acid loss by vomiting. The respiratory acidosis may be compensatory, via chemoreceptors depressing respiration, but may also be due to respiratory failure in a very sick chronic bronchitic. The problem is to resuscitate him for surgery.

Question. Should we infuse acid?

Answer. No. This man's main problems, in fact, are loss of sodium, water and potassium. Infuse normal saline with 25 mEq potassium per litre, and the acid-base disturbance will sort itself out. (It is almost *never* necessary to infuse acid. The author in sixteen years of practice has never done so. His senior colleague, over a larger time span, has done so once.) Repeat blood gases after 12 hours, and 4 litres normal saline with 100 mEq potassium, are

Arterial PCO_2 43 mmHg (5·8 kPa), pH 7·51, PO_2 60 mmHg (8 kPa).

Clinically the patient is improved, and is now starting to talk sense, but the pH has increased a little, while PCO_2 is now normal. Clearly the respiratory acidosis was *not* compensatory, but reflected respiratory failure.

Further infusion of saline and potassium over the next 48 hours restored the plasma electrolytes to normal.

3 A man aged 48 with ulcerative colitis has an acute attack, and is admitted after four days of profuse bloody diarrhoea. He is dehydrated and obviously severely ill. There is an irregular tachycardia and the blood pressure is 90/50. There is no evidence of heart failure. Urinary output is probably, from the history, diminished. E.C.G. shows multifocal ventricular ectopics, with one run of five, and evidence of old infarction. Hb. is 8.OG/100 ml.

Blood gases: PCO_3 40 mmHg (5·3 kPa), PO_2 60 mmHg (8 kPa); pH 7·25.

Question. He clearly needs fluid, including blood.
Does he need bicarbonate?

Answer. Yes, I think so. The arrhythmia is sinister, and bicarbonate can be added to the intravenous regime without danger of fluid overload.

Question. How much and how fast?

Answer. This question brings us to the fundamental difference between the approach to acid-base disturbances described here, and the more traditional attempt to predict bicarbonate requirements using the concept of base deficit.

FAREWELL, STANDARD BICARB.—GOODBYE, BASE EXCESS?

These terms have not been defined or explained here. They have four major disadvantages.

First, it is necessary to calculate bicarbonate from the Henderson–Hasselbalch equation, using an assumed value for pK and that pK may be wrong in those very circumstances where acid-base physiology is most deranged. We prefer to use a diagram which plots the actual measurements made, pH and PCO_2. No calculations are required. For that matter, knowledge of the Henderson–Hasselbalch equation is not required either.

Second, predictions on base deficit lines assume an *in vitro* dissociation curve which is frankly not applicable, and may mislead [6].

Third, the calculations require some estimate of the volume of a 'compartment' into which bicarbonate is infused. Although no such compartment really exists, it is said that some reasonable guess may be made from a knowledge of the body weight. This is certainly untrue in severe metabolic acidosis, where bicarbonate requirements may be two to three times the figure calculated by the standard formula [7]. In any case, in many acute clinical problems, the body weight is not known, and has to be guessed by eye, a procedure more appropriate to the village fête than the hospital emergency room. The result is that a doubtful number is placed in a doubtful formula and gives a doubly doubtful answer in terms of the number of milli-equivalents of bicarbonate 'needed' by the patient.

We prefer to follow lines suggested by Kappagoda and colleagues [6]. They showed, in dogs, that the amount of bicarbonate needed to correct an acute metabolic acidosis depended on the rate at which it was given. This is the fourth, final, and fatal blow to the base-deficit approach. If bicarbonate was infused at 0·2 mEq/Kg/minute, much of it was 'wasted' in that it spilled over into the urine. With infusion at 0·1 mEq/Kg/min, this did not occur. There is no similar information in acute metabolic acidosis in patients.

In view of the above difficulties with the calculation of bicarbonate requirements, we prefer to take a more flexible approach, which may be summed up as

TITRATE—DON'T CALCULATE

If a proper clinical appraisal suggests that bicarbonate is needed, and pH is greater than 7·1, start the infusion at 50 mEq/hour, and repeat the measurments in one hour. If initial pH is less than 7·1, start at 100 mEq/hour. Base further bicarbonate administration on serial measurements.

REFERENCES

1. DAVENPORT H.W. (1969) *The ABC of Acid-Base Chemistry*. 5th Ed. Revised. The University of Chicago Press, Chicago.
2. CUMMING G. & SEMPLE S.J.G. (1973) *Disorders of the Respiratory System*. Ch. 6. Blackwell Scientific Publications, Oxford.
3. FLENLEY D.C. (1971) Another non-logarithmic acid-base diagram? *Lancet* i, 961–965.
4. BRACKETT N.C. Jr., COHEN J.J. & SCHWARTZ W.B. (1965) Carbon dioxide titration curve of normal man. *New Eng. J. Med.* **272**, 6–12.
5. STOKER J.B., KAPPAGODA C.T., GRIMSHAW V.A. & LINDEN R.J. (1972) A new method for assessing states of acute acidaemia in man. *Clin. Sci.* **42**, 455–463.
6. KAPPAGODA C.T., LINDEN R.J. & SNOW H.M. (1970) An approach to the problems of acid-base balance. *Clin. Sci.* **39**, 169–182.
7. GARELLA S., DANA C.L. & CHAZAN J.A. (1973) Severity of metabolic acidosis as determinant of bicarbonate requirements. *New Eng. J. Med.* **289**, 121–126.

Chapter 5. The Respiratory Control System

THE MEANING OF CONTROL

In ordinary life, we use the word control to denote the influence of one body on the action of another. Thus 'the driver controls the car', 'the teacher controls the class', and 'Parliament controls the people'. In the simplest form, the action of the first body affects the action of the second without any further interaction. The first body is entirely independent of the actions of the second, while the actions of the second are clearly highly dependent on those of the first, controlling body.

In real life, both at sociological and physiological levels, true independence of the controlling body is rare. Parliament controls legislature, and legislature affects the people, which may not receive it with approval and can vote accordingly at the next election, thus affecting the composition of Parliament and subsequent legislature.

Similarly, if the level of CO_2 in the body increases above normal levels, it causes an increase in ventilation which tends to decrease CO_2 levels towards normal.

Such interaction is called by the ugly but expressive word feedback. In the second example above the CO_2-ventilation interaction is an example of negative feedback, which causes the influence of a disturbance, such as an increase in inspired CO_2 concentration, to be minimised by the accompanying increase in ventilation. Positive feedback tends to maximise the influence of a disturbance. For example if increased CO_2 caused a decrease in ventilation, the decrease in ventilation would cause a further increase in CO_2, which would further depress ventilation, which would further increase CO_2, and so on. This is the type of interaction known as a 'vicious circle'.

In the presence of feedback a simple statement '*A* controls *B*' is basically wrong and usually confusing. A true statement would be '*A* controls *B*, and *B* controls *A*'. Thus the statement that 'CO_2 levels control ventilation' might imply that if ventilation increases there must be an increase in CO_2 to cause it. If then as in exercise CO_2 levels do not rise, whereas ventilation does, it may be thought that CO_2 levels are *not* controlling ventilation. One of the purposes of this chapter is to show that they may be.

A major problem about the use of the word control is that it tends to imply that one or other of two parties has the whip-hand, or should have. In the teacher-class example, while feedback from class to teacher is recognised and may be thought desirable, it is also desirable that the teacher, and not the class, should be 'in control'. In the CO_2-ventilation example we might agree that the overall function of the organism depends importantly on the CO_2 levels, whereas ventilation is merely the exhaust mechanism which enables CO_2 levels to be maintained relatively constant and the organism to continue to function. While CO_2 levels control ventilation and ventilation controls CO_2 levels, it would be reasonable to think that CO_2 levels should have the whip-hand. In the government-people example no such generalisation is possible. The possession of the whip-hand will depend on the type of government. A despot will have it, but a democratically elected parliament may not. Indeed the design of suitable feedback circuits between government and people is the basis of one branch of political theory.

A second difficulty with the word control is that control implies purpose. We should distinguish immediately between two types of problem, that of design and that of interpretation. An engineer designing an amplifier or a lawyer designing a constitution will incorporate certain feed-back circuits, or 'checks and balances', intended in the first case to make an electrical signal larger without distorting its shape beyond certain defined limits, and in the second to safeguard certain human rights while allowing government sufficient power to take action in the general interests of the people. These feedback circuits are included to produce effects known from experience or intended by hypothesis, but they are incorporated for a definite purpose. The physiologist on the other hand is presented with an organism in which a very large number of variables are all varying at once. Inspection reveals that some of these variables are apparently connected in the sense that varying one of them by experiment will be consistently accompanied by systematic changes in some of the others. The physiologist does not have a design problem since the organism already exists and he did not design it. His problem is one of interpretation. There are two approaches to this, the first being descriptive, and an example of information thus obtained would be the compliance curve of the lung. The question answered is 'How does it behave?'. The second approach is speculative and attempts to answer the question 'What is it for?'. At this stage physiologists tend to exclaim 'teleology' and stop listening. Speculation, teleology and intuition are the three dirty words of fashionable medical science, and like all dirty words they have magic properties since the use of them in criticism proves the worthlessness of whatever is criticised without need for further argument or justification. In fact most users of the word teleology seem to use it in a sense other than that defined by the Oxford dictionary—'the view that *developments* are due to the purpose or design that is served by them'. A statement that giraffes have developed long necks in order that they may reach the branches of tall trees is teleological. Water does not grow on trees but occurs in pools at ground level or below, and in order to drink it the giraffe stretches his neck down, not up. There is an obvious problem of venous return from the head in this position. It is a curious fact that the giraffe has a highly developed pterygoid plexus of veins. What is it for? To act as a venous pump under these circumstances, perhaps. If this is teleology then teleology is the basis of the investigation of control mechanisms.

Take, for example, this Martian, who has just emerged from his UFO somewhere on Salisbury Plain. There is a lot of grass, a few butterflies, and an old Model T Ford car, in the front seat of which is a bag of oranges. The starting handle is in position, and the car in reverse gear. Our Martian examines this contraption with some care, draws certain conclusions, and finally grasps the starting handle with two tentacles and turns it. He is supernaturally powerful, of course, and the car moves backward at about 10 m.p.h. The Martian goes back into the UFO and takes off. Subsequently an article appears in a distinguished Intergalactic Journal entitled 'A primitive orange transporter; an interesting example of translation of rotational motion into longitudinal mass transport'. Where did he go wrong? First, his observation was poor. He did not find out how to open the bonnet, or the petrol tank, or what was in the petrol tank. Second, his curiosity was too limited. He saw a steering wheel, several pedals on the floor and a number of dials and switches on the dashboard. He did not bother to ask himself what they were for. Third, and this is the new point, he assumed that because he could drive a system in a certain way, that was the way that the system was designed to be driven. Thus he grasped a basic principle of the machine, which was that when the engine crank rotated the car moved, but he failed to realise that what he was looking at was an engine. Four marks out of ten for him.

To summarise, we need to interpret and explain the workings of a mechanism that we did not design. In order to do this we need
1   accurate observations of its structure and behaviour;
2   a hypothesis—when considering control, this hypothesis will be based on the idea that the control mechanisms subserve some sort of purpose (no need to say Whose) and will essentially be an attempt to answer the question 'What is it for?'; and
3   an experiment. All experiments involve changing some input to the system or variable within it. These variables can be changed in a natural way (e.g. exercise) in which the system is being driven naturally, or in an unnatural way (e.g. CO_2 breathing). Interpretation of the natural behaviour of a system based on information of the second type may be difficult or misleading as we shall see.

SYSTEMS OR CONTROL THEORY [1]

Feedback is a universal phenomenon. Any event which can be represented as an interaction between two or more molecules, cells, structures, organs, organisms, people or groups of people can in theory be described by a system containing one or more feedback loops. Systems theory seeks to describe interactions, to classify them and to quantify their effects. It owes no allegiance to any single discipline, and it has its own terminology, which is applicable to subjects as diverse as business studies and medicine. Its powers of description and classification permit considerable interdisciplinary communication. It does not solve problems, but it enables problems to be set down in a form in which they can be solved, and may have already been solved in a parallel problem in an entirely different field. Scientifically its approach and importance are Linnaean not Newtonian.

A numerical description of the behaviour of a system can only be set down systematically in terms of a set of equations. Such a set of equations is called a mathematical model.

INPUT, OUTPUT, AND BLACK BOXES

A pressure manometer is connected to an arterial catheter (Fig. 5.1). The desired signal (output) is the continuous record of arterial blood pressure. Pressure waves are transmitted along the fluid-filled catheter, but will be

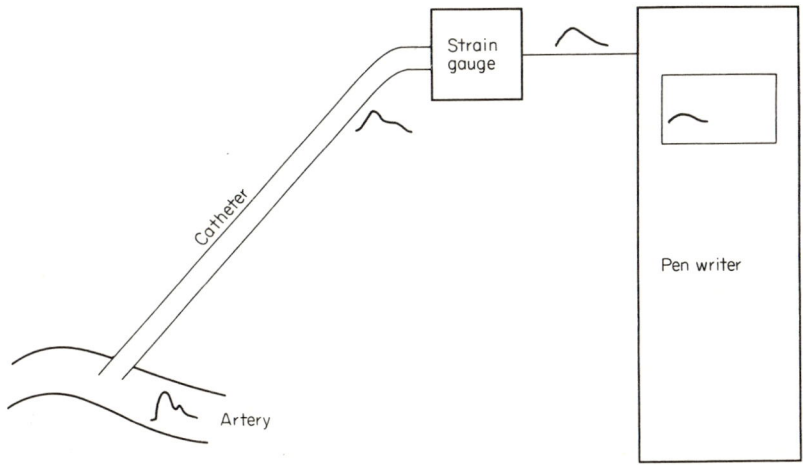

Fig. 5.1. Progressive distortion of an arterial pressure wave by a catheter-transducer-recorder system.

distorted depending on its length, calibre and constitution. Arriving at the manometer the signal is transduced from one form of energy (hydrostatic) to another (electrical). If the transduction is exact the shape of the electrical signal will be exactly correspond to the shape of the pressure wave, but in practice there will be some further distortion of the signal, depending on transducer design. The signal then goes to the penwriter which contains amplifiers and galvanometers designed to reproduce the signal on paper. Further distortion occurs.

It is clearly vital that a physiologist should know to what extent his recording (output) resembles the true pressure waveform (input). Fortunately in order to do so he does not have to be an expert in the behaviour of plastic under stress, and the design of transducers, amplifiers and galvanometers. The only signals he need consider are the true input waveform and the observed output. He considers the system as a 'black box'. There is nothing on the outside of the black box except two connectors labelled input and output. Inside the black box is the catheter, the transducer, the amplifiers, the galvanometers, and the pen.

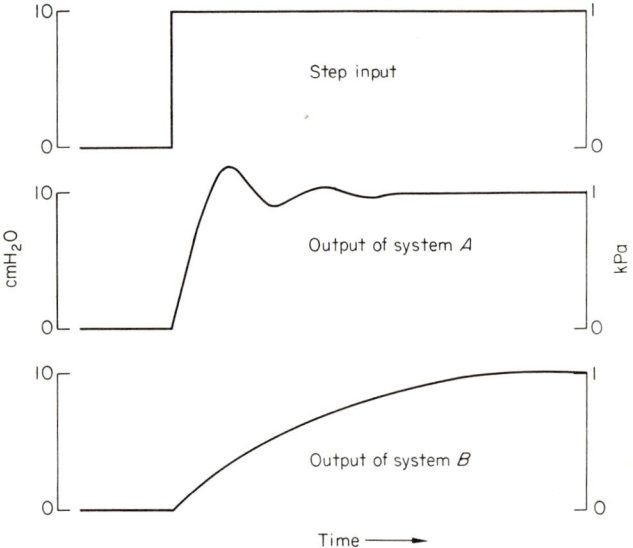

Fig. 5.2. Output of underdamped (A) and overdamped (B) systems for a step input.

The tip of the catheter is placed in a fluid filled chamber in which known pressure changes may be accurately generated. Step changes in calibrating pressure are applied (input) and compared with the recorded results (output). System A (Fig. 5.2) responds rapidly but overshoots and oscillates before reaching its steady-state value. System B responds more sluggishly and creeps up to the steady state reading. System A is described as under-damped; system B is overdamped. These responses can be represented by second-order linear differential equations of no great complexity, but we shall not follow the mathematics here. As the degree of damping is increased, for a system that oscillates after a step input (System A), a point is reached where the response just fails to overshoot. This system is then described as 'critically damped', a term which has a precise mathematical meaning and does not reflect some vagary of the operator. ('There is a knob marked damping and you are the critic': D. Mendel.)

We are now capable of defining the response of our catheter-recorder system to a step input in mathematical terms, but cannot say what might happen to an arterial pressure wave-form, which is of course a repetitive phenomenon.

Suppose then that we put a sinusoidal pressure wave into our system with amplitude identical to the size of the previous input, and again record the

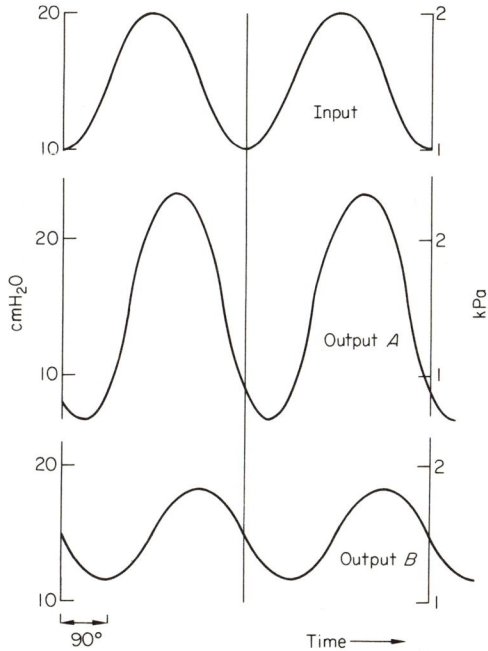

Fig. 5.3. Outputs of systems A and B (Fig. 5.2) for a sine wave input. System B lags by one quarter of a cycle, or 90°.

output. It might be found (Fig. 5.3) that for the underdamped system A, the output oscillations were larger than predicted from the previous 10 cm step steady state outputs, and that they were lagging slightly behind the input, whereas for system B the output amplitude was diminished but the lag was even more pronounced. These lags are sometimes called phase shifts and expressed as fractions of a cycle. For system B the phase shift or phase lag is one quarter of a cycle and since output lags input is defined as negative, i.e. − 90°. Note that we have only described the behaviour of our two systems at

one input frequency. Clearly for a more complete description we should
investigate their response to a large number of frequencies, and we then find
(Fig. 5.4) that for system A as frequency is increased from zero the output
amplitude at first accurately reproduces the input, but then increases to a
peak. This finding of increase in output amplitude with increasing frequency is
called resonance. After the peak, amplitude falls off rapidly. For system B

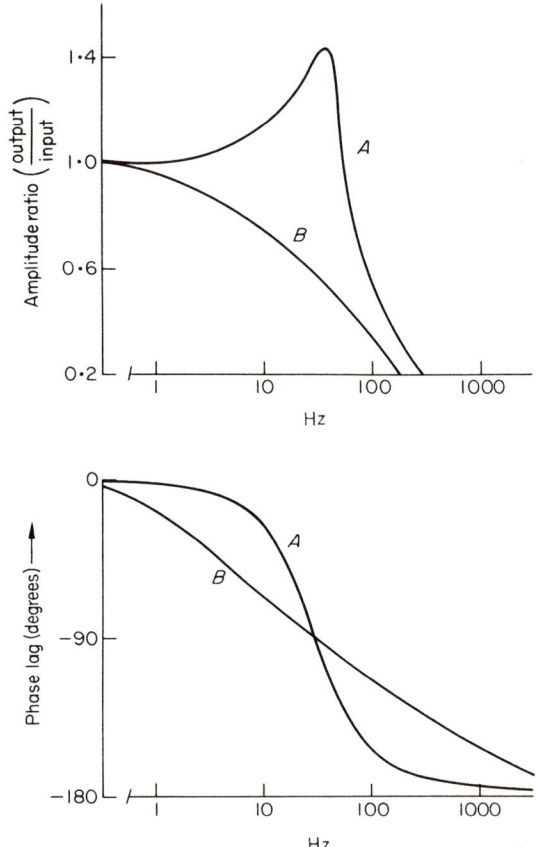

Fig. 5.4. Frequency response of Systems A (underdamped) and B (overdamped). Note log scale
on abscissa. 1 Hz = 1 cycle per second.

amplitude begins to fall off at a lower frequency and there is no resonant peak.
Turning to the phase plot we find that for system A there is very little phase lag
until frequency exceeds 10 Hz, when phase lag rapidly becomes more
pronounced. For system B there is a rather gradual and progressive phase lag
as frequency increases.

These two plots for amplitude and phase define the 'frequency response' of a system. Similar graphs of the same data but with units on the axes expressed differently are called Bode plots. We can now define graphically or if necessary mathematically what our two systems will do to any sine wave when it is transmitted from catheter tip to paper.

The arterial pressure pulse however is not a sine wave, so we cannot yet predict what would happen to it. Here we make use of Fourier analysis the basis of which is the statement that any continuous repetitive wave-form of whatever shape may be described as the sum of a number of sine waves of varying amplitude and phase. The more precise the description the greater the number of sine waves needed. The principle of the analysis may be understood by anyone with an intuitive feeling for least-squares regression.

Take an arterial pressure trace, with pulse rate say 60/min (fundamental frequency 1 Hz). Do a sinusoidal least-squares regression through the pulse wave-form—i.e. find the best fitting sine wave. This sine wave will have a certain amplitude, which is the amplitude of the 'fundamental' component of the pressure record. Subtract this best-fit sine wave from the original signal and some form of pulsatile signal will remain. Do a second sinusoidal regression for a sine wave of frequency 2 Hz. Another sine wave of certain amplitude and certain phase relation to the fundamental will be obtained, and this is the first harmonic. Subtract this first harmonic from the signal and some form of pulsatile signal will still remain. Repeat the regression with a sine wave at 3 Hz (second harmonic), subtract that sine wave from the signal, repeat for a sine wave of 4 Hz (third harmonic) and subtract, and so on. At each subtraction the signal will become less and less pulsatile until eventually it becomes almost a straight line, and this straight line is the mean (or 'd.c. level') of the original signal. We could now reconstitute the original signal by taking this mean and adding to it all the sine waves we have obtained by regression. The accuracy of the reconstitution will depend on the number of harmonics which are taken which determines the degree to which the pulsatility is removed, or alternatively the straightness of the final approximation to the straight line of the mean. Thus we can describe, to any desired degree of accuracy, any continuous repetitive wave-form as the sum of the mean plus a series of sine waves of varying amplitude and phase. Now we are in a position to say what our catheter-recorder system will do to an arterial pressure wave-form. If we know the true shape of the input wave-form we can predict what the recording system will do to it, since we can dissect the pressure pulse into its Fourier components, see from the known frequency response (Fig. 5.4) what will happen to each of them, correct them accordingly, and then reconstitute the wave-form by adding them all up again. Alternatively we can take the distorted output signal, dissect that, work backwards from the frequency and phase plots to correct each component, and reconstitute to find the original true input signal. All this can be done conveniently by computer techniques and there are much more efficient ways of calculating the Fourier components than that described above. This approach also enables us to define the desired performance of a catheter-recorder system. In general we would like the amplitude response to be uniform ('flat') $\pm 5\%$ to about ten times the fundamental frequency of the input wave-form. Thus for pulse rates of up to 180/min or 3 Hz, the response should be flat $\pm 5\%$ to 30 Hz. We would obviously like no phase lag at all, or say less than 5°, up to 30 Hz, but it will be equally satisfactory if phase lag varies linearly with frequency. (Why?) If however the final signal is to be treated mathematically, especially by differentiation, much more precise reproduction is required.

We have now seen two types of input–output analysis, for step and sine wave inputs respectively, applied to the catheter-transducer-recorder system. Underlying the entire discussion is a very large assumption, namely that the system is linear.

LINEARITY, ALINEARITY AND LINEARISATION

We can describe a linear system as one defined by linear differential equations of motion, but many readers may find this profoundly unhelpful. It is better perhaps to point out some of the useful implications of linearity, some of the disadvantages of alinearity, and one of the ways of getting round difficulties raised by the latter.

In a linear system, an analysis of the input-output relation for a single type of input allows in theory the prediction of the output for any type of input. In our previous example we could predict frequency response (Fig. 5.4) from the transients observed after a step input (Fig. 5.2). It follows for example that in a linear system frequency response is independent of input amplitude. If one started with a low frequency amplitude of 10 cm H_2O and plotted out the frequency response as in Fig. 5.4, and then repeated the procedure with double the initial amplitude, the amplitude vs frequency plot would be identical, provided that the amplitude was expressed as an output/input ratio.

No physical system is expected to be linear over more than a certain range, which will differ according to the design and purpose of the instrument, for which the working range, which is the range over which the instrument behaves linearly, should always be quoted. Similarly when a biological system is described as linear the range over which this is reasonably demonstrable should be stated.

Superposition is a basic property of linear systems (Fig. 5.5). This states that for two or more differing inputs to a linear system, the sum of the inputs will result in the sum of the outputs, both in the transient and in the steady state. This principle lies behind the simple definition of linearity which is

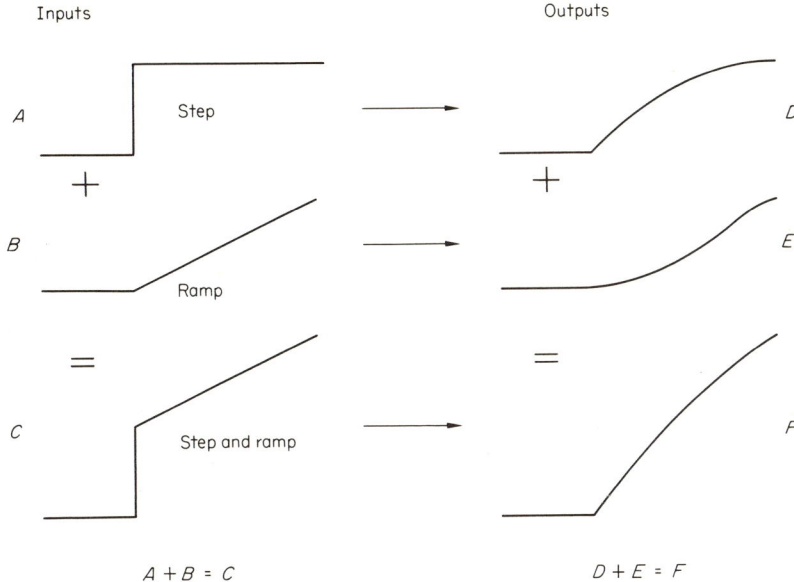

Fig. 5.5. In a linear system the sum (*C*) of two inputs (*A* + *B*) gives an output (*F*) which is the sum of the outputs generated by each separate input (*D* + *E*). The principle of superposition.

implied when manometers are calibrated in the laboratory, when a series of different steady state pressures are applied, say from a sphygmomanometer. Then if the steady output of a 10 mmHg (1·3 kPa) signal is 2 cm deflection on the chart, by superposition the steady state output from a $10 + 10 = 20$ mmHg input is $2 + 2 = 4$ cm.

It should be clear that linearity confers useful properties of simple description and prediction upon a system, but that the limits within which the system behaves linearly must always be defined.

Unfortunately no physiological system is linear. With alinearity all the convenient simplicities described above disappear. Whereas before we could plot the frequency response at one amplitude and know the frequency response at all amplitudes within the linear range, we can no longer do so. We are in a strange town and do not know what lies around the corner. A stranger in a North American chess-board city can easily travel from 3rd and 8th to 5th and 10th, since the system is known, logical, and predictable ('linear'), but if a stranger in Piccadilly Circus needs to get to Marble Arch, he needs a map, since there is no logic behind the London street plan.

This mapping is exactly what has to be done with alinear systems. If frequency response varies with amplitude, there is no help for it but to test the frequency response at varying amplitudes. The result will not be a single plot like Fig. 5.4 for system *A*, but a very large number of plots indeed, maybe one for every amplitude tested. Here is the major difficulty with alinearity. The general shapes of the plots in Fig. 5.4 are not difficult to memorise, but the shapes of a large number of such plots cannot be so comprehended. Rules we can remember, maps we cannot.

Linear equations can be solved analytically, that is with pencil, paper and brain. A large body of operational mathematics exists which was designed to assist such solutions rapidly, concisely and elegantly (e.g. the Laplace transform). A second problem is that alinear equations cannot ordinarily be solved by these means.

Fortunately alinearity is not a bugbear to be borne by biologists alone, and a very great deal of attention is being given to alinear mathematics, particularly to mapping techniques which may give useful and intuitively helpful answers, and prediction within limits.

One standard technique is that of linearisation in sections. Fig. 5.6 shows an alinear relation between y and x, which has been divided into small

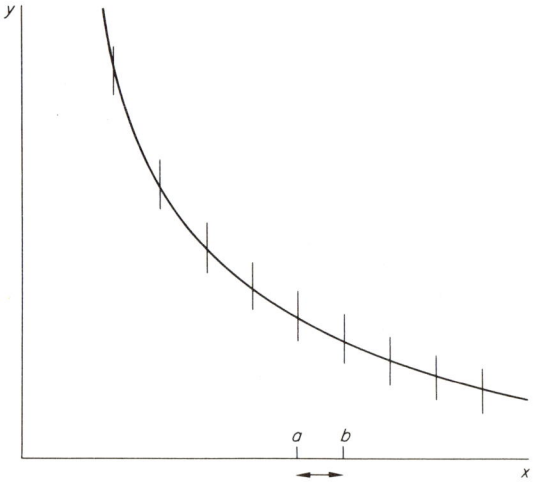

Fig. 5.6. Linearisation by segments. See text.

segments. Each individual segment is rather like a straight line, indeed no great harm may come if we assume it to be so, and say that within limits $a < x < b$ the system behaves linearly. This implies that our input function must not be of greater amplitude than distance $a–b$. If we wish to map this system we must take this very small input function and apply it at intervals along the range on the x-axis.

The problem of solution of equations is also not so bad as it appears at first sight, for alinear equations may be solved by the iterative methods of digital computing. This implies that anyone interested in the numerical description of alinear systems will need either to compute, or to know someone who can.

TRANSIENTS AND STEADY STATES

If we suddenly apply some input to a system, it will take some time to settle down—the on-transient—before reaching a steady state condition (Fig. 5.2). If the input is then removed, an off-transient occurs before the initial situation is restored. The steady state is not necessarily a straight horizontal line; it normally is so only for a step input. The steady state result for a ramp input will normally be a ramp, and for a sine wave the steady state will normally be sinusoidal. In one sense the steady state result tells us about the shape of the input, which we already knew. It is the transient which tells about the system. In Fig. 5.2 the steady state output is the same, a constant, but the transients characterise two very different systems.

Traditionally physiologists have been interested almost entirely in steady state results. The experimenter will set up a preparation, wait for it to settle down, take serial measurements of the important variables to make sure there is no progressive trend away from constant values, and then apply some input. The immediate events following the onset of the stimulus are usually ignored, indeed special care is taken to exclude events during the transient, until a new steady state is obtained, when further measurements are taken.

This is not to say that steady state measurements are of trivial importance. Indeed the plot of steady state input v. output measurements gives primary information concerning linearity, and steady state information from a periodic input (Fig. 5.3) can be used to obtain the frequency response (Fig. 5.4) which in turn can be used to predict the form of transient events (Fig. 5.2), within the bounds of linear behaviour.

It seems clear that classical physiology ignored transient phenomena not through lack of interest but through lack of the mathematical and data-handling techniques needed to analyse them. This has now changed, and properly so, for after all in life a steady state never occurs. On the contrary life can be described as the sum of a large number of simultaneous transients.

SERVOSYSTEMS AND REGULATORS

In engineering feedback control is especially used in servosystems where the usual purpose is to produce an output ('controlled variable') which follows precisely changes in the input, as in a physiological recording system. Regulators on the other hand are designed to keep some output constant in the presence of disturbances. In the sense that the respiratory system appears

designed to maintain certain variables (P_{CO_2}, P_{O_2}, pH) constant despite
disturbances, it behaves like a regulator.

In engineering systems, the feedback often works through a comparator,
that is some mechanism for comparing the actual output to the desired output.
Thus in Fig. 5.7 if actual rev/min is less than desired, the comparator or

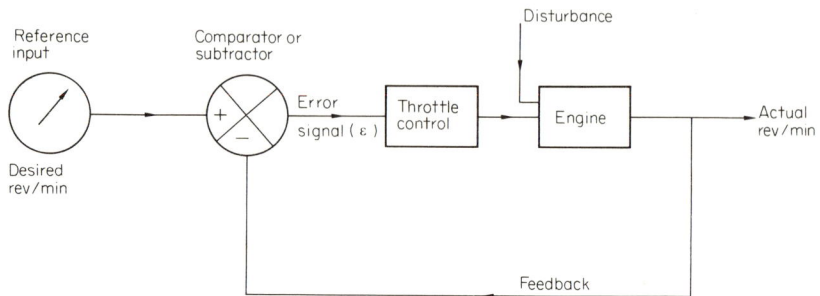

Fig. 5.7. A regulator for revolutions per minute (rev/min) from an engine.

subtractor will allow a positive signal to go to throttle control, and the engine
will go faster; the throttle will continue to move until actual rev/min equals
desired rev/min, when throttle position is fixed, for the error signal is zero. The
intervention of a disturbance such as a minor engine malfunction will at first
cause a decrease in engine rev/min., but the feedback mechanism acting as a
regulator will minimise this.

In biological control systems we do not find comparators as such, but we
do find mechanisms which minimise disturbances. This is commonly associated with the interaction of two functions with slopes of opposite sign
(Fig. 5.8). In the respiratory system, if CO_2 concentration increases it will

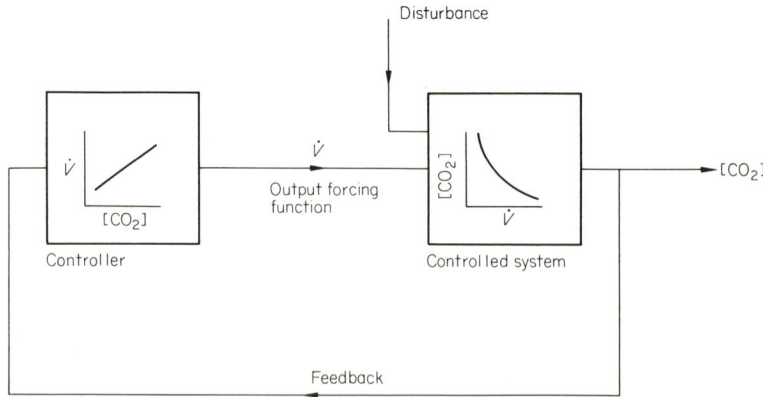

Fig. 5.8. A respiratory regulator. Note the absence of a comparator. The signal from controller
to controlled system is the output forcing function. A disturbance (e.g. increased concentration
of CO_2 in inspired air) may be another input to the controlled system.

cause an increase in ventilation (left-hand function, positive slope), which in turn is associated with a decrease in body levels of CO_2 (right-hand function, negative slope). The final steady-state result is obtained as the solution of the two simultaneous equations, which can be found by superimposing the two graphs and noting the point of intersection of the two functions.

OPEN AND CLOSED LOOPS

Taking a generalised feedback loop (Fig. 5.9) in a linear system, the overall steady state gain of the system is given by the change in output divided by the change in input.

Steady state gain $= \Delta C / \Delta R =$ 'closed loop gain'

If the feedback loop is broken, and the gain of the system is again measured we obtain the 'open loop gain', which is a frequently quoted system

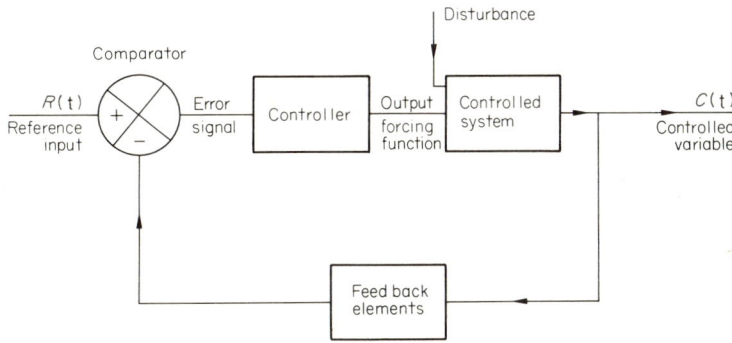

Fig. 5.9. A more general configuration for a regulator.

characteristic, for the higher the open-loop gain the better the compensation by a regulator. The steady state response to a disturbance supplies a method of calculating open loop gain. A disturbance of given magnitude is applied to the system in both open and closed loop conditions and the steady state change of output (ΔC) recorded for both. Then [1]

$$\text{Open loop gain} = \frac{(\Delta C_{\text{open}})}{(\Delta C_{\text{closed}})} - 1 \qquad (5.1)$$

It follows that for better compensation for a disturbance the ratio between effect of disturbance with loop open and effect with loop closed should be high, and the higher the open loop gain, the better the compensation.

Rearranging equation 5.1 we obtain the 'minification' of the system

$$\text{minification} = 1/(1 + \text{open loop gain}) = \frac{(\Delta C_{\text{closed}})}{(\Delta C_{\text{open}})} \qquad (5.2)$$

Thus if it is said of a system that the open loop gain is 3, it implies that for a disturbance of magnitude 1 in open loop conditions, when the loop is closed the steady state output disturbance will only be $\frac{1}{4}$. Similarly for open loop gain 10, minification is $1/11$, for 100, $1/101$ and so on. For perfect regulation, that is zero change in output in response to a disturbance, an open loop gain of infinity is theoretically required.

PROPORTIONAL, DERIVATIVE AND INTEGRAL CONTROL

In Fig. 5.9. we see that the error signal ε goes to the controlling system, whence the output forcing function goes to the controlled system.

In its simplest form the controlling system might be a simple gain change such that

$$\text{output forcing function} = k\varepsilon \qquad (5.3)$$

The higher the gain k the larger the effect of the error signal. This simple type of manipulation is called 'proportional control'. One problem with it is that it tends to 'hunt', that is to oscillate excessively around the desired value before settling. Performance may be improved by incorporating a component for the first derivative of the error signal—'proportional plus derivative control'.

$$\text{output forcing function} = k_1\varepsilon + k_2\, d\varepsilon/dt \qquad (5.4)$$

This type of control will settle down faster to the steady state, but the steady state value will not be altered since at steady state $d\varepsilon/dt$ is zero.

A third type of control incorporates an integration of the error signal—'proportional plus integral control'.

$$\text{output forcing function} = k_1\varepsilon + k_2 \int \varepsilon\, dt \qquad (5.5)$$

This may be used to reduce steady state error.

In a sense derivative control, which responds to rate of change of an error signal, can be thought of as anticipatory. It assumes that since the error signal is changing fast it is going to change a long way, and compensates on this basis. The major disadvantage of derivative control is high-frequency noise.

Contrariwise, the characteristics of integral control resemble not anticipation but memory, for an error signal once integrated must be compensated for, though not necessarily instantaneously. The integrated error signal can be regarded as a debt which must be repaid—some time. The major disadvantage of integral control is low-frequency noise, or drift.

THE LEAD-LAG SYSTEM AND UNIDIRECTIONAL RATE SENSITIVITY

A lead-lag system responds to derivative information in the input signal as well as to its instantaneous value. When applied to a step input (Fig. 5.10a) there is a sharp overshoot followed by a slower decay to steady state (Fig. 5.10b). The off-transient undershoots symmetrically. The shape of this response shows obvious similarities to the behaviour of biological receptors

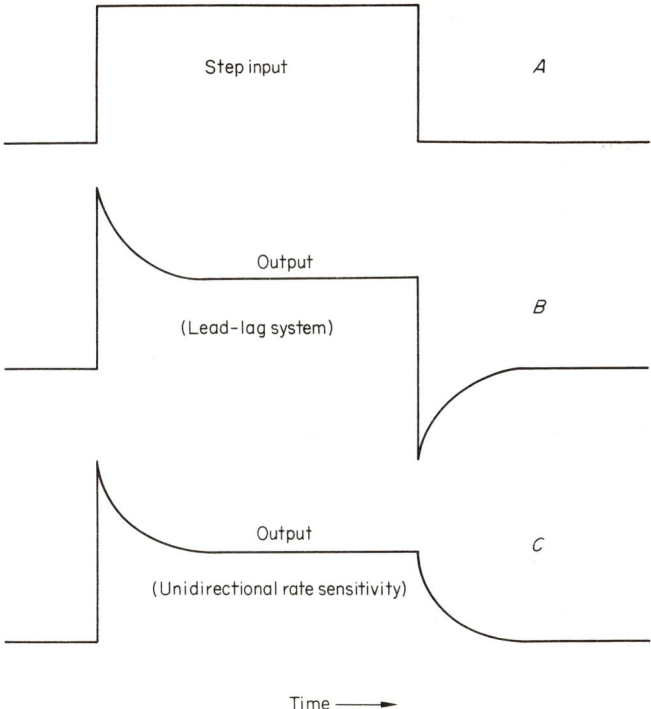

Fig. 5.10. On- and off-transients for a step input (a) to a lead-lag system (b), and to a lead-lag system showing unidirectional rate sensitivity (c).

which show what physiologists call 'adaptation'. Note that systems engineers use that word in an entirely different sense.

If a system responded to rate of change only when it was positive, then there would be no under-shoot on the off-transient (Fig. 5.10c), and this phenomenon is called unidirectional rate sensitivity. A more interesting characteristic of this assymetrically-responding system lies in its response to an oscillating signal (Fig. 5.11), for the resulting output oscillations have a mean value which is higher than the steady state level achieved by a step input of magnitude equal to the mean of the input oscillation.

THE CONTROL OF RESPIRATION

The peripheral chemoreceptors (carotid bodies) respond to changes in arterial P_{CO_2}, pH, and P_{O_2}, in such a way that hypoxia, hypercapnia and acidosis tend

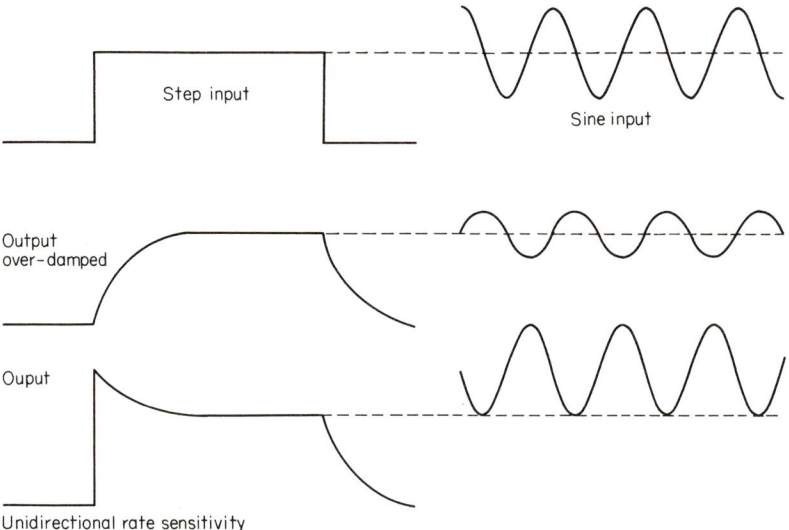

Fig. 5.11. On the left, outputs and transients for a step input to an overdamped system (e.g. Fig. 5.2b), and for a system with unidirectional rate sensitivity (UDRS). On the right, steady state sinusoidal outputs for a sine wave input with mean identical to the height of the step input. Output from the overdamped system has the same mean value as the height of the output to the step; but output from the UDRS element has a *higher* mean. Thus UDRS produces a higher mean signal from an oscillating signal than it does from a step signal with height equal to the mean of the input oscillation.

to stimulate respiration, whereas hyperoxia, hypocapnia and alkalosis tend to depress respiration. The aortic bodies seem to have little or no chemoreceptor action in man.

The central chemoreceptor is sited in the brainstem and responds similarly to P_{CO_2} and pH, but whereas hypoxia stimulates breathing by its action at the peripheral chemoreceptor, it probably depresses ventilation centrally.

THE PERIPHERAL CHEMORECEPTOR: ANIMAL EXPERIMENTS

The signal to the chemoreceptor

The cardiovascular system is a circulatory pump, whereas the lung is a reciprocal (in-and-out) pump. During inspiration alveolar CO_2 concentration is lowered and O_2 concentration increased by dilution of alveolar with inspired gas; during expiration CO_2 output and O_2 uptake proceed, and alveolar CO_2 concentration increases while O_2 concentration falls. The result is that the partial pressures of O_2 and CO_2 (P_{A,O_2}, P_{A,CO_2}) in alveolar gas oscillate in time with respiration, with an amplitude of the order of 2–3 mmHg (0·3–0·4 kPa). These oscillations are transmitted to the arterial blood, where P_{a,O_2} and pH oscillations [2, 3] have been measured by indwelling electrodes.

The signal from the chemoreceptor

A single chemoreceptor fibre fires at random intervals (Poisson distribution) and rather slowly, but the mean frequency of the random pulse train can be modulated, for example increased by arterial hypoxia and decreased by hyperoxia. Although a single fibre fires rather slowly, each sinus nerve contains several hundred chemoreceptor fibres. The total output of these is difficult to measure for some method must be found of inactivating the accompanying baroceptor fibres from the carotid sinus. If however the output of a single fibre or of a few fibres is bin-averaged over 40–50 breaths (Fig. 5.12) it is found that the output, in terms of instantaneous average impulse frequency (Fig. 5.12e), itself oscillates with the fundamental frequency of tidal breathing. The assumption here is that the output of one fibre averaged over many cycles is the same as the output of many fibres averaged over one cycle, i.e. that the system is ergodic. The main point is that the oscillatory input signals of P_{a,CO_2} and P_{a,O_2} are transduced into an oscillatory output signal of impulse frequency in the sinus nerve, and this has been repeatedly demonstrated [4, 5].

Steady state response to hypoxia and hypercapnia [6, 7, 8]

In a series of experiments where arterial PO_2 and PCO_2 could be varied and the resulting mean frequency of chemoreceptor impulses measured it was found that (Fig. 5.13):
1   frequency fell rather hyperbolically as P_{a,O_2} rose, P_{a,CO_2} being constant;
2   frequency rose rather linearly with increasing P_{a,CO_2}, P_{a,O_2} being constant, and the relation was displaced to the left by decreasing pH for the same P_{a,CO_2};
3   the steepness of the CO_2 response lines, found on this occasion to be rather curvilinear, was increased by hypoxia and decreased by hyperoxia.

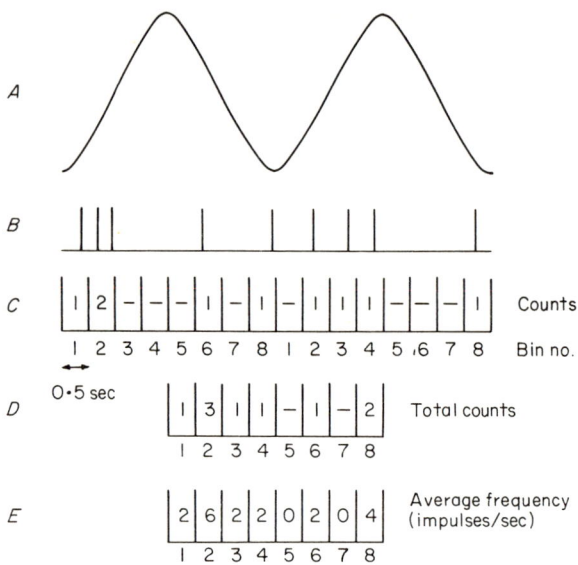

Fig. 5.12. Bin-averaging. Two cycles of a tidal volume signal (a) correspond with a recording of impulses from a single chemoreceptor fibre (b). Each cycle is divided into 8 bins of 0·5 sec width, and the occurrence of an impulse recorded in the relevant bin (c). The counts for each bin are then summed (d) and converted to average frequency in impulses/sec (e).

These results are attractively similar to those found in CO_2 and O_2 breathing experiments in intact man, when ventilation is plotted in place of frequency.

The frequency response of the chemoreceptor

Black and colleagues [9] examined the effect of large step changes in Pa,O_2 and Pa,CO_2 on the rate of firing of chemoreceptor fibres (Fig. 5.14). After a step change in Pa,O_2 firing rate rose rather slowly to a steady state, and declined similarly to control levels when the stimulus was removed. In contrast when Pa,CO_2 was suddenly increased the firing rate rose abruptly and then fell more gradually to a steady state. On the off-transient there was an undershoot, but this was necessarily smaller than the overshoot on the on-transient, for the control firing rate of chemoreceptors was slow, much less than the magnitude of the overshoot.

The transient response of the chemoreceptor to CO_2 resembles that of a lead-lag system, that is a system which responds in part to the derivative of the input signal. The smaller size of the undershoot gives an effect of uni-directional rate sensitivity, here caused by a simple threshold alinearity. The undershoot cannot equal the overshoot because negative impulse frequency

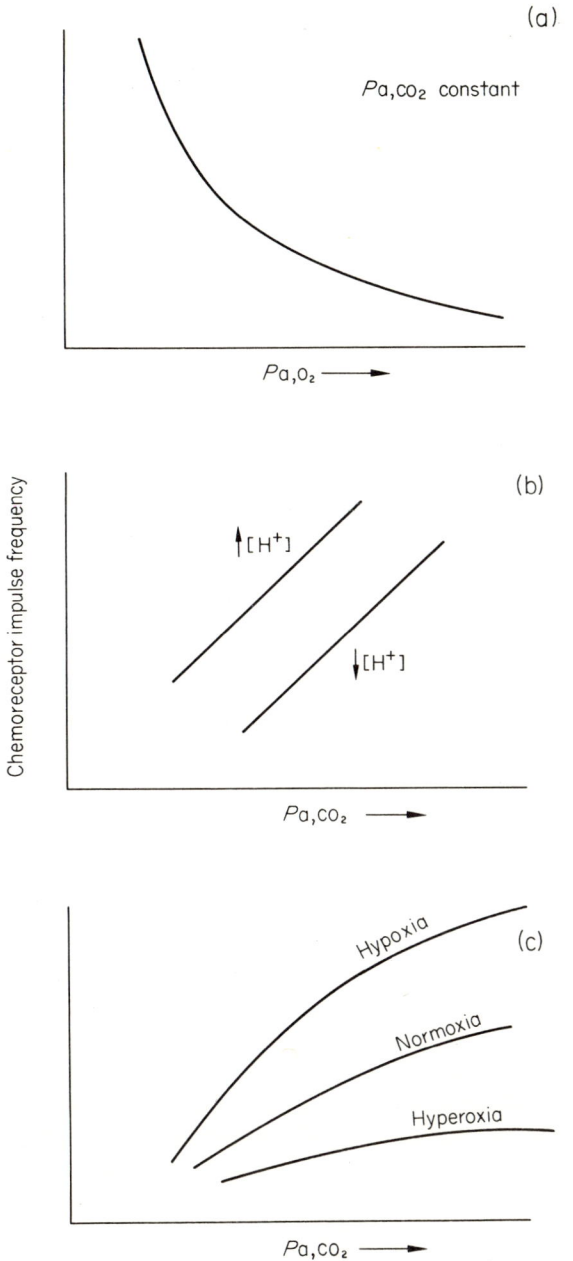

Fig. 5.13. Chemoreceptor activity recorded from the sinus nerve [6, 7], (a) when Pa,o_2 is changed, Pa,co_2 constant; (b) when hydrion concentration is varied independently of Pa,co_2; and (c) when Pa,co_2 is varied and Pa,o_2 is kept constant at various levels.

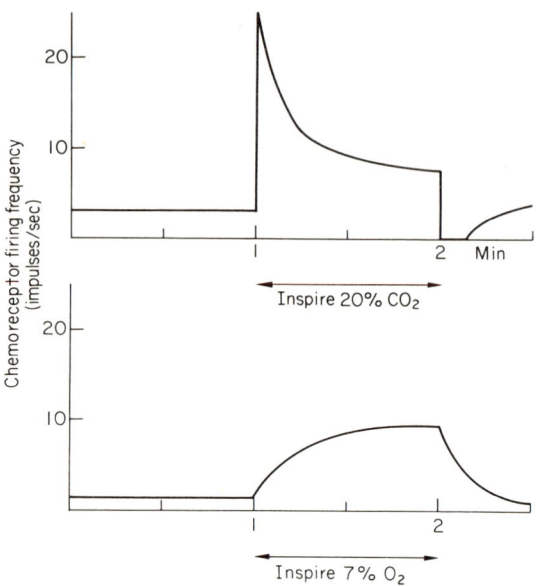

Fig. 5.14. The response of the chemoreceptor in the cat to a sudden increase in $Pa,{CO_2}$ (breathing 20% CO_2) or sudden hypoxia (breathing 7% O_2) [9].

cannot exist. If the system does indeed respond to rate-of-change of CO_2, but responds more to increasing than to decreasing rate-of-change, two predictions can be made. First the oscillating changes in frequency should lead the cycle of chemical oscillations, but by not more than one-quarter of a cycle, and this has been observed [10]. Second, the mean frequency of firing produced by an oscillatory signal should be greater than the mean frequency of firing produced by a steady state input equal in magnitude to the mean of the input oscillations (Fig. 5.11).

In a series of experiments relating step changes in $Pa,{CO_2}$ in the carotid artery to transient changes in ventilation (Fig. 5.15) Dutton and colleagues [11, 12, 13] showed that there was a sharp overshoot in ventilation in the on-transient, that ventilation then adapted, and that there was no undershoot on the off-transient. These results are perfectly compatible with the presence of a response to rate of change of CO_2, which has more effect when CO_2 is increasing than when it is decreasing. Furthermore when CO_2 was applied in a series of pulses (Fig. 5.15) the steady state ventilation was higher than that produced by a step input with $Pa,{CO_2}$ equal to the mean of the pulsed input, agreeing with the second prediction above.

Turning to the effect of hypoxia we find that the peripheral chemoreceptor appears to respond more slowly than for hypercapnia, with little or no adaption [9, 14]. In agreement with this, the chemoreceptor output was found

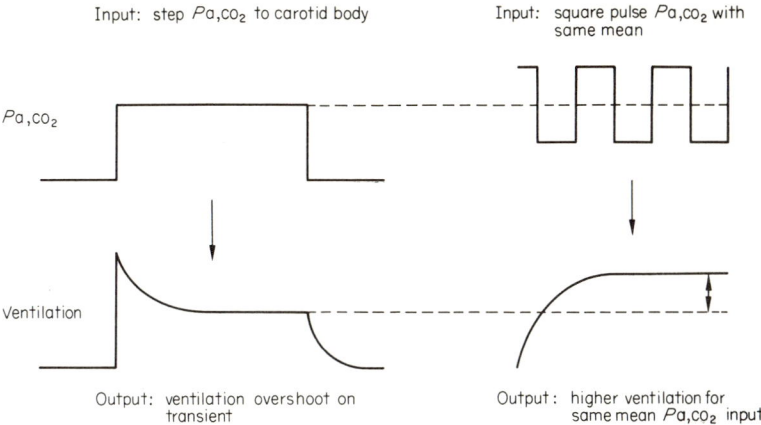

Input: step Pa,CO_2 to carotid body

Input: square pulse Pa,CO_2 with same mean

Pa,CO_2

Ventilation

Output: ventilation overshoot on transient

Output: higher ventilation for same mean Pa,CO_2 input

Fig. 5.15. Ventilatory response to step and square pulse input changes of Pa,CO_2 in the carotid artery of the cat [11, 12, 13].

to follow experimental oscillations of CO_2 input at up to 70 cycles/min, whereas it could only follow O_2 oscillations up to 30 cycles/min [15].

In summary there is evidence that the chemoreceptor responds to rate of change of Pa,CO_2 as well as its instantaneous value, and that its response is greater for an increase in rate of change than for a decrease, perhaps for the simple reason that impulse frequency cannot be less than zero. Observed changes in ventilation are compatible with these results and in particular with the prediction that an oscillating input should produce a higher steady state ventilation than a step input equal to the mean of the oscillations, but these particular observations were not made in man. It should be noted that if the unidirectional rate-sensitive effect is due to the intrinsic low firing rate of the chemoreceptor fibres, it should diminish in importance if that firing rate is increased, for example by large increases in mean Pa,CO_2, for then large decreases in firing rate towards zero would be possible. Thus the effect would be more easily demonstrated at normal Pa,CO_2 with hyperoxia, in theory.

Efferent signals to the chemoreceptor [16, 17, 18, 19]

If recordings are made from the central cut end of the sinus nerve an efferent signal can be detected with impulse frequency increased by hypoxia. If recordings are first made from an efferent slip of an otherwise intact nerve, this hypoxic increase in frequency can be almost abolished by cutting the nerve. If on the other hand the distal end of the cut nerve is stimulated the impulse frequency of the afferent chemoreceptor impulses is decreased. If afferent impulses are recorded from a slip of the otherwise intact nerve, and the nerve is then cut, removing the influence of efferents, chemoreceptor impulses increase.

A feedback loop therefore exists. Hypoxia in the chemoreceptor causes an increase in afferent impulse frequency which itself causes an increase in efferent impulse frequency, which decreases chemoreceptor frequency. It is not possible to say what importance this loop has in the intact organism, and there is no information about its dynamic responses. It should be noted first that all experiments on chemoreceptor neural output described in previous sections were done with the nerve cut, and the loop open, and second that this is a mechanism whereby in theory the central nervous system might modulate the behaviour of the peripheral chemoreceptor, which makes any attempt to separate peripheral and central chemoreceptor effects extremely difficult.

The importance of timing

Using an intra-arterial electrode to follow instantaneous changes in pH, Band and colleagues [20] injected various substances to produce abrupt changes in

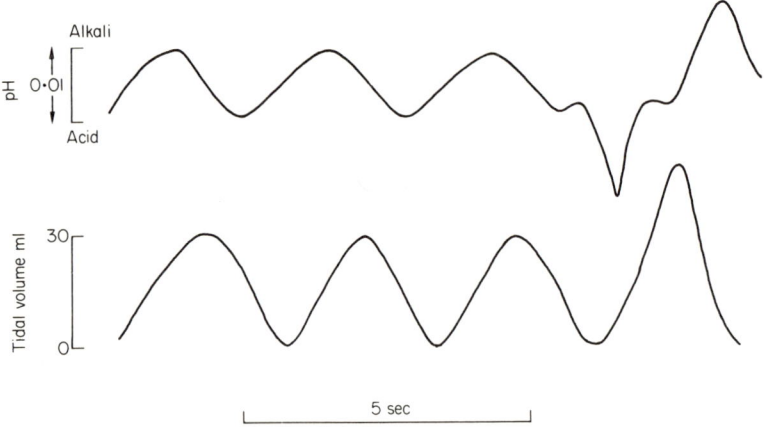

Fig. 5.16. Effect of an abrupt increase in PCO_2 of carotid arterial blood on ventilation [20]. The PCO_2 change is reflected in the transient decrease in pH.

carotid artery pH and PCO_2 in the cat. An injection of saline equilibrated with 100% CO_2 was followed by a small transient decrease in pH. Some, but not all, of these injections were followed by an increased tidal volume in the next breath (Fig. 5.16). It was found [20, 21] that to produce a consistent change in tidal volume the injection had to be timed so that the resulting afferent volley from the chemoreceptor arrived at the medulla in late inspiration. In other phases of the tidal volume the respiratory centre appeared insensitive to the stimulus. Injections of acid to produce similar transient falls in pH had no effect whatever the timing, suggesting that the chemoreceptor could follow rapid changes in P_{CO_2} but not pH.

This finding considerably complicates the understanding of breath-to-breath chemical control of respiration, for the timing of any naturally produced perturbation in P_{CO_2} in relation to medullary events depends primarily on the circulation time between lung and chemoreceptor and it becomes difficult to predict the behaviour of such an arrangement in any systematic and simple way [21, 22].

Summary

Animal experiments show that the neural output of the chemoreceptor to steady state changes in perfusing CO_2 and O_2 concentrations bears a strong resemblance to the steady state ventilation response to hypercapnic and hypoxic stimuli in man.

In response to transient events, the chemoreceptor output can follow the chemical oscillations in the blood, and there is some evidence that there is a response to rate of change of CO_2 as well as to instantaneous values of CO_2 and O_2, and that the rate-sensitivity may be greater for CO_2 increasing than decreasing. However it appears that for very rapid transients the brain only reads information arriving in late inspiration, and the effect of signals of this type will therefore depend on the lung to carotid body circulation time.

THE CENTRAL CHEMORECEPTOR

Somewhere in the brainstem exists tissue which can detect changes in P_{CO_2} or pH so that ventilation is appropriately adjusted.

Two major difficulties complicate the investigation of the central chemoreceptor function. First specific receptors have not been histologically identified, and their exact position can be suspected only by inference. Second, the chemical milieu of these hypothetical receptors cannot be directly sampled for analysis, since it consists presumably of brain extracellular fluid (ECF). This contrasts with the relative ease with which arterial blood can be analysed with reference to the carotid body. Much work has been based on the assumption that cerebrospinal fluid (CSF) composition, which can with difficulty be measured, is identical to that of brain ECF, but this assumption can only be justified in the steady state. Therefore the exact shape of input signals applied to the central chemoreceptor cannot be determined, and much potentially useful information from transient analysis is unavailable.

The physiology relevant to central chemoreceptor function is concerned with the processes of ionic homeostasis and their relation to cerebral blood flow and metabolism. Expertise in this field is rare in applied physiologists, and many clinicians, including the author, find it the most difficult of all fields of respiratory physiology. We shall not go into great detail, attempting rather to abstract from a complicated literature some of the major points. A particularly lucid review of the complexities is given by Cameron [23], and a clear account of the effects of acid-base disturbances by Semple [24].

Some basic principles

When describing the function of the peripheral chemoreceptor we considered as input the partial pressures of O_2 and CO_2 in the arterial blood. We now make a basic and common assumption, namely that the central chemoreceptor responds to the chemical environment of brain ECF, in particular to its hydrion concentration. It follows that we must now take account of not only the concentrations of O_2, CO_2 and hydrion in arterial blood, but also

1 the delivery and removal rates of these substances to and from the brain,
2 their transport across membranes, and
3 the generation of CO_2 and consumption of O_2 by brain tissue.

1. Cerebral blood flow varies with blood gas tensions. If Pa,CO_2 rises or Pa,O_2 falls, cerebral vascular resistance decreases and brain blood flow increases, thus bringing more O_2 to the brain and removing more CO_2. If Pa,CO_2 falls or Pa,O_2 rises, the reverse occurs. Thus there are two important fast mechanisms which regulate brain PCO_2 and pH, namely ventilation and brain blood flow of which ventilation has by far the most potent effect. The situation for oxygen is more complicated and will be discussed separately below.

2. While CO_2 can pass rapidly from blood to brain ECF, and from brain to CSF, the blood-brain barrier seems to impede the passive transport of bicarbonate (Fig. 5.17). Thus if Pa,CO_2 rises rapidly, for example following CO_2 inhalation, arterial and CSF pH will both fall as CO_2 rapidly reaches the CSF. During acute metabolic alkalosis however the rise in blood bicarbonate is not accompanied by an equal rise in CSF bicarbonate.

3. It is a common and worrying assumption that the metabolic production and consumption of CO_2 and O_2 are unchanged during experimental procedures which alter acid-base and cerebral blood flow. Thus changes in cerebral flow are sometimes inferred to be proportional to changes in cerebral arterio-venous differences for CO_2 and O_2 [29].

Finally, the effect of anaesthesia on the performance of the central chemoreceptor may be profound. In general observations on conscious animals and man are of far greater value.

The hydrogen ion; Loeschke's areas, Mitchell's pledgets, and Pappenheimer's goats

It is generally accepted that CO_2 affects the central chemoreceptor through the production of hydrion, the concentration of which determines the output of the respiratory centre.

Although individual chemoreceptor cells cannot be identified, chemosensitive areas are known to exist near the medullary surface of the fourth ventricle, away from the classically described respiratory centres of medulla and pons. Mitchell and coworkers [25] extended some of Loeschke's previous work [26] referring to the chemosensitive areas on the ventrolateral surface of the medulla, using techniques designed to apply chemical stimuli to small areas, such as the application of tiny pledgets of filter paper impregnated with test solutions. They found that respiration was stimulated by application of

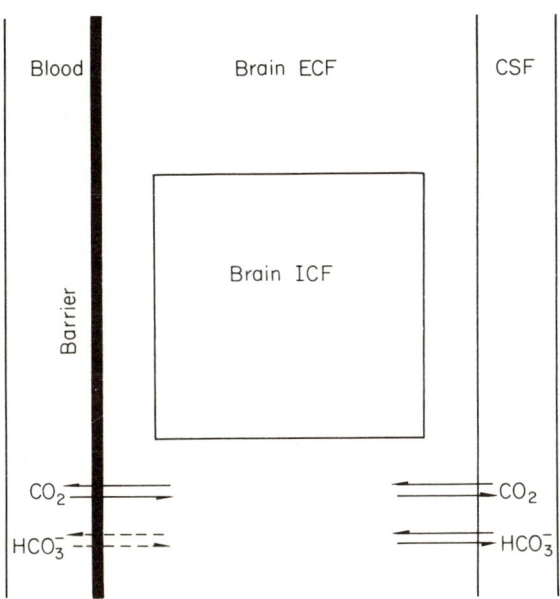

Fig. 5.17. CO_2 can pass easily between blood, brain and CSF, but the passage of bicarbonate ions across the blood-brain barrier is impeded. ECF—extracellular fluid, ICF—intracellular fluid.

solutions of high P_{CO_2}, low pH, nicotine or acetyl choline, and depressed by low P_{CO_2}, procaine, lobeline or sodium cyanide. They noted first that the responses occurred almost instantaneously and concluded that the receptor must be superficial, and second that procaine regularly produced apnoea, and concluded that all the central chemoreceptive properties must have resided in the area studied. It appeared that the central chemoreceptor might respond primarily to changes in CSF pH.

It is always easy to criticise in retrospect, but this theory never seemed to carry much weight, for changes in CSF composition could only occur secondarily to changes in the composition of brain ECF (Fig. 5.17) unless the generation of CSF, which is a matter of some mystery, were particularly purposively arranged. Since CSF changes are thought to lag transiently behind ECF changes, the effect of such CSF changes could only be to damp or slur the changes at the chemoreceptor. It is difficult to see how CSF composition could primarily affect ventilation unless receptors were so superficial that they were in contact with CSF but not with brain ECF. The case bears a striking similarity to that of the Martian and the starting handle (p. 116), in that although the respiratory system can be driven from the CSF compartment, it does not follow that the system must normally be driven in that way.

Pappenheimer and colleagues [27] developed a new experimental preparation, using conscious goats with access to the ventricular system for perfusion and sampling of CSF. They used CO_2 inhalation to alter CSF pH acutely under different conditions of background CSF $[HCO_3^-]$, changing the latter by infusing bicarbonate solutions of differing concentrations into the CSF. It was found that the relation between ventilation and CSF pH (Fig. 5.18a) varied according to the concentration of bicarbonate infused into the CSF. Under these conditions a bicarbonate concentration gradient should exist in brain ECF (Fig. 5.18b). If the chemoreceptor were located some distance along such a concentration gradient, the $[H^+]$ driving it would be different from the CSF $[H^+]$, for the P_{CO_2} in both places would be the same, whereas the $[HCO_3^-]$ would be lower in the ECF than the CSF for high $[HCO_3^-]$ infusion, and higher in the ECF than in the CSF for low $[HCO_3^-]$ infusion. If we were to plot a calculated chemoreceptor $[H^+]$ against ventilation the left hand high $[HCO_3^-]$ infusion line in Fig. 5.18a would move to the right and the right hand low $[HCO_3^-]$ line to the left. It was found possible to calculate a position along the $[HCO_3^-]$ gradient at which ventilation was a single function of chemoreceptor $[H^+]$. For this calculated point on the gradient the goat behaved 'as if' ventilation were entirely determined by chemoreceptor $[H^+]$ (Fig. 5.18c).

This work was in direct disagreement with that of Mitchell and colleagues in that ventilation was *not* solely controlled by CSF pH (Fig. 5.18a) and that the chemoreceptor did *not* behave as though it were superficial.

Further evidence both in goats and medical students [28, 29] confirmed that in metabolic acidosis or alkalosis, once a steady state had been reached when brain ECF and CSF composition was identical, ventilation could again be expressed as a single function of 'chemoreceptor $[H^+]$', now identical to CSF $[H^+]$.

The stabilisation of $[H^+]$ at the chemoreceptor

It was initially thought that in the steady state CSF pH was maintained within normal limits in metabolic acidosis and alkalosis, and there was therefore a

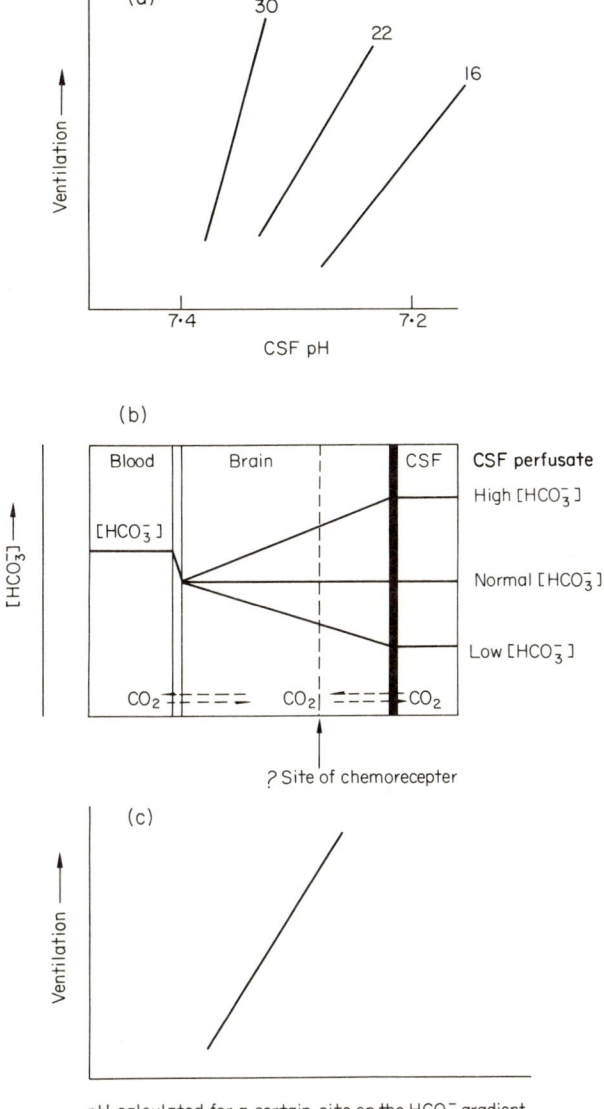

pH calculated for a certain site on the HCO$_3^-$ gradient

Fig. 5.18. (a) Relation between CSF pH and ventilation while CSF is perfused with bicarbonate solutions of concentration 30, 22, and 16 mEq/L [27].

(b) Hypothetical [HCO$_3^-$] gradients during perfusion of solutions with high, normal and low [HCO$_3^-$]. pH along the gradients will be different from CSF pH for high and low [HCO$_3^-$] perfusates, since P_{CO_2} is everywhere the same (Diagram after I. R. Cameron [23]).

(c) A hypothetical point on the gradient could be calculated where ventilation was a single function of pH.

tendency to ascribe changes in ventilation to the peripheral chemoreceptors. Because CSF is a very poorly buffered fluid, measurement of its pH is very difficult, and cannot be performed with the same accuracy as in arterial blood. Another important finding in the conscious goats was that very small changes in central pH of the order of 0·01 units could produce large changes in ventilation, that is that the central chemoreceptor was exquisitely sensitive to changes in $[H^+]$. In the goats small changes in steady state CSF pH were found in metabolic acidosis and alkalosis, although only one tenth as large as the changes in arterial blood. When observations in man from the literature were pooled and re-examined, this was confirmed. Previous small changes in CSF pH in metabolic acidosis and alkalosis had been un-noticed because of scatter in the measurements and the small number of observations in individual studies.

In respiratory alkalosis the change in CSF pH is also less than that in arterial blood, but in respiratory acidosis the brain ECF seems less well protected, and changes in arterial and CSF pH are approximately the same. The reason for the differential behaviour in respiratory and metabolic disturbances is not known, but we should now consider the mechanisms responsible for homeostasis of the brain ECF $[H^+]$.

Apart from the mechanisms of

1   ventilation and

2   renal compensation which affect all tissue compartments, the brain as we have seen

3   changes its blood flow to stabilise its CO_2 load. Other mechanisms include

4   intracellular buffering. The ECF has a low protein content and poor buffering powers. The intracellular fluid however does contain proteins and can buffer H^+ rather like haemoglobin with the production of bicarbonate. A second process involves the generation of NH_3^+ ions by the brain during respiratory acidosis [31] which then take up hydrions.

5   The blood-brain barrier. Barriers to ionic transport may be either passive, due to mechanical impediment to diffusion, or active, when the gradient for an ion across a membrane is maintained by active transport. In the brain it is known that the blood-brain gradient for certain ions (e.g. K^+) is maintained by active transport, but there is considerable argument about whether an active transport mechanism exists for bicarbonate. A major difficulty is that present techniques do not allow the separation of bicarbonate ions in a given compartment into those which have been generated there from hydration of CO_2 and those which have been transported thither as HCO_3^-.

6   There is normally a potential difference (PD) of about 4 mv between brain CSF and blood, such that CSF is positive to blood. In both respiratory and

metabolic acidosis this potential difference increases. In metabolic alkalosis the potential falls and may be reversed. The mode of generation of the potential, and the reasons for its change in magnitude with acid-base disturbances are obscure, but it does exert a stabilising influence in metabolic disturbances. Thus in metabolic acidosis plasma $[HCO_3^-]$ decreases below brain ECF $[HCO_3^-]$ but there is an increased potential difference with ECF positive, tending to prevent transfer of HCO_3^- from ECF to plasma and of H^+ in the reverse direction.

7 Under certain conditions the brain cells may produce ions other than HCO_3^- which alter pH, particularly lactate. Lactate ions are generated for example during respiratory alkalosis, partly by a direct effect on cellular metabolism, partly because hypocapnia causes tissue hypoxia by cerebral vasoconstriction.

The effect on brain ECF of acid-base disturbances depends on the complicated interaction of these seven factors, and will now be separately considered as occurring in a series of steps, with initially no HCO_3^- exchange across the blood-brain barrier (BBB).

Respiratory acidosis

	Blood	Brain ECF
Step 1 Acute	P_{CO_2} increases.	P_{CO_2} increases, but not so much due to increased brain blood flow.
	$[HCO_3^-]$ increases (CO_2 dissociation curve). $[H^+]$ increases.	$[HCO_3^-]$ unchanged (BBB). $[H^+]$ increases, more than in blood.
Step 2 Renal adjustment	$[HCO_3^-]$ increases (metabolic alkalosis).	$[HCO_3^-]$ increases (tissue buffering, plus NH_3^+ generation, plus transfer of HCO_3^- from blood to brain along PD).
	$[H^+]$ tends towards normal.	$[H^+]$ tends towards normal.
Step 3 General result	P_{CO_2} increased. $[HCO_3^-]$ increased. $[H^+]$ increased.	P_{CO_2} increased. $[HCO_3^-]$ increased. $[H^+]$ increased.

An attempt at this stage suddenly to decrease P_{CO_2} to normal by artificial ventilation may lead to disastrous results, for

	Blood	Brain ECF
	P_{CO_2} decreased to normal.	P_{CO_2} decreased to normal.
	$[HCO_3^-]$ decreases, but not to normal, for renal metabolic alkalosis still present.	$[HCO_3^-]$ stays high.
	$[H^+]$ now decreased, i.e. alkalotic.	$[H^+]$ even lower than blood, i.e. severe alkalosis.

The severe alkalosis in brain ECF may be associated with cerebral vasoconstriction with further impairment of oxygen delivery and cerebral function, leading in turn to lactic acid production. The respiratory and metabolic disturbances now present are sufficient in number and variety to preclude any useful prediction of events—but the organism is certainly more sick than before the rapid artificial hyperventilation.

Respiratory alkalosis

	Blood	Brain ECF
Step 1 Acute	P_{CO_2} decreases.	P_{CO_2} decreases, but not so much due to cerebral vasoconstriction.
	$[HCO_3^-]$ decreases (CO_2 dissociation curve).	$[HCO_3^-]$ unchanged (BBB).
Step 2 Renal adjustment	$[H^+]$ decreased. $[HCO_3^-]$ decreases further.	$[H^+]$ decreased. $[HCO_3^-]$ decreases due to production of lactate, and active transport (?).
Step 3 General result	P_{CO_2} decreased. $[HCO_3^-]$ decreased. $[H^+]$ decreased.	P_{CO_2} decreased. $[HCO_3^-]$ decreased. $[H^+]$ decreased, but less than in blood.

The effect of sudden relief of the respiratory alkalosis which would occur if it had originally been produced by artificial hyperventilation which was then stopped, is also seen in respiratory alkalosis due to altitude acclimatisation, if the subject is suddenly brought to sea level, when

	Blood	Brain ECF
	P_{CO_2} increases.	P_{CO_2} increases.
	$[HCO_3^-]$ increases.	$[HCO_3^-]$ stays low initially.
	$[H^+]$ increases.	$[H^+]$ increases and is higher than in the blood.

Therefore the central $[H^+]$ drives ventilation at a lower than normal P_{CO_2}, since central $[HCO_3^-]$ is low, and hyperventilation with low PCO_2 persists after return to sea level, until central $[HCO_3^-]$ eventually rises to normal.

Note however that ideas about the movement and generation of HCO_3^- in respiratory alkalosis and acidosis are rapidly changing [30, 31, 32, 33].

Metabolic acidosis

	Blood	Brain ECF
Step 1 Acute	P_{CO_2} no change.	P_{CO_2} no change.
	$[HCO_3^-]$ decreases.	$[HCO_3^-]$ no change (BBB).
	$[H^+]$ increases.	$[H^+]$ no change.
Step 2 Adjustment at BBB.		$[HCO_3^-]$ decreases slowly, since PD acts to prevent transfer from brain to blood. $[H^+]$ increases slightly and ventilation increases.
Step 3 General result	P_{CO_2} decreases. $[HCO_3^-]$ further decreases, (CO$_2$ dissociation curve). $[H^+]$ tends to decrease.	P_{CO_2} decreases. $[HCO_3^-]$ slightly decreased. $[H^+]$ tends to decrease.
Step 4 Final Result	$[H^+]$ increased.	$[H^+]$ increased little, by one-tenth of plasma change in pH.

The effects of rapid bicarbonate infusion at this stage may not be as intended. Thus $[H^+]$ concentration in the plasma may be rapidly corrected, or overcorrected, but the HCO_3^- will not rapidly reach the brain ECF, and hyperventilation will continue since central $[H^+]$ is still high. Hence the plaxma may be alkaline while the brain ECF is still acid.

Metabolic alkalosis

	Blood	Brain ECF
Step 1 Acute	P_{CO_2} no change. [HCO_3^-] increased. [H^+] decreased.	P_{CO_2} no change. [HCO_3^-] no change (BBB). [H^+] no change.
Step 2 Adjustment at BBB		[HCO_3^-] increases slowly, since reversed PD tends to prevent transfer from blood to brain. [H^+] decreases slightly and ventilation decreases.
Step 3 General result	P_{CO_2} increases. [HCO_3^-] increases further. [H^+] tends to increase.	P_{CO_2} increases. [HCO_3^-] small increase. [H^+] tends to increase.
Step 4 Final result	[H^+] decreased.	[H^+] decreased very little; one-tenth of plasma pH change.

The reader might like to work out what *might* now happen after a rapid infusion of acid.

It must be stressed that the steps described above are stated only to illustrate the interactions of the seven processes affecting brain ECF [H^+]. None of these steps occur independently. All are happening simultaneously with different time courses. The dynamics of the interactions are largely unknown, though some processes are known to be slower than others. The reasons why some processes are slower than others are not invariably clear. The main effect on the author is to induce, on prescription of a bicarbonate infusion or of artificial ventilation, a feeling of uncharacteristic humility.

Two major principles can be clung to:
1   CO_2 leaves and enters the brain easily and quickly; and
2   HCO_3^- leaves and enters the brain with difficulty, and more slowly.

Two major observations should be remembered:
1   a chronic change in arterial [H^+] due to respiratory disturbance produces a similar change in brain ECF [H^+]; and
2   a chronic change in arterial [H^+] due to metabolic disturbance produces a relatively small change in brain ECF [H^+].

Two major deductions seem plausible:

1   for a given change in arterial pH there will be a larger change in ventilation for a respiratory than for a metabolic disturbance; and

2   a new steady state will be reached more quickly for a respiratory than for a metabolic disturbance.

These deductions are in general borne out by the facts.

SENSITIVITY TO CARBON DIOXIDE

Step changes in the concentration of inspired $CO_2 (F_{I,CO_2})$

If man breathes gas mixtures which are hypoxic or contain CO_2, ventilation increases. The interaction between hypoxia and hypercapnia is not simply additive in that the steady state ventilation achieved for a mixture of 15% O_2, 4% CO_2 in nitrogen is greater than the sum of the steady state ventilations reached for 15% O_2 and 4% CO_2 in separate experiments. This multiplicative interaction between hypoxia and hypercapnia was known to Haldane and further explored by Nielsen, but demonstrated with particular detail and clarity more recently by the Oxford School of Physiology [34].

In these experiments subjects breathed various CO_2 mixtures to reach different steady state levels of ventilation. The inspired fraction of O_2 (F_{I,O_2}) was manipulated so that steady state alveolar P_{O_2} (P_{A,O_2}) was constant for varying F_{I,CO_2}. Then for any chosen P_{A,O_2} it was found that the relation between ventilation ($\dot{V}$) and P_{A,CO_2} was rather linear (Fig. 5.19), and that the lines when extrapolated appeared to converge on a single point on the P_{A,CO_2} axis. This fortunate coincidence enabled these steady state relations to be described by the simple equation

$$\dot{V} = S(P_{A,CO_2} - B) \tag{5.6}$$

where $\dot{V}$ is the steady state ventilation, S is the slope, CO_2 sensitivity, or gain of the CO_2 response at a given P_{A,O_2}, and B is the theoretical intercept on the P_{A,CO_2} axis, which occurs at about 38 mmHg (5 kPa). Note first that S depends on P_{A,O_2} – the higher the P_{A,O_2}, the lower the CO_2 sensitivity –, and second that B is a purely theoretical extrapolation which enables us to write a relatively simple equation. B does not exist, biologically, for if it did all ventilation would cease at any P_{A,CO_2} less than 38 mmHg (5 kPa).

In this section we shall continue to consider CO_2 sensitivity, putting to one side temporarily the questions of sensitivity to hypoxia and of the interaction. Practically, this involves experiments where the inspired gas contains high concentrations of O_2 so that there is no hypoxic stimulation of ventilation. It should be realised that this manoeuvre does not in fact separate the CO_2 and O_2 factors, and that when workers refer to CO_2 or hypercapnic response, they are usually referring to the combined response to hypercapnia and hyperoxia, or if preferred to hypercapnia without hypoxia. There would be much to be

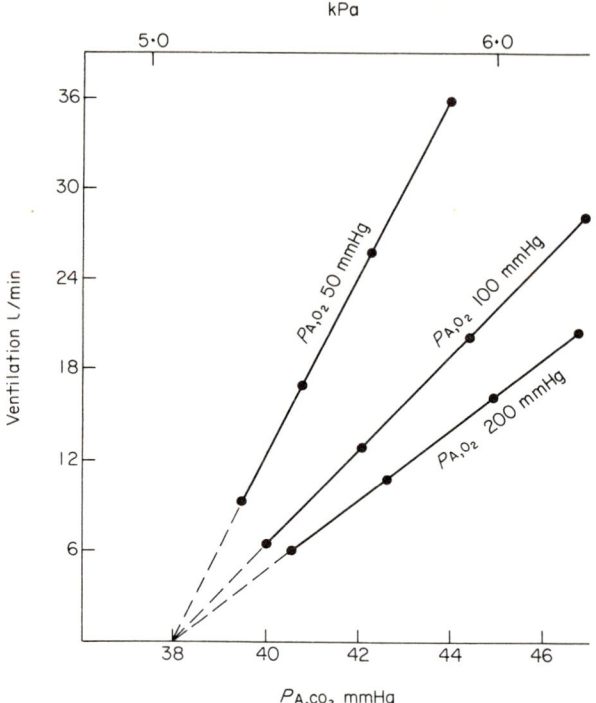

Fig. 5.19. The fan of CO_2 response lines obtained by maintaining P_{A,O_2} constant at various levels while varying inspired CO_2 concentration [34].

said for using the words 'CO_2 response' to refer only to experiments where P_{A,O_2} has been maintained at normal, rather than hyperoxic, levels but such experiments are much more difficult to do.

The transients in ventilation and P_{A,CO_2} which results from a sudden step change in F_{I,CO_2} (Fig. 5.20) have been best described by Reynolds and Milhorn [35]. Ventilation rises rather slowly on the on-transient to reach a steady state at about 20–25 minutes for F_{I,CO_2} less than 5%. The higher F_{I,CO_2}, the longer it takes to reach a steady state. On the off-transient the ventilation falls much more rapidly to normal. It has been said that the slow on-transient is due to the time needed for chemical equilibration at the central chemoreceptor, but there is no explanation on these grounds for the assymetrically rapid fall in the off-transient. P_{A,CO_2} in contrast rises more rapidly than ventilation, with an overshoot at lower values of F_{I,CO_2}, and falls almost instantaneously on the off-transient, with an undershoot.

To a physiologist this type of experiment is simple, but from the standpoint of systems theory it is highly complex, for although the input is a step change in F_{I,CO_2}, it is not a step change in CO_2 input to the system. Increasing F_{I,CO_2} increases ventilation, but the more the ventilation the more

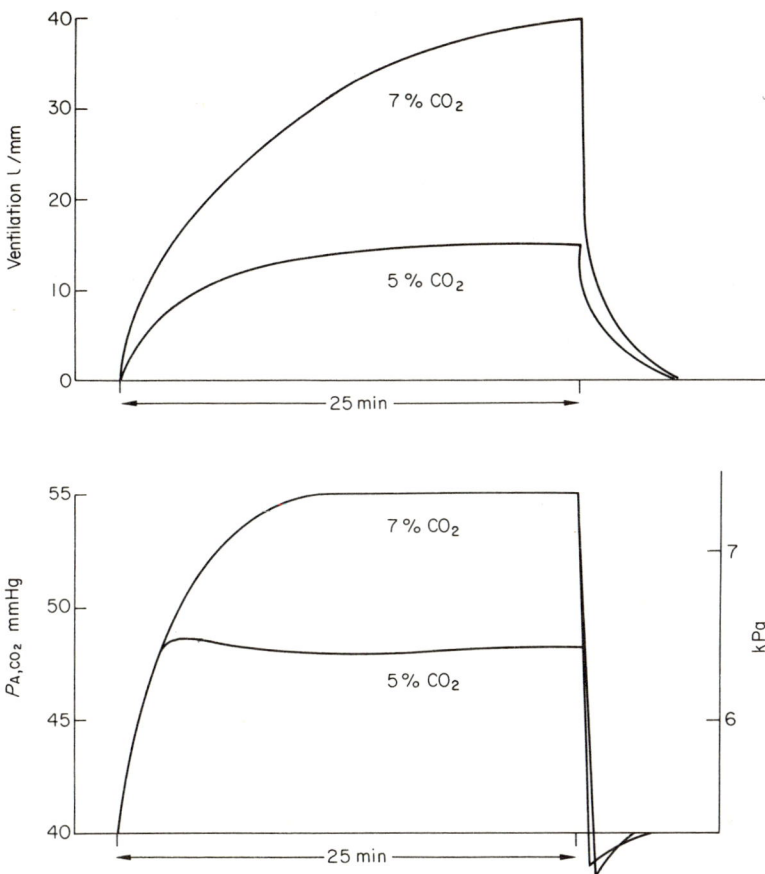

Fig. 5.20. On- and off-transients for ventilation and P_{A,CO_2} for a 25 minute period of breathing CO_2 (5% and 7%).

the CO_2 input in terms of L/min CO_2 input to the system. Note the profound asymmetry between breathing hypoxic and hypercapnic gas mixtures. Both increase ventilation. With a hypoxic mixture, the more the subject breathes, the more oxygen he gets. This is good. With a hypercapnic mixture, the more he breathes, the more CO_2 he gets. This is bad.

Step changes in CO_2 inflow in inspired gas

Fenn and Craig saw this problem early [36] and examined the effect of a constant flow of CO_2 applied into the mouth-piece of the breathing valve. They were looking, for reasons which will be later apparent, for changes in the relation between P_{A,CO_2} and ventilation as compared with the relation found for changes in F_{I,CO_2}, and did not find them. Chambille and colleagues [37] in similar experiments published tantalisingly few results but the illustrated on-transients suggest that steady state ventilation is reached much more rapidly than for a step change in F_{I,CO_2}. This makes excellent sense, for in the latter procedure the stimulus of CO_2 loading is constantly increasing with increasing ventilation. Therefore one would expect that steady state ventilation would be reached slowly, if at all, but that the off-transient would be much more rapid. The important implication is that equilibration at the central chemoreceptor is reached much more rapidly than classical CO_2 inhalation experiments suggested. Feedback diagrams for CO_2 inhalation experiments with step changes in F_{I,CO_2} often show changes in F_{I,CO_2} as a simple disturbance to the controlled system. Fig. 5.21 shows such changes for what they are, namely a good example of positive feedback.

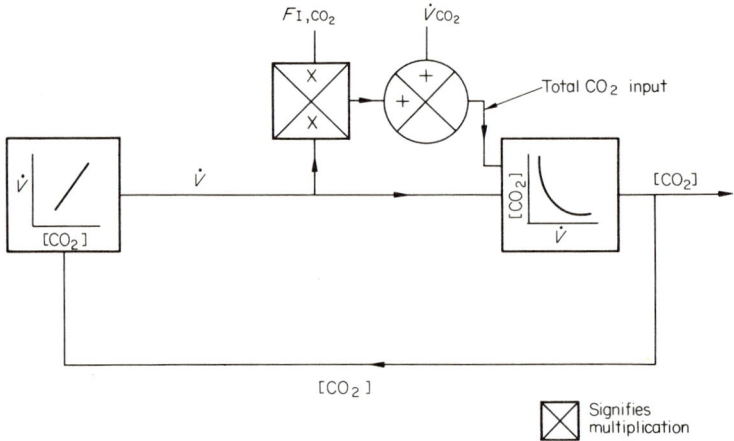

Fig. 5.21. A feedback diagram (cf. Fig. 5.8).
The product of ventilation ($\dot{V}$) and F_{I,CO_2} is added to the metabolic output of CO_2 ($\dot{V}_{CO_2}$) to give the total load, or disturbance, to the controlled system. Thus the disturbance causes an increase in ventilation which in turn increases the magnitude of the disturbance. This is positive feedback.

The rebreathing method

The classical method for measuring CO_2 response by making step changes in F_{I,CO_2} is extremely tedious, for a steady state has to be attained for each gas mixture inspired. A rapid and convenient method consists of rebreathing from a small (6 L) bag with an initial concentration of about 7 % CO_2 in O_2. [38, 39] After initial equilibration CO_2, measured instantaneously at the mouth, rises linearly at about 6 mmHg/min (0·8 kPa/min) and ventilation naturally increases. Mean ventilation and mean end-tidal CO_2 are calculated for thirty-second periods, ignoring the first thirty seconds of the procedure, to obtain a CO_2 response curve which differs little from that obtained by the steady state technique. The key to the method lies in the simple fact that CO_2 cannot be expelled from the lung-bag system, whatever the ventilation. The implications of this are

1   that the section of the feedback loop whereby normally increased ventilation decreases CO_2 input to the chemoreceptors is broken;
2   that when the rebreathing bag is small, and there is an initial CO_2 concentration such that inspired $P\text{CO}_2$ is about equal to mixed venous, CO_2 exchange across the alveolar membrane virtually ceases after a brief equilibration period;
3   that thereafter arterial and brain ECF $P\text{CO}_2$ rise at identical rates;
4   that the gradient between arterial and brain ECF (or brain venous) $P\text{CO}_2$ is very small, perhaps as small as 1 mmHg (0·13 kPa);
5   that because of the small arteriovenous difference, increases in cerebral blood flow which accompany rising $P\text{CO}_2$ have only a minor effect;
6   and that therefore arterial $P\text{CO}_2$, and since there is no transalveolar gas exchange, end-tidal $P\text{CO}_2$, may be taken as closely representative of brain chemoreceptor $P\text{CO}_2$ [39].

If the central chemoreceptor is rather slow to respond to inspired CO_2, how is it that we can plot simultaneous values of end-tidal CO_2 and ventilation from the rebreathing procedure? The reason is that the delays in ventilation response in the steady state method, even with a constant CO_2 inflow, result from delay in equilibration of the brain ECF together with delays from the lung and circulation when the CO_2 input is outside the brain, whereas the CO_2 input to the chemoreceptor during rebreathing arises inside the brain, being the brain's metabolic CO_2 production. ECF equilibration under these conditions seems to be rapid, and no circulatory or lung delays are involved.

While the reasonable agreement between CO_2 response slopes obtained by both methods gives some indirect support to this notion, two discrepancies should be noted. First, we have seen that arterial $P\text{CO}_2$ approximates closely to brain ECF $P\text{CO}_2$ during rebreathing, but during the steady state procedure arterial $P\text{CO}_2$ must be less than brain ECF $P\text{CO}_2$ by several mmHg (perhaps 1 kPa). One would expect the rebreathing $P\text{CO}_2$ response therefore to be shifted to the right of the steady state slope and this is in fact the case. The slope is not changed, if there is no acid-base disturbance. Second, if there is a metabolic acid-base disturbance there is indeed a systematic difference in results obtained by the two techniques. In metabolic acidosis and alkalosis, the slope of the CO_2 response by the steady state method is unchanged, but the line is shifted to the left and right respectively with changes in intercept B (Fig. 5.22). With the rebreathing technique for reasons which are not known the slope is increased in metabolic acidosis and decreased in metabolic acidosis, with no change in intercept [40].

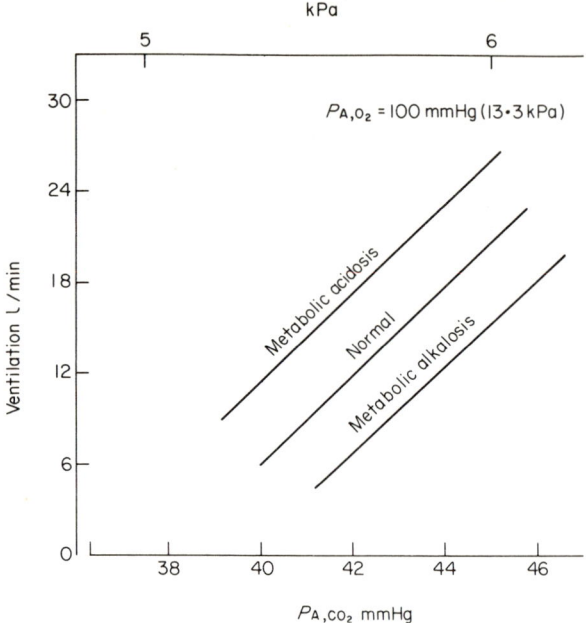

Fig. 5.22. Effect of metabolic acidosis and alkalosis on the CO_2 response by the steady-state technique.

Despite this important reservation, the simplicity and rapidity of the rebreathing technique account for its popularity and indeed in patients who cannot undertake long sessions of steady state measurements and where severe abnormalities of lung function preclude the assumption that end-tidal equals arterial P_{CO_2}, it may be the only practical way of assessing the CO_2 response.

Sinusoidal changes in F_{I,CO_2}

It was predictable that when exponents of systems theory became interested in respiratory control a sinusoidal input would sooner or later be employed. Stoll [41] analysed the ventilation response to a sinusoidally changing F_{I,CO_2} at various frequencies. He fitted the data to a second order linear equation (his Equation 4) with a transfer function (his Equation 3) which suggests that total response was half accounted for by a component of the system which had a pure time delay of a few seconds and a time constant of about 30 seconds, and half by a component which had the same pure time delay but a time constant of 400 seconds. The scatter from repeated experiments, especially from the phase measurements, was very large. Stoll points out an important moral when he shows that the amplitude data could also be well fitted by a transfer function derived from step transient analysis by Lambertsen and colleagues

[42]. This transfer function had three components, one with a 4 second delay and a fast 6 second time constant, and two with 16 second delays and longer time constants of 11 and 155 seconds. It had been suggested that the fastest of these three components had represented peripheral chemoreceptor function while the other two represented the behaviour of well and poorly perfused portions of the central chemoreceptor. Yet Stoll's transfer function gave two entirely different components.

In this type of analysis where the scatter is large and the equations to be fitted are complicated, any number of equations can be found which fit the data quite well. Any attempt to interpret obtained parameters in terms of separate body compartments or functions must be highly suspect without additional rigorous experimental evidence.

Daubenspeck [43] provided such evidence by applying sinusoidally varying F_{I,CO_2} to the unanaesthetised decerebrate cat, and repeating the experiment after cutting the sinus nerves, the vagus nerves, or both. Selecting some of his important findings, we find that with the neural input intact, his data was best fitted by a transfer function with two components. The first accounted for about one fifth of the steady state gain with a pure time delay of 2·5 seconds, and a time constant of 9 seconds. The second accounted for about four-fifths of the steady state gain, with a pure time delay of 2·5 seconds and a time constant of about 2 minutes. When the sinus nerve was cut, the first component disappeared, in the sense that the data could now be fitted by a transfer function consisting solely of the second component. Thus the first component could be attributed to the peripheral, and the second to the central chemoreceptor.

Note first that even with the sinus nerve cut, the pure time delay between alveolar P_{CO_2} stimulus and central chemoreceptor response was short, about 2·5 seconds, a finding confirmed by Borison and McCarthy [44] in the same experimental preparation using step inputs. Second, a time constant of two minutes for the central chemoreceptor implies that after a step input 95% of the steady state output value should be reached in 4 minutes. Overall, the central chemoreceptor is much faster than classical CO_2 breathing experiments had suggested.

Both Stoll and Daubenspeck [43, 44] used tests of system linearity to justify their application of linear theory. They applied input sine waves of varying amplitude and mean value to see whether the frequency response was altered, for in a linear system it should not be. Another characteristic of a linear system is that a sine wave input gives a sine wave output, differing perhaps in mean, amplitude and phase, while in an alinear system the output wave form will be distorted from the sinusoidal shape. They used Fourier analysis to see whether the output was distorted, in which case harmonics of the fundamental frequency would be found. In general the application of linear theory was justified.

Step changes in alveolar or end-tidal P_{CO_2}

Complex experimental technology is required to produce a true step in alveolar or end-tidal P_{CO_2} [45, 46]. The advantage of such a procedure is to remove from the CO_2 response the dynamics concerned with the ventilatory process, examining more precisely the relation between controller input and response. However the arterial P_{CO_2} does not necessarily follow the measured input of alveolar or end-tidal P_{CO_2}, so some of the dynamics of the controlled system still remain.

Experiments of this type in man [45] show that the ventilation response approaches a steady state in 5 minutes, and that the on-transient is now faster than the off-transient, in sharp contrast with the results for the classical CO_2 breathing method (Fig. 5.20). Analysis of the response into fast and slow components cannot with confidence be referred to central and peripheral chemoreceptors, but are of great importance in the consideration of $CO_2:O_2$ interaction, to which we shall return.

Single breaths of high CO_2 concentration

The plan is that a very brief input of CO_2 will cause a peripheral chemoreceptor response (fast) which will be over before any central response (slow) and will thus separate peripheral from central components.

Bouverot and colleagues [47] gave single breaths of 6% CO_2 to anaesthetised dogs and noticed a transient increase in ventilation after a lag of 5–10 seconds. After the sinus nerve was cut, a smaller transient increase was produced, and occurred later than 15 seconds. The two responses were attributed respectively to peripheral and central chemoreceptor activity. A similar transient response with a lag of a few seconds may be observed in man after a vital capacity breath of 15% CO_2 [48]. Note the basic disagreement between these findings and the results of Daubenspeck [43] and Borison and McCarthy [44] in the cat.

Voluntary hyperventilation

All previous stimuli have caused an increase in P_{CO_2} at the controller. We should now consider how the controller behaves when CO_2 decreases. Is there for example a threshold below which apnoea occurs? Early experiments suggested that after voluntary hyperventilation there was indeed such a threshold but in retrospect it seems probable that the subjects of the experiments knew too much respiratory physiology. Eldridge has shown that if the subjects are truly unaware of what might or should happen ('physiologically naive') there is no apnoea after voluntary hyperventilation, whereas there is if hyperventilation is produced passively during anaesthesia [49, 50].

Animal experiments suggested that this is due to a remaining central neuronal drive which is induced by voluntary muscle movement accompanying the hyperventilation, a kind of residual neuronal afterglow [51, 52].

Normal variation of CO_2 response in man

The slope of the CO_2 response, obtained usually by the rebreathing procedure, varies ten-fold in normal subjects. Some of this variation is due to differing body size; one would expect the change in ventilation for 1 mmHg (0·13 kPa) change P_{CO_2} to be greater for the elephant than for the mouse. Therefore if ventilation is expressed as vital capacities or total lung capacities per minute the variation in slope diminishes. Still, it is wide. There is considerable argument as to whether it is under genetic control [53, 54]. Cortical influences also produce variation, as experiments on the effects of hypnosis show [55].

Abnormal variation of CO_2 response in man

CO_2 sensitivity may be diminished by opiates, barbiturates, pethidine, pentazocine, and flurazepam (for references see [56]). Small changes may also be seen after the administration of diuretics and bronchodilators [57, 58].

Many patients with chronic lung disease show an apparently low sensitivity to CO_2. This finding is difficult to interpret since we do not know if their CO_2 response has always been low, or has become low because of their disease; and since they may have severe abnormalities of mechanical function such that their respiratory centre output might be normal, but incapable of translation into ventilatory performance. These major questions are considered in the chapter on respiratory failure.

SENSITIVITY TO OXYGEN

The steady state method

We have previously noted that the slope S of the CO_2 response varies systematically with P_{A,O_2} [34]. If the slope S is plotted against P_{A,O_2}, a rather hyperbolic relation is established (Fig. 5.23), which may be conveniently summarised by the equation

$$S = D \left\{ 1 + \frac{A}{(P_{A,O_2} - C)} \right\} \tag{5.7}$$

This function is not defined for values of P_{A,O_2} less than or equal to C. By inspection, as P_{A,O_2} decreases to approach the value of the constant C the expression $A/(P_{A,O_2} - C)$ increases without bound, and so also does slope S, and so, therefore, does ventilation. If P_{A,O_2} is allowed to increase without bound the expression $A/(P_{A,O_2} - C)$ approaches zero, and slope S approaches the value D. Constants C and D define the asymptotes of the hyperbola, and its position on the graph. Like intercept B in Fig. 5.19, they are extrapolated values of theoretical interest. With C and D fixed, increases in A give a greater slope S for all P_{A,O_2} values above C (Fig. 5.23), for the hyperbola is displaced up and to the right. The constant A is sometimes described as the 'shape

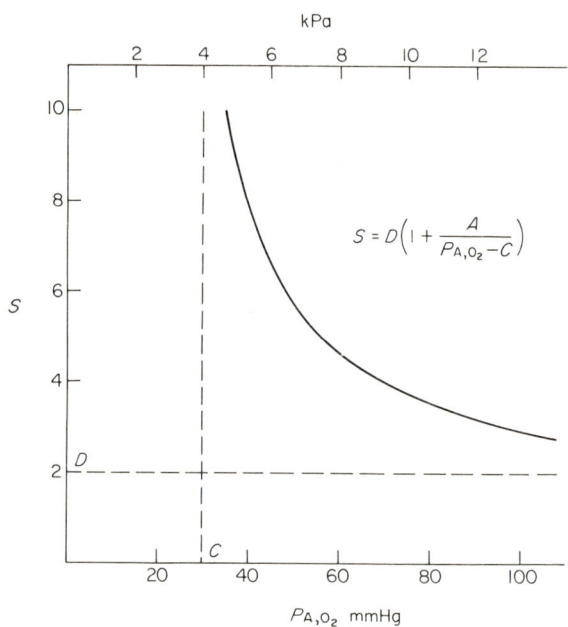

$$S = D\left(1 + \frac{A}{P_{A,O_2} - C}\right)$$

Fig. 5.23. The relation between slope of CO_2 response (S) and P_{A,O_2} is hyperbolic, with asymptotes C and D.

factor' with larger A implying greater sensitivity to hypoxia. Note particularly however that increases in C and D will also shift the hyperbola, respectively to the right and upwards. Increases in these two variables will also give a larger slope S for all P_{A,O_2} greater than C.

Progressive isocapnic hypoxia

If classical methods for CO_2 response were tedious, the method of assessing response to hypoxia was even less adapted to clinical work, for an entire fan of CO_2 response lines (Fig. 5.19) had to be obtained, the slope of each line giving one point only to plot S against P_{A,O_2} and obtain the constants A, C and D of the hyperbola. Therefore more rapid methods were devised whereby the ventilatory response was measured during progressive hypoxia (e.g. from rebreathing) while P_{A,CO_2} was kept normal.

Then a plot of P_{A,O_2} against ventilation gave a hyperbolic response and the question was how to characterise the response in terms of numbers.

Combining equations 5.6 and 5.7, and eliminating S we obtain

$$\dot{V} = (P_{A,CO_2} - B) . D . (1 + A/(P_{A,O_2} - C))$$

or

$$\dot{V} = D' . (1 + A/(P_{A,O_2} - C)) \tag{5.8}$$

where $D' = (P_{A,CO_2} - B) . D$

Thus if steady state results can be equated with those from progressive hypoxia the hyperbola obtained by plotting ventilation against P_{A,O_2} during isocapnic progressive hypoxia has two constants, A and C, identical from those obtained from the S v. P_{A,O_2} plot, with the third, D', now a function of P_{A,CO_2} (here constant), B, and D.

Weil and colleagues [59] used the method of progressively decreasing the concentration of O_2 in inspired gas while increasing the CO_2 concentration to keep end-tidal P_{CO_2} constant. They used a slightly different form of equation 5.8 and took A as the 'shape-determining parameter', the magnitude of which defined the response to hypoxia. Rebuck and Campbell [60] used rebreathing to produce the progressive hypoxia, removing CO_2 by a variably bypassed absorber. Rather than handle the rather awkward hyperbolic response, they measured O_2 saturation (S_{a,O_2}) continuously by ear oximeter. If S_{a,O_2} is plotted against ventilation the response is linear, and the hypoxic response was defined by the slope of the line. These techniques raise a number of questions. Can the response obtained by a continuously changing stimulus of P_{A,O_2} be fairly compared to steady state results? Weil and colleagues [59] found that steady state ventilation after a step change in F_{I,O_2} was reached only about 20 seconds later than steady state P_{A,O_2}, and suggested that the differences due to a continuously changing input would therefore be small. Is end-tidal P_{O_2} a reasonable approximation to mean alveolar P_{A,O_2}? In normal lungs probably it is, but in abnormal lungs the assumption is not justified. One of the great advantages of the CO_2 rebreathing technique was that since CO_2 exchange was impeded, partial pressures of end-tidal gas could be assumed equal to alveolar, or arterial, even in abnormal lungs, but this advantage does not apply to progressively hypoxic rebreathing. The use of an ear oximeter to measure saturation gets round this problem and simplifies analysis of the response, but ear oximeters are almost impossible to calibrate, certainly without simultaneous blood sampling, which spoils the simplicity of the procedure. Finally the use of 'shape-determining parameter A' to characterise response disguises the fact that ventilation for a given P_{A,O_2} depends also on C, the theoretical P_{A,O_2} at which ventilation becomes impossibly large, and D, the theoretical ventilation when P_{A,O_2} is very high.

These things said, the techniques of isocapnic progressive hypoxia have given useful information from subjects for whom the classical steady state methods were patently impractical.

Single breath tests

A single tidal breath of nitrogen in man may be followed by a transient increase in ventilation [61], but the effect is more obvious if a vital capacity breath is taken [48].

Single-breath tests have major advantages, both for CO_2 and O_2 sensitivity testing, in that

1 the transient nature of the stimulus should give a response uncontaminated by secondary adaptive changes, for example in cerebral blood flow;
2 they are rapid to perform; and
3 in the case of hypoxia, are less risky than steady state methods.

On the other hand, it may be difficult or impossible to pick a small transient response out of the naturally noisy signal of tidal breathing. To get round this, the stimulus can be repeated many times and the signals averaged, in which case the rapidity of the test is lost and complex data-handling apparatus may be required; or the procedure may be carried out during exercise, in which case additional neural inputs to the respiratory centre may be involved; or the concentration of CO_2 in the test breath may be increased, in which case the subject will taste it; or the test breath may be increased in size, say to vital capacity, in which case the subject must recognise the test breath, and additional neural input arrives from the chest wall and the vagus. Thus single-breath tests have major advantages and give interesting qualitative information, but as usually performed do not purely test the peripheral chemoreceptor.

The main problem with progressive hypoxia and the steady state method lies in the maintenance of isocapnia, for while alveolar P_{CO_2} may well be kept constant, the presence of hypoxia alters both the buffering capacity of the blood (Haldane or CDH effect) and the cerebral blood flow, so that brain ECF P_{CO_2} may change while alveolar P_{CO_2} is constant. The cerebral blood flow effect is probably eliminated in the single breath method. A good comparison of steady state, progressive, and single-breath hypoxia testing is given by Kronenberg and colleagues [62].

Transient responses to breathing hypoxic gas mixtures [63]

These depend whether P_{A,CO_2} is allowed to fall, or maintained at the normal level by addition of CO_2 to the inspired gas. In the former case small overshoots in the ventilation on-transients are observed, whereas in both cases small undershoots occur on the off-transient. Ventilation invariably lags P_{A,O_2}. Steady state ventilation is reached within 4 minutes for the hypocapnic procedure.

Normal values for hypoxic response

As with the CO_2 response there is wide variation among apparently normal nonathletic subjects, whatever the method of assessment. On the whole, subjects with a low sensitivity to CO_2 tend to have a low sensitivity to hypoxia, though the correlation is not strong [64, 65, 66].

Factors affecting hypoxic response

1   Exercise apparently increases the gain of the hypoxic drive. While it is tempting to ascribe this to the increase in circulating catecholamines, for adrenaline is known to increase hypoxic drive, the effect of exercise in this respect is not diminished by blocking the beta-adrenoceptors [67], nor is it abolished by stellate ganglion block [68].
2   Long-term exposure to hypoxia either at altitude or in children with congenital cyanotic heart disease appears to induce a relative insensitivity to hypoxia.
3   Highly-trained athletes may be insensitive to hypoxia [69]. It is not clear whether this is acquired during training, or whether a congenitally small response allows these subjects an advantage in achieving athletic distinction.

4   A patient with asthma who had particularly profound hypoxia during severe attacks was found to be very insensitive to hypoxia, as were some other members of his family [70].
5   Patients with severe chronic airways obstruction were studied [71] using the classical method of CO_2 breathing at two levels of P_{A,O_2}. In some patients the CO_2 response slope was increased in hypoxia as in normals (multiplicative); in some the slope was unchanged, but the line shifted in a parallel fashion (additive); and in some there was apparently no effect of hypoxia (insensitive). The response slopes were obtained necessarily from few steady state measurements, and it was not possible to assess repeatibility. The difficulty of applying the classical technique to sick patients thus leads to results which are difficult to interpret.
6   Some patients with tabes dorsalis have been found to be insensitive to hypoxia [72]. It is assumed that their peripheral chemoreceptors have been denervated.
7   Morphine diminishes ventilatory response to hypoxia [73].

THE CENTRAL EFFECT OF HYPOXIA

While it is certain that hypoxia stimulates the peripheral chemoreceptor, its effect centrally is not quite so clear-cut. Original evidence that hypoxia depressed ventilation centrally could be questioned on the grounds that the animals were anaesthetised. Moreover the vasodilator effect of hypoxia on the cerebral circulation, and the increased buffering power of hypoxic blood (Haldane or CDH effect) would tend to reduce cerebral P_{CO_2} and severe hypoxia would be expected to cause lactate production.

More recent evidence has on the whole supported the classical concept of central hypoxic depression. Thus in dogs exposed to progressive hypoxia [74], ventilation increases as Pa,O_2 falls until a Pa,O_2 of about 20 mmHg (2·7 kPa) is reached, when ventilation decreases. If the peripheral chemoreceptors are denervated, the hypoxic rise in ventilation is abolished, and ventilation is unchanged until Pa,O_2 falls to 20 mmHg (2·7 kPa) when again ventilation decreases. These findings were not affected by anaesthesia. In support of this, Lee and Milhorn [75] found in dogs that when they maintained peripheral chemoreceptor drive constant, by perfusing the carotid sinuses with blood at constant P_{O_2} from a donor animal, and then obtained CO_2 response lines at differing alveolar (and cerebral arterial) P_{O_2}, they obtained a fan of CO_2 response lines which differed from that obtained in the intact animal in that the fan was reversed. The slope of the CO_2 response was progressively *decreased* by hypoxia. Moreover this hypoxic depression of the CO_2 response was made less by increasing the chemoreceptor drive, that is by decreasing P_{O_2} at the carotid sinuses from the donor dog. Rigatto and colleagues [76] found a similarly reversed fan in preterm infants in whom peripheral chemoreceptor function might not be fully developed.

In this literature it is important to define what is meant by hypoxic depression. Weiskopf and Gabel [77] noted that in man the off-transient following a step change decrease in FI,O_2 was faster than the on-transient. They described this phenomenon as due to 'depression of ventilation during hypoxia', but deduced that it might well be caused by a fall in cerebral P_{CO_2} during hypoxia accompanying increased cerebral blood flow. Their 'hypoxic depression' does not refer to a direct effect of hypoxia on the respiratory centre. Second, possible influences of species variation and of anaesthesia must be considered. For example, in conscious cats with denervated peripheral chemoreceptors, Miller and Tenney [78] found that hypoxia induced a remarkable tachypnoea, in contrast to the findings of Morrill and colleagues in awake dogs [74].

HYPEROXIA

In man breathing pure O_2, cardiac output decreases slightly, peripheral resistance increases, and blood pressure remains about the same [79].

From our previous findings (Fig. 5.19 [34]) it would be expected that breathing pure O_2 would depress ventilation. In fact in man there is a transient fall, followed by a recovery to about the normal level. This is most likely due to the accompanying decrease in cerebral blood flow, and diminised blood buffering power due to the Haldane effect, which both tend to raise cerebral P_{CO_2}.

If it is assumed that the transient depression in ventilation is due to suppression of peripheral chemoreceptor activity, what is the central chemoreceptor doing? In intact conscious cats, hyperoxia causes a transient decrease in ventilation as in man, but if the carotid bodies are denervated, there is hyperventilation by increased tidal volume [80]. Rather similar results have been obtained in the decerebrate preparation [81]. The implication of these findings in human physiology is not clear.

THE SEPARATION OF CENTRAL AND PERIPHERAL CHEMORECEPTOR ACTION, AND THE SITE OF INTERACTION BETWEEN CARBON DIOXIDE AND OXYGEN

We have tried as far as possible to consider the effects of hypercapnia, hypoxia and hyperoxia as separate events, for the reason only that this is a useful way to start. It is very clear that there is a complicated interaction between several variables, the most important being the partial pressures of O_2 and CO_2 in alveolar gas and arterial blood and their effect on the peripheral chemoreceptors; the blood flow to the brain, which with its metabolic activity determines the concentrations of O_2 and CO_2 in brain tissue; and the properties of the blood brain barrier, all of which affect the hydrion concentration at some central chemoreceptor which has not yet been precisely located.

The analytic processes which are used to separate the various components have been illustrated in the previous section, but in no particular order. We shall now attempt

1   to list in logical order the possible experimental approaches;
2   to describe some very recent work which seems to give unusually clear-cut results; and
3   to point out the major difficulties in interpretation which the reader should bear in mind when reading any paper on this subject.

Possible experimental approaches

Frequency response of the intact animal

A variety of methods are based on the fact that the peripheral chemoreceptors respond faster than the central chemoreceptors. It is assumed that both the lag time (circulation delay) and the speed of response, analysed in terms of time constants, are shorter for the peripheral chemoreceptor.

Possible inputs are;

1 *Step change in F_{I,CO_2} or F_{I,O_2}.* Disadvantage—positive feedback in case of F_{I,CO_2}.

2 *Step change in CO_2 load.*

3 *Step change in alveolar P_{CO_2} or P_{O_2}.* Disadvantage—both 2 and 3 require complex apparatus.

4 *Sinusoidal change in F_{I,CO_2}.*

Both the above disadvantages apply. It is not a true sinusoidal load in terms of inflow to the system.

All these inputs are accompanied by secondary adaptive changes in cerebral blood flow which mask the primary response of central chemoreceptors. Analysis in terms of components with differing time constant is possible, but it is extremely risky to assign these components to the function of differing anatomical structures.

5 *Sinusoidal change in alveolar P_{CO_2} or P_{O_2}.* We will now introduce the most penetrating work in this particular field. Swanson and Bellville [82] devised apparatus to deliver inspired CO_2 and O_2 in varying concentrations such that the end-tidal concentrations of either CO_2 or O_2 could be varied sinusoidally or held constant. They then examined the frequency response to sinusoidal end-tidal CO_2, with end-tidal O_2 held constant, first at 125 mmHg (17 kPa), then at 60 mmHg (8 kPa). They found (Fig. 5.24) that hypoxia increased the gain and decreased the phase lag at all frequencies studied, that the ratio of hypoxic to normoxic gain increased with frequency, and argued as follows. Assume only that the peripheral chemoreceptor has a faster frequency response than central, i.e. acts as a relatively high pass filter. Then

(i) If hypoxia increases the gain of the CO_2 response at the central chemoreceptor ('interaction central') the ratio of hypoxic to normoxic gain should decrease with frequency. This was not so.

(ii) If hypoxia increases the gain of the CO_2 response equally at both peripheral and central chemoreceptors the ratio of hypoxic to normoxic gain should not change with frequency. This was not so.

(iii) If hypoxia increases the gain of the CO_2 response at the peripheral chemoreceptor, the ratio of hypoxic to normoxic gain should increase with frequency, and this was so. Therefore the multiplicative interaction between hypoxia and hypercapnia occurs at the peripheral chemoreceptor.

All this was done in intact, unanaesthetised man, at levels of P_{O_2} which do not markedly affect cerebral blood flow, and represents a very remarkable technical achievement.

6 *Brief transient changes in inspired CO_2 or O_2.* These techniques have the advantage of removing the cerebral blood flow problem, and may separate peripheral and central effects both in time, if the peripheral sensor has a

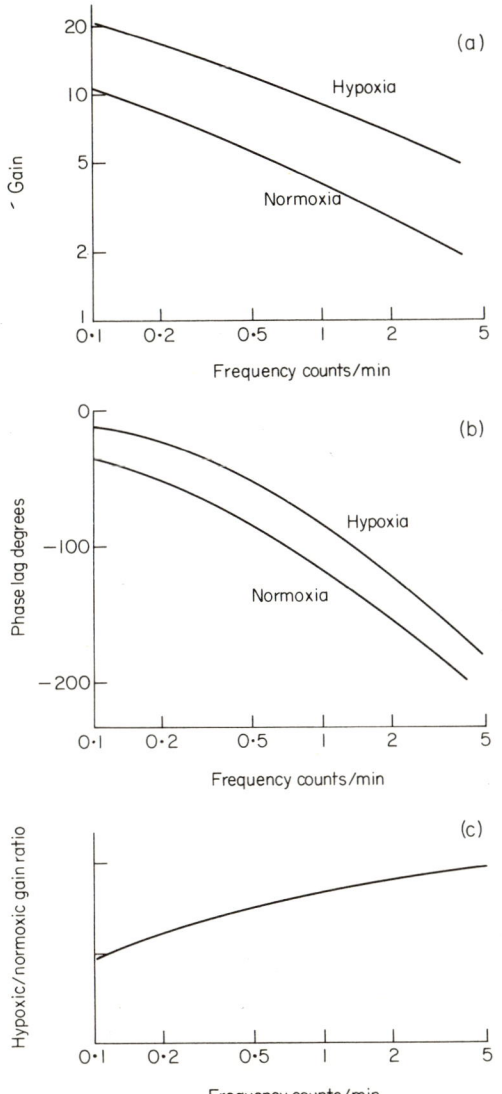

Fig. 5.24. Frequency response in normal man for a sinusoidal change in end-tidal P_{CO_2} at two levels of P_{A,O_2}, with ventilation as output [82].

(a) Amplitude response. Gain is calculated by dividing the amplitude of the oscillations in ventilation by the amplitude of the input oscillation of end-tidal P_{CO_2}.

(b) Phase response.

(c) The ratio of hypoxic to normoxic gain increases with frequency.

shorter time delay, and because of the greater damping effect of the central chemoreceptor. Unfortunately the output in terms of ventilation is difficult to analyse quantitatively because of the inherently noisy tidal breathing signal.

Excluding the peripheral chemoreceptor

1   *Chemical exclusion, by hyperoxia.* The assumption here is that hyperoxia abolishes the firing of the peripheral chemoreceptor, whatever the P_{CO_2}. This cannot be rigorously defended from the literature, since some (not all) chemoreceptor fibres continue to fire at high P_{O_2}. Nevertheless results such as those of Miller and colleagues [83] support the concept. They found that in hypercapnic, slightly hypoxic man, a sudden decrease in F_{I,CO_2} was followed by a decrease in ventilation 2–3 breaths later, whereas in hyperoxic hypercapnia a decrease in F_{I,CO_2} caused a fall in ventilation 3–5 breaths later.

2   *Surgical denervation of the carotid body.* We have already considered work in anaesthetised or decerebrate preparations and will now examine some results from conscious animals and man, and in particular work on dogs [84], ponies [85] and asthmatic subjects whose carotid bodies had been exercised for therapeutic reasons. A series of careful studies on these patients is summarised in the most recent publication [86].

Is the removal of the carotid body followed by a rise in $Pa,_{CO_2}$, which would imply that a drive from the peripheral chemoreceptor contributes to normal ventilation? In dogs, yes; in ponies, yes; in man $Pa,_{CO_2}$ was within the normal range, but the preoperative levels were not known, so that a small rise could have occurred.

In ponies, the initial rise in $Pa,_{CO_2}$, 12–25 mmHg (1·6–2 kPa) at 1–2 weeks postoperatively, falls to about 6 mmHg (0·8 kPa) at 4 weeks and thereafter. Simultaneously a hypoxic response returns in parallel with the changes in $Pa,_{CO_2}$. Therefore in ponies some sensitivity to hypoxia is recreated at some unknown receptor site.

In the asthmatics with carotid bodies exercised,

(i) ventilation, arterial blood gases and acid-base variables were normal at rest and in moderate steady state exercise.

(ii) Breath holding time was prolonged.

(iii) The ventilatory response to hypercapnia was reduced by about one third.

(iv) The response to hypoxia was eliminated. Note the unimportance of the aortic bodies in this respect.

(v) There was no effect on the immediate hyperpnoea of exercise, but the subsequent change of ventilation towards steady state at moderate work loads was slower.

(vi) at high work loads with lactic acid production, the subjects failed to hyperventilate in response to the metabolic acidosis.

In general when interpreting work on the interaction of peripheral and central chemoreceptors, the following factors should be considered.

(i) Species difference; cats in particular tend to behave in a manner peculiar to cats.

(ii) Anaesthesia may disturb central function.

(iii) Although the central chemoreceptor responds more slowly than the peripheral, it is not *that* much slower [43, 44].

(iv) Whereas the input to the carotid body has been considered to be $Pa,{CO_2}$ and $Pa,{O_2}$, which can be controlled experimentally with relative ease, such as by keeping $PA,{CO_2}$ constant in isocapnic experiments, a similar approach does *not* guarantee a constant $[H^+]$ in brain ECF, since brain $P{CO_2}$ may change when $Pa,{CO_2}$ and $PA,{CO_2}$ are constant if there are secondary changes in blood buffering power (Haldane effect) or cerebral blood flow. This point has been mentioned purposefully several times.

(v) Although we have taken the input to the peripheral chemoreceptor as $Pa,{CO_2}$ and $Pa,{O_2}$, there is argument about the importance of O_2 content and arterial $[H^+]$ (see for example [65, 87]).

(vi) No way exists of examining the effect of the peripheral chemoreceptor on ventilation in the absence of central activity.

(vii) Removal or denervation of the carotid body does not impair the function of the aortic chemoreceptors, though these seem unimportant in man.

(viii) We have throughout taken ventilation to be the output of the respiratory control system. This is only fair when lung mechanics are normal.

EXERCISE

During light or moderate exercise at constant load, ventilation increases at first abruptly, then more gradually to reach a steady state in 4–5 minutes (Fig. 5.25). In the early on-transient the blood gases may deviate slightly from

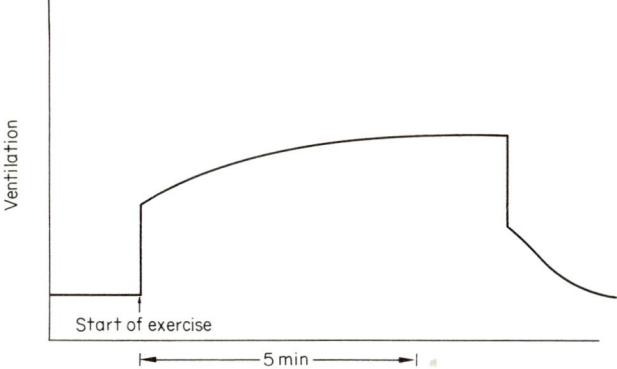

Fig. 5.25. Time course of increase in ventilation during moderate exercise.

normal, but such changes are small and not sufficiently consistent for systematic description. In the steady state, in almost all studies (but see, for example, [88]), $Pa,\mathrm{CO_2}$, $Pa,\mathrm{O_2}$ and arterial pH are normal.

There are two problems. First why does ventilation increase at all? This is one of the larger mysteries of physiology. Second, what causes the initial abrupt increase?

There are two intellectual approaches to the subject. The first, in classical physiology, states that since CO_2 concentrations in the arterial blood are normal during moderate exercise, CO_2 cannot be the stimulus responsible for the increase in ventilation. Similar arguments are adduced for O_2 and pH. Therefore some other mechanism, independent of CO_2, O_2 and pH, must be responsible. Note the one-sided approach to the feedback loop. The second, in systems theory, starts from the precept that if the purpose of respiratory control is to maintain CO_2 concentration at a certain normal level, then the more efficient the control, the less the CO_2 will deviate from normal in response to a change in CO_2 input to the system. If the control is perfect, CO_2 concentration will not change at all. If man breathes CO_2 mixtures, $Pa,\mathrm{CO_2}$ rises: if man increases metabolic production of CO_2 by exercise, $Pa,\mathrm{CO_2}$ does not change. Therefore the respiratory system is completely efficient in eliminating metabolically produced CO_2, but not in eliminating an inspired load. In an alinear system the apparent efficiency may vary if it is loaded at different points, even though the controller equations are unchanged. This possibility has received little attention, though calculations based on alinear modelling suggest it is not of major importance [89]. If not, there must be a change in controller tactics, but this need not mean that CO_2 is uninvolved, for the CO_2 signal may be processed in a different and more efficient way. Alternatively, or additionally, there may indeed be entirely separate control mechanisms which are brought into play during exercise.

Neurological mechanisms

There seem to be three main possibilities.
1   When the motor cortex generates signals to the spinal motoneurones during exercise, collateral impulses pass into the reticular formation which excite the respiratory centre.
2   Joint proprioceptors transmit excitatory impulses to the respiratory centre.
3   Joint proprioceptors transmit signals which increase the sensitivity of the peripheral chemoreceptor via connections in the sympathetic nervous system.

The first two hypotheses are plausible, but the third must be extensively modified. Initial suggestive evidence that passive hind-limb movements in the anaesthetised cat increased the rate of firing of chemoreceptor fibres, and that this was abolished if the sympathetic outflow to the carotid body was interrupted, [90] has not been confirmed [91, 92]. In the dog, when carotid sinus Po_2 and Pco_2 are controlled by cross perfusion from a donor animal, leg muscle exercise does not increase the chemoreceptor output [93]. In man with chemoreceptors surgically removed [86] steady state ventilation at low or moderate levels of exercise is normal, albeit with a slower ontransient. Those subjects however lacked the increase in ventilation associated with lactic acid production in heavy exercise. Finally beta-blockade or stellate ganglion block in man do not affect the steady state exercise response [67, 68].

In considering the initial abrupt increase in ventilation, it is difficult to exclude the participation of a neurological drive at cortical level. If the subject anticipates the onset of exercise, his initial ventilatory response is likely to be affected by the anticipation. Even if the exact time of onset of the exercise in unknown to the subject the fact that he has been placed on a bicycle ergometer or treadmill must arouse a certain anticipatory speculation. The nature of the initial response can however be altered by preliminary manoeuvres which change arterial blood gases [94]. In the study on chemodenervated asthmatics [86] compared with normal controls, some in both groups showed an abrupt increase, and some did not.

INCREASING CARBON DIOXIDE OUTPUT WITHOUT EXERCISE

One way of artifically increasing CO_2 output is to infuse CO_2 into mixed venous blood. Ventilation then increases, but the question is what happens to Pa,co_2. Earlier experiments were conflicting, but it now appears that in rat [95], rabbit [96], and dog [97, 98], infused CO_2 is eliminated without a rise in Pa,co_2. A single recent piece of work in the awake but highly restrained baboon does not conform [99].

The potential importance of these experiments lies in the fact that there could be no neural input to the respiratory centre due to exercise, since the preparations were at rest. Therefore it seems that at any rate in some animals, an increased metabolic output of CO_2 could be sensed in some way and the information used to increase ventilation so that Pa,co_2 is normal in the steady state. A simple hypothesis would be that there are CO_2 receptors on the mixed venous side, but there is no supporting evidence for that at all.

A new way of handling old signals?

We have previously seen that Pa,co_2 oscillates with the frequency of the breathing cycle, and that a similarly oscillating signal of impulse frequency is dispatched from the carotid body to the brain stem. (It may now be helpful to read again the section on the peripheral chemoreceptor).

Yamamoto [100] calculated that if CO_2 was loaded into the system via the inspired gas, the amplitude of these oscillations would diminish, whereas if the metabolic output of CO_2 increased, their amplitude would increase, and this has been confirmed experimentally. Was there some way in which these larger oscillations could generate a larger ventilation for the same mean Pa,CO_2? Here are three hypotheses.

1 One general possibility depends on the presence of a threshold type of alinearity (Fig. 5.26). Then if the input signal oscillates partly below the threshold, it will generate a larger mean output for the same mean input.

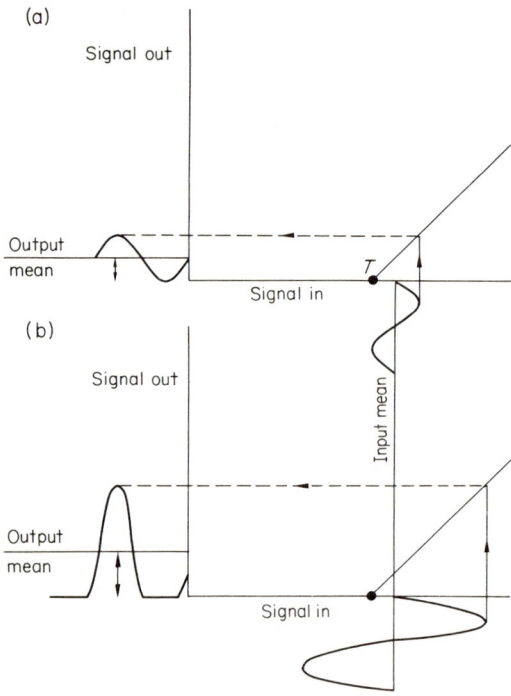

Fig. 5.26. Where there is a threshold (T) an oscillating signal will be completely transmitted only if all the oscillation is above threshold. If part of the oscillation is subthreshold, it will produce a higher mean output signal for the same input.

2 Since for a metabolic increase of CO_2 production the amplitude of CO_2 oscillations in arterial blood increases, the rate of change of the signal must also increase, unless breathing frequency decreases, which it does not. To an extent therefore the rate of change of the oscillations carries instantaneous information about the magnitude of metabolic CO_2 production. There is indeed some evidence that the peripheral chemoreceptor responds to the rate of change of CO_2, but if the amplitude of the oscillation increased, a pure derivative signal would not be expected to produce a higher mean output for the same mean input, for although the absolute value of the rate of change is invariably increased with increased amplitude, the increase in positive rate of change is balanced by the opposing negative excursions. If however the sensor responds more to rate of change in a positive than in a negative direction, showing the properties of unidirectional rate sensitivity, then if oscillations increase in magnitude they will indeed generate a greater mean output for the same mean input (Fig. 5.11). The attractive features of this type of hypothesis are

(a) that the oscillations carry in their first derivative information about the magnitude of metabolic production of CO_2;

(b) that the peripheral chemoreceptor may respond to the first derivative;

(c) that if so, to generate extra ventilation there should be unidirectional rate sensitivity;

(d) that one way of doing this is to use a transmission system with a low natural firing rate, which can therefore respond to increases more than decreases; and

(e) that a naturally low firing rate is what the peripheral chemoreceptor fibres do indeed have.

It all fits very nicely, but experimental evidence in its favour is less systematic than the hypothesis.

3   In some animal experiments (p. 136) it appears that abrupt changes in Pa,CO_2 are transmitted by the carotid body, but only influence ventilation if they arrive at the brainstem at a certain phase of the respiratory cycle. If the respiratory system selects information in this way, then the magnitude of the perceived signal will depend on the phase relation between the oscillating neural frequency signal arriving at the brainstem and the oscillating output signal leaving the respiratory centre (Fig. 5.27). In these circumstances the mean of the perceived signal may be quite different from the mean of the signal from the carotid body.

The difficulty with interpreting such a system is that the relevant phase relation depends critically on the lung to carotid body circulation time, and it is hard to see, intuitively, how variation in circulation time could produce any sensible form of control.

The present situation may be summarised as follows.

1   During light or moderate exercise Pa,CO_2 is normal.

2   Therefore (a) neurological mechanisms are involved, or (b) the chemical signal is differently handled, or (c) both.

3   After carotid body resection in man, steady state ventilation in light or moderate exercise is normal, although the on-transient is slower.

4   Therefore (2a) may be true, and (2b) may be true, but if the steady state increase in ventilation is really due to a subtle treatment of the chemical signal, it must be sensed by some chemoreceptor other than the carotid body.

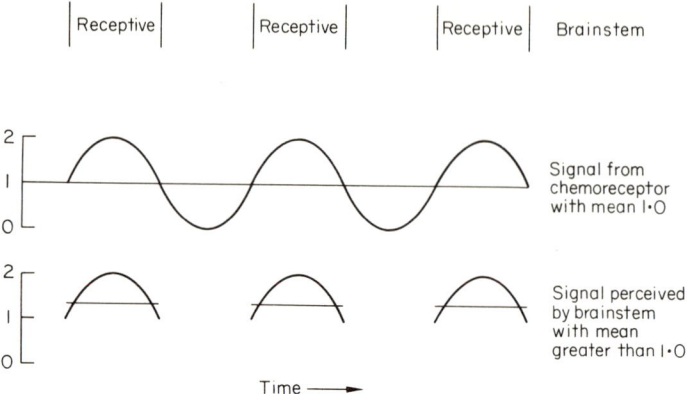

Fig. 5.27. If only part of a signal is perceived, the mean of the perceived part may be higher than the mean of the original. The nature of the perceived mean will depend on the time relation between the oscillations and the receptive period.

5   Note however the mysterious recovery of chemosensitivity by the denervated ponies [85] and the absence of observations immediately before and after carotid resection in man.

6   Increasing CO_2 output by infusing CO_2 into mixed venous blood also increases ventilation, and in some preparations Pa,CO_2 remains normal. Here increased neural input associated with muscle work cannot be responsible.

7   Therefore a mechanism does exist for matching increased ventilation to increasing CO_2 output with Pa,CO_2 kept normal.

8   In normal exercising in man the relative importance of neural and chemical signals cannot as yet be determined.

9   The possibility that the so-called 'slow' central chemoreceptor also responds to the CO_2 oscillations cannot be excluded.

The words tidal volume and frequency have so far hardly appeared in the text, since we have in general been concerned with overall ventilation, rather than control of breath-to-breath events.

The study of the possible importance of oscillations in chemical variables in time with the respiratory cycle clearly has implications in the control of tidal volume and frequency. A series of studies from Cunningham's laboratory has shown that in conscious man manoeuvres designed to alter the shape of the oscillations in alveolar PCO_2 may produce systematic changes in the respiratory pattern (see for example [101]). However it is difficult to assess the importance of fast chemical control in determining breath to breath events when the way in which oscillatory neural signals are handled by the brain is a matter of so much debate and speculation. We shall leave the matter here, and turn to the neural control of tidal volume and frequency.

RECEPTORS IN THE LUNG [102, 103]

1   Stretch receptors are located in the bronchi and bronchioles. They are stimulated by inflation and are slowly adapting.
2   Cough receptors lie in large airways and are stimulated by particulate or chemically irritant matter.
3   Irritant receptors lie under the endothelial lining of the bronchioles and are rapidly adapting.
4   J-receptors lie predominantly in the alveoli.
The first three types are supplied by medullated, the fourth by non-medullated fibres. Stimulation of irritant and J-receptors has been held responsible for disturbance of the breathing pattern in a large number of pathological conditions.

Inflation

Maintained inflation of the lungs inhibits inspiration and promotes expiration. This can be blocked by cutting, cooling, or anaesthetising the vagus nerve. The duration of apnoea is secondarily affected by the consequent changes in blood gases, depending on the depth of inflation and the nature of the inflating gases [104].

Deflation

A sudden complete deflation of one lung causes a tachypnoea which comes on too quickly to be accounted for by blood gas changes. Tidal volume is unchanged or slightly diminished. Alveolar ventilation is surprisingly increased and Pa,co_2 falls. It is not clear whether stretch or irritant receptors are responsible for the deflation reflex [105].

    The threshold is set high for the inflation and low for the deflation reflex in man, and neither plays any part in normal breathing. Thus in man alone, section of the vagus nerve does *not* cause slow deep breathing.

Irritants

Irritants such as SO_2, dust and smoke; *histamine* and rapid *changes in bronchial calibre* caused by cough, rapid breathing or rapid expansion of airways all stimulate irritant receptors [106].

    The role of J-receptors is more problematic. It is tempting because of their site to ascribe to them the tachypnoea of pulmonary embolism, congestion and oedema. Since they are served by non-myelinated fibres, their function may be separated by anodal-blocking techniques which prevent conduction in the myelinated fibres, which run from the stretch and irritant receptors. It is then found [107] that the tachypnoea of pulmonary oedema is probably due to stimulation mainly of irritant receptors, but stretch and J-receptors are also involved. Pulmonary embolism also probably stimulates all three types [108].

In experimental pneumonia in cats and rabbits, the tachypnoea during the first week after induction of pneumonia depends on the presence of an intact vagus nerve on the same side as the lesion [109]. In dogs with experimental pneumonitis, overall ventilation was normal at rest, but increased more than normally on exercise. This excessive increase was abolished by blocking the vagus [110].

Inhalation of local anaesthetic in dogs and rabbits [111, 112] blocks inflation, deflation and cough reflexes. The effect of histamine is partially blocked, but that of phenyl diguanide, which stimulates J-receptors, is unaffected. This is reasonably explained by the failure of the aerosol to reach the more peripheral receptors.

Stimulation of pulmonary receptors also affects the smooth muscle of airways. Stimulation of stretch receptors tends to cause bronchodilatation whereas stimulation of irritant or J-receptors causes bronchoconstriction. One important theory of the causation of asthma states that the known hyperreactivity of the bronchi could be due to an increased sensitivity of the irritant receptors, either innate or associated with epithelial erosion by infection. In normal subjects with upper respiratory tract infections, airways show an increased reactivity to histamine and citric acid inhalation, which can be blocked by atropine [113].

RESPIRATORY SENSATION AND DYSPNOEA

This is the first time we have used the word dyspnoea, as opposed to tachypnoea which can be measured, for it refers to a subjective experience, a feeling of awareness of respiratory events and discomfort due to them. No more precise definition will be attempted.

Guz has drawn attention to a number of different aspects of dyspnoea. It is relatively easy to separate first the feeling of irritation, with cough and lacrimation, which accompanies tracheitis or stimulation of large airways during mechanical aspiration of secretions. Considering the more usual implications of dyspnoea, a normal person breathing 7% CO_2 will feel dyspnoeic, yet if CO_2 is given to a paralysed patient the subject would eventually lose consciousness as Pco_2 rises, but there is no sensation of breathlessness. Therefore dyspnoea is not caused by a rise in the concentration of CO_2 in some body compartment, but the presence of the motor events of increased ventilation is essential. Campbell refers to the 'imbalance' or 'inappropriateness' between the volume demanded and the forces required to meet this demand [114].

One much studied type of respiratory discomfort occurs on breath-holding. If a normal subject holds his breath, eventually the discomfort becomes so great that at the 'breakpoint' inspiration (often following expiration if the breath is held above residual volume) becomes mandatory. It has been long known that the drive to breathe is not purely due to falling Po_2 and rising Pco_2, for the sensation may be temporarily relieved by an inspiration of gas with concentrations of CO_2 and O_2 identical to those in the lung at the breakpoint. On the other hand if breath-holding is preceded by hyperventilation to lower Pa,co_2 or O_2 breathing to raise Pa,o_2, the breath-holding time is prolonged.

Breath-holding time in man is much prolonged by vagal blockade, suggesting that afferent impulses from the lungs are required to induce the sensation of discomfort. If the subject is curarised, breath-holding causes no discomfort, suggesting that some motor event is also required. If the chest wall motor system is blocked by spinal anaesthesia to the level of the first thoracic segment, breath-holding time and sensation are unchanged [115]. If the phrenic nerve alone is blocked, breath-holding time is prolonged [116]. Therefore both an intact efferent pathway to the diaphragm and an intact afferent pathway in the vagus are required for the normal breath-holding sensation.

If the diaphragmatic EMG is recorded during breath-holding, bursts of activity are recorded with increasing frequency as the breakpoint approaches. A patient with cervical cord transection at the level of C3, whose breathing was performed entirely by contraction of the sternomastoid muscles, had no sensation of discomfort on breath-holding, but bursts of sternomastoid EMG activity were recorded as breath-holding proceeded [116]. It appears that the feeling of discomfort at the breakpoint of the breathhold can be equated with the feeling of the diaphragm being driven.

In a group of 8 patients with diaphragmatic paralysis [117] significant alveolar hypoventilation was found in 5 when supine and in 6 when asleep. (Breath-holding time was not measured.) It is possible therefore that the role of the diaphragm in breath-holding sensation may have more implication in the general control of respiration than might at first seem likely. In particular, patients with severe airways obstruction have diaphragms which, while not paralysed, are flattened to the point of severe mechanical disadvantage.

THE CONTROL OF TIDAL VOLUME AND FREQUENCY

Clark and Von Euler [118] compared the effect of CO_2 rebreathing on tidal volume V_T and frequency in cat and man. In the cat, V_T was inversely related to the length of the inspiratory period T_I, in a hyperbolic form (Fig. 5.28a). In man as ventilation increased, there was at first no change in frequency (F), or

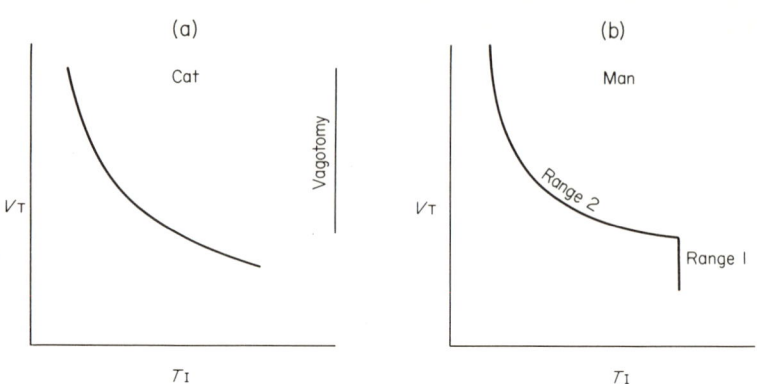

Fig. 5.28. In the cat, as ventilation increases with rebreathing, tidal volume (V_T) increases and inspiratory time (T_I) decreases in a hyperbolic fashion. Vagotomy is followed by slow deep breathing with T_I fixed. In man, as ventilation increases, T_I at first does not change, the increased ventilation being entirely due to increased V_T. (Range 1). Subsequently V_T and T_I take a hyperbolic relation (Range 2).

T_I, but then at a certain tidal volume T_I began to shorten, and the T_I/V_T relation was again hyperbolic (Fig. 5.28b). In both species T_I and the length of the expiratory period T_E seemed linearly related.

In a vagotomised cat rebreathing CO_2, T_I is fixed, hence it is fair to assume that the signal which cuts off inspiration is carried in the vagus. In man, blocking the vagus by local anaesthetic does not cause any change in resting ventilation, but the increase in frequency which occurs in CO_2 breathing is abolished. Thus it is probable that during normal breathing and as ventilation increases up to a certain point (about twice normal V_T), impulses from the lung receptors have no effect, but as ventilation increases further, signals from receptors start to cut off inspiration with a hyperbolic relation between V_T and T_I. Since it was found that T_I and T_E were linearly related it was tempting to assume that the vagal cut-off of inspiration also sets the expiratory time. Note that the threshold for inspiratory cutoff, in terms of V_T, falls with time in the sense that the longer T_I, the smaller the V_T needed to end T_I (Fig. 5.28). This appears to be a basic characteristic of the bulbopontine rhythm generator.

These observations have been extended, in the cat, by studying the relation between V_T and T_I when V_T is smaller than normal due to the imposition of an elastic load during inspiration [119] (Fig. 5.29). The wider span of observations suggest that the relation between V_T and T_I does not have quite the hyperbolic form suggested by Clark and Von Euler, but rather that there is an intercept on the T_I axis, which represents the intrinsic rate set by the bulbopontine pacemaker, and so coincides with the fixed rate seen after vagotomy. Moreover when the T_I–T_E relation was examined over this wider range, it was found to be systematic but not linear.

The curvilinear relation between V_T and T_I, according to which the vagal mechanism terminates inspiration, has been called the 'inspiratory characteristic'. The relation between T_I and T_E has been called the 'timing relationship'.

Which receptors are responsible for the inspiratory characteristic? It was natural to feel that the slowly adapting stretch receptors which subserve the Hering–Breuer inflation reflex were also involved in the termination of inspiratory time. Phillipson and colleagues [120, 121] attempted to differentiate between stretch and irritant receptor activity by using a vagal cooling technique. Myelinated fibres from stretch receptors are larger than those from irritant receptors, and will be blocked first during cooling. In conscious dogs with the vagus nerves exteriorised in skin loops, as the nerves were cooled, the

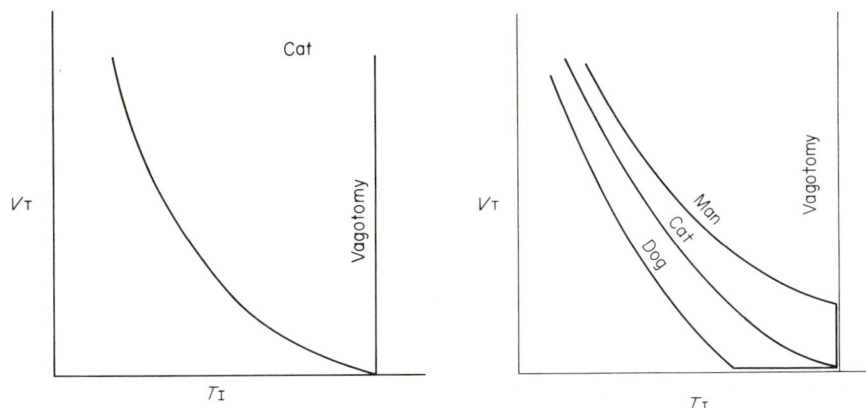

Fig. 5.29. The V_T/T_I relation in the cat extended by applying elastic loads to diminish V_T below normal.

Fig. 5.30. A schematic comparison of the $V_T - T_I$ relation in man, cat, and dog.

first reflex to go was the Hering–Breuer inflation reflex. But when this could not be elicited, V_T and T_I were normal. T_E in contrast was shortened, ventilation was increased because of the increase in rate, Pa,co_2 was low, and the ventilation response to inspired CO_2 was abnormally large. As cooling proceeded, V_T, T_I, and T_E all increased to give the slow deep fixed-rate breathing typical of complete vagotomy. Pa,co_2 was normal and the ventilation response to inspired CO_2 was low because frequency did not increase.

From these elegant experiments in the dog it was suggested that the stretch receptors were in general inhibitory to breathing, and the irritant receptors stimulatory, and that the latter were responsible for the inspiratory characteristic. However a paradoxical effect of partial blockade of stretch receptors cannot be excluded.

In further experiments in conscious dogs it was shown [122] that when phasal vagal input was prevented by total airway occlusion for one breath, T_1 was increased, but not so much as when all vagal input was blocked by cooling. This is in contrast to the anaesthetised cat (Fig. 5.29), where T_1 during complete occlusion is the same as T_1 post-vagotomy, and may be accounted for either as species variation, or as the effect of anaesthesia. A schematic comparison between cat, dog and man is given in Fig. 5.30. The 'dog' pattern

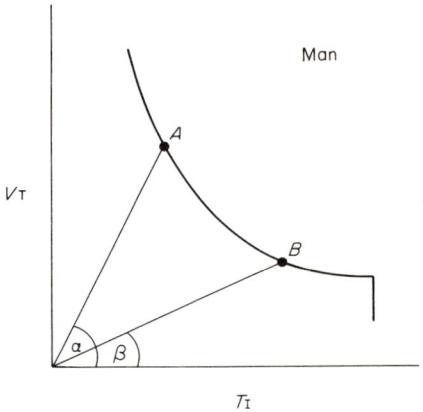

Fig. 5.31. For breath A, the slope α is V_T/T_1, which is the mean inspiratory flow rate, and similarly for breath B and slope β. The higher the inspiratory flow rate (dependent on respiratory drive) the higher V_T, in Range 2.

implies that the vagus exerts both a phasic and a tonic influence on the control of respiratory rhythm; the 'cat' pattern implies a phasic influence only; and the 'man' pattern implies no influence at all at small tidal volumes, with a phasic influence only when tidal volume increases above twice normal.

The inspiratory characteristic

In Fig. 5.31 slope α, which is V_T/T_1 for the line intercepting the inspiratory characteristic at point A, represents the mean gas flow during inspiration, and similarly for slope β and point B. It can be seen that the higher the mean flow, the higher the V_T achieved.

Thus where the hyperbolic $V_T - T_1$ relation obtains and the vagal cutoff mechanism is operative, the point on the inspiratory characteristic which determines the V_T for any given breath depends on mean rate of inspiratory flow. An increase in respiratory drive, or any unloading manoeuvre, increases mean inspiratory flow and thus increases V_T. A decrease in respiratory drive, or an additional mechanical load, decreases V_T.

After vagotomy, or when the phasic vagal information is abolished by preventing change of lung volume by airway occlusion, T_1 in cats appears to be fixed by the bulbopontine rhythm generator, a situation which also obtains in man during normal tidal breathing, where phasic vagal information exists but is apparently ignored by the respiratory centre. The afferent input from the peripheral chemoreceptor appears to have no specific effect on the tidal volume—frequency relation, serving rather to increase or decrease the level of respiratory centre output [123].

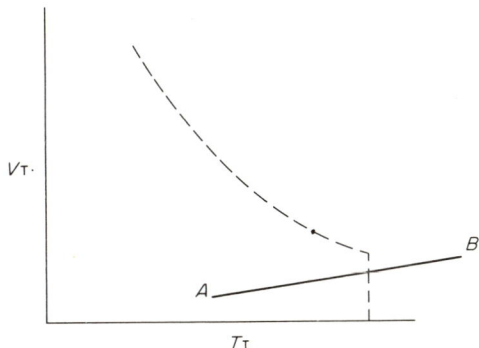

Fig. 5.32. During normal breathing at rest the $V_T - T_I$ relation is shown by the line AB, which is V_T Range 1 for breathing driven by CO_2 (inspiratory characteristic—dotted line).

Breath-to-breath variation in tidal volume and frequency during the 'steady state'

In Figs 5.28–31 we have considered the relation between V_T and T_I when the system is driven by CO_2 rebreathing. If we now consider the relation which occurs in man, at rest, breathing air, in a steady state, we find a totally different relation due to spontaneous breath-to-breath variation (Fig. 5.32) [124].

Now V_T and T_I are directly and linearly related, and the line if extrapolated tends to go through zero. Its slope therefore represents mean inspiratory flow.

Note first that these results are obtained with tidal volumes in the range where vagal feedback is unheeded by the respiratory centre, and have not been extended to the curvilinear part of the inspiratory characteristic. Second, it looks as though two very different control mechanisms apply. At rest, the larger V_T, the larger T_I and the slower the rate, and it looks as though the system is set to hold mean inspiratory flow constant. When however the respiratory system is driven by CO_2 breathing into the curvilinear range, the larger V_T, the smaller T_I and the faster the rate. In the first case the system tends to maintain constant ventilation by balancing rate against tidal volume. In the second case the system achieves increased ventilation by increasing both rate and tidal volume.

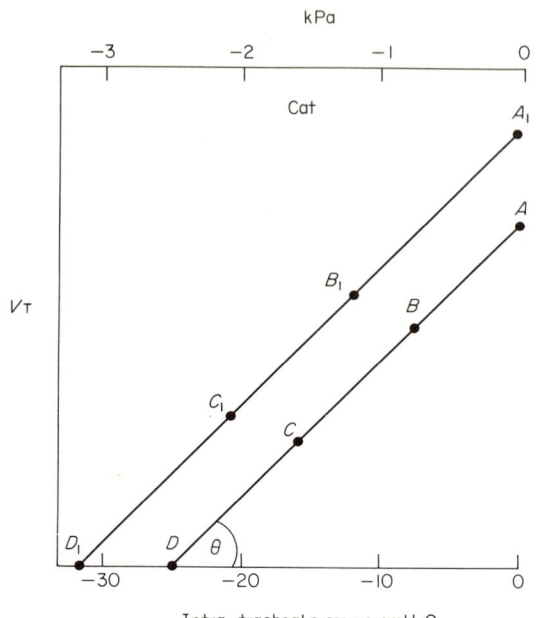

Fig. 5.33. Tracheal pressures and tidal volume during elastic loading in cats [125]. Point *A* represents a normal unloaded breath, when tracheal pressure is effectively zero. Point *D* represents the tracheal pressure generated during a complete occlusion, with zero tidal volume. Points *B* and *C* are obtained by graded elastic loads. The relation is linear, and the effective elastance E'_{rs} is given by $\Delta P/\Delta V$, or the reciprocal of the slope θ. When ventilation was increased by added deadspace (points A_1, B_1, C_1, D_1) E'_{rs} was not changed.

LOADED BREATHING

One way of investigating the control of the mechanical aspects of ventilation is to load the system mechanically. An elastic load can be applied by causing the subject to breathe from a drum or jar: the smaller the container, the higher the load. A resistive load may be applied by placing a narrow orifice in the breathing circuit: the narrower the orifice the higher the load. Loads may be applied in inspiration, expiration, or both. One complicating feature of expiratory loading is that functional residual capacity increases, whereas in inspiratory loading it does not.

A third method is to apply an expiratory threshold load, by placing the expiratory pipe in the experimental circuit under water. Before expiration can begin a threshold load equal to the depth of the pipe below the water must be overcome.

The largest interference of all may be applied by blocking the airway completely, which can be regarded as an infinite resistive and an infinite elastic load.

Inspiratory elastic loads

In the anaesthetised cat breathing spontaneously, if an inspiratory load is suddenly switched into the circuit, the next breath has a smaller tidal volume than control [125]. The passive elastance (E_{rs}) of the cat's respiratory system can be measured during muscular paralysis by inflating the chest, pausing at different volumes, and plotting airway pressure against volume. If the elastance of the added load is also known, it might be thought that the size of the next breath could be calculated, for by definition,

$E_{rs} = \Delta P/\Delta V$

$\Delta V = \Delta P/E_{rs}$

ΔV here is tidal volume, V_T, so

V_T,unloaded $= \Delta P/E_{rs}$
V_T,loaded $\quad = \Delta P/(E_{rs} + \Delta E)$,

where ΔE is the elastance of the added load. Then by combining the last two equations,

$$V_T \% \text{control} = (E_{rs}/(E_{rs} + \Delta E)).\,100 \tag{5.9}$$

It is invariably found that the actual tidal volume of the first loaded breath is greater than that calculated by equation 5.9. Under these conditions the effective elastance E'_{rs} of the respiratory system is greater than the passive elastance E_{rs}, for when the muscles of inspiration are contracted the system behaves as if it were stiffer. E'_{rs} can be measured by applying a series of graded loads (jars of decreasing size) and finally by totally occluding the airway during one breath. When tracheal pressure is plotted against tidal volume (Fig. 5.33) the relation is linear. The reciprocal of the slope of this line

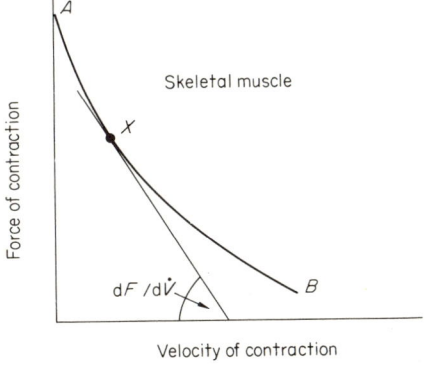

Fig. 5.34. Hyperbolic force-velocity curve AXB of skeletal muscle. dF/dV is the slope of the curve at point X.

$(\Delta P/\Delta V)$ is the effective elastance of the respiratory system E'_{rs}. If the cat's ventilation is increased by adding deadspace to the respiratory circuit and the experiment repeated, a different line is obtained, but the slope, and E'_{rs}, are unchanged. The linear behaviour of this experimental preparation has considerable convenience in that E'_{rs} can be calculated if necessary from two points, A and D in Fig. 5.33, requiring only the measurement of control V_T, and of the tracheal pressure during total airway occlusion.

The cause for this compensatory behaviour of the respiratory system cannot be ascribed to an increased chemical drive, for during the first breath it is too early for any changes in blood gas tensions to affect ventilation. It is partly due to the intrinsic behaviour of the chest wall muscles, in that in general, when loaded, inspiratory airflow is slower. Since there is a reciprocal relation between force produced and velocity of muscle contraction (Fig. 5.34), the muscles of inspiration will automatically produce a bigger force, and

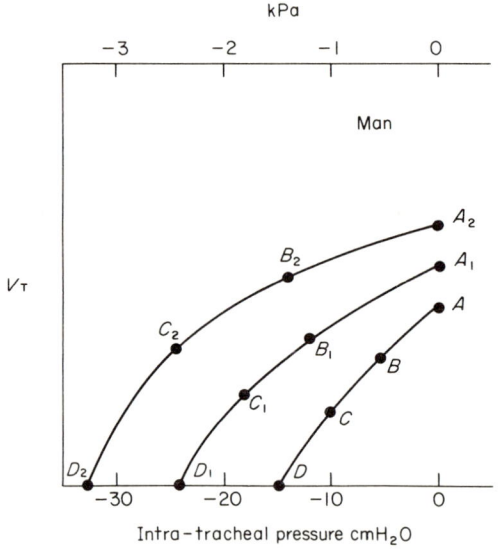

Fig. 5.35. Tracheal pressure and tidal volume during elastic loading in man [126]. Conventions as for Fig. 5.33. Lines A_1–D_1 and A_2–D_2 were obtained by increasing overall ventilation by adding deadspace.

will behave more stiffly. Second, the application of an elastic load diminishes the output of lung stretch receptors, which are active during normal tidal breathing in the cat, and this prolongs inspiration. Note that in this analysis, only elastic forces are considered.

In man the situation is more complicated [126]. In general compensation in the first loaded breath is less marked than in the cat, for vagal reflexes do not operate during normal tidal breathing. It is found that when graded loads are applied, the relation between tidal volume and tracheal pressure is not linear (Fig. 5.35), so that no single value of E'_{rs} exists. Moreover if ventilation is increased by adding deadspace, the slope of the V_T-tracheal pressure lines decreases, implying that E'_{rs} measured at any particular tracheal pressure increases. Pengelly and colleagues [126] derived model equations which took into account both E'_{rs} and the 'effective resistance' R'_{rs} of the respiratory system, and concluded that both should increase with increased frequency of breathing.

We have already suggested that the more strongly a muscle contracts, the stiffer it becomes, thus increasing E'_{rs}. R'_{rs} is intuitively much more difficult to understand, but referring again to a muscle force-velocity curve (Fig. 5.34), we see that the slope of the curve $dF/d\dot{V}$ is much steeper at low velocities. In the sense that force of contraction is related to alveolar driving pressure, and velocity of contraction to rate of airflow into the lung during inspiration, dF/dV in $G/(mm/sec)$ is a parallel measurement to airflow resistance in $cmH_2O/(L/sec)$, or $kPa/(L/sec)$. It is in this sense, I think, that the term effective resistance is used. Its relation to airflow resistance is the complicated relation whereby muscle contraction is coupled to airflow.

It was concluded that in man breathing at rest, the compensatory response, in the first breath after an elastic load was applied, was accounted for by intrinsic mechanisms of the chest wall. At higher ventilation, where tidal volume increased sufficiently to bring vagal mechanisms into play, and increased frequency itself gave evidence of vagal modulation, the intrinsic compensatory response was augmented by a vagal mechanism, as in the cat.

So much for the first loaded breath. What happens next? Total ventilation returns to normal gradually, and it seems clear from animal studies that this secondary compensatory process is achieved by chemical drive, since if the changes in blood gases consequent upon the initial decrease in ventilation are prevented, by cross perfusion techniques, the rapidly progressive secondary compensation is not seen [127–129].

Thus within a few breaths there is complete compensation for inspiratory elastic loading, with no decrease in ventilation, and this is true for breathing at rest and when ventilation is stimulated by exercise, CO_2 breathing or hypoxia [130, 131].

Resistive loading

Zechman and colleagues [132] applied resistive loads either in inspiration or expiration to anaesthetised cats, and examined the first loaded breath where chemical drive was unchanged. When the load was presented during inspiration V_T was reduced and T_I prolonged according to the inspiratory characteristic of Clark and Von Euler. T_E was unchanged, whereas according to the 'timing relationship' it should have increased. Vagotomy was followed by a fixed prolonged T_I and T_E. When the load was presented during expiration, V_T decreased, and therefore FRC increased, and T_E was prolonged. Thus whereas it had previously appeared that T_E was automatically set by T_I, under these conditions T_E could vary independently suggesting separate control of both phases of respiration, both dependent on vagally mediated volume feedback.

Considering events after the first breath, in contrast to elastic loading, resistive loading causes some decrease in ventilation at rest, and when ventilation is stimulated by exercise, CO_2 breathing or hypoxia [133].

Expiratory threshold loading (ETL)

Grunstein and colleagues [134] examined in cats the effect of ETL on the inspiratory characteristic, varying V_T for each value of ETL by imposing an elastic load during inspiration and examining the first loaded breath. Although FRC increased, the inspiratory characteristic was not changed, suggesting that regulation of T_I is determined by lung volume changes above FRC, whatever the value of FRC. This in turn suggests that discharge of pulmonary stretch receptors is adapted to new end-expiratory levels, and single-fibre vagal recordings confirmed this.

In dogs [135] a positive end-expiratory pressure causes an increase in FRC and an increased response to brief progressive hypercapnia and hypoxia, while a negative end-expiratory pressure causes a decrease in FRC and a decreased response. However in steady state hypercapnia or hypoxia, the response gradually returns to normal, and there is evidence that this adaptation occurs both at the stretch receptors and centrally [135].

WHAT IS THE INPUT TO THE RESPIRATORY CONTROL SYSTEM?

It is frequently convenient to consider arterial blood gases or pH as input to the respiratory control system, and much useful and important information has been obtained with this approach. Clearly it is limited by the fact that the quantity of CO_2, O_2, and hydrion present in the circulating blood is of no importance whatsoever, except that those quantities both reflect and affect the quantities of CO_2, O_2 and hydrion in the metabolising tissues. We are always in grave danger of examining the messenger and not the message. If the purpose of the respiratory system and circulation is to maintain optimal conditions for metabolism in the tissues, then the input to the respiratory centre should reflect those metabolic needs. The fact that Pa,CO_2 for example does *not* reflect metabolic needs is shown by the finding that it remains constant during moderate exercise. We should now stop thinking of the relation between Pa,CO_2 and ventilation, and keep thinking in terms of the relation between metabolism and ventilation, a statement which as such is remarkably unhelpful since it does not say what aspects of metabolism should be measured.

It seems likely that the relevant index is instantaneous CO_2 production ($\dot{V}\text{CO}_2$), as delivered to the lung, and that this is the most relevant input to the respiratory centre. We do not know how the brainstem centre is advised about $\dot{V}\text{CO}_2$. Is the information obtained from the magnitude of oscillations of Pa,CO_2, and if so how much of this translation is done by the carotid body, and how much elsewhere, and if elsewhere, where? To be blunt, we still cannot be certain if the oscillations are a subtle signal, or merely the result of the juxtaposition of circulatory and reciprocal pumps, a piece of sloppy design work by The Great Physiologist in the Sky. Does the brainstem alternatively or additionally respond to neural signals from working muscles? If so, how does it respond to increased $\dot{V}\text{CO}_2$ produced by infusion in the resting animal?

WHAT IS THE OUTPUT OF THE RESPIRATORY CENTRE?

It is frequently convenient to consider ventilation as the output of the respiratory centre, but this is quite unfair if the ventilation is limited by a mechanical load, whether experimental or due to disease.

Note first that the input and output most frequently used are arterial blood gases and expired ventilation, and that it just so happens that these variables are relatively easy to measure; and second that in any case ventilation cannot be regarded as the directly controlled variable, for its magnitude is quite irrelevant to the organism, apart from the fact that it affects conditions for metabolism in the tissues.

In conditions of mechanical loading when respiratory centre output or drive might be normal, but ventilation diminished because of mechanical hindrance, one approach is to measure some neural output, say in the phrenic nerve. The handling of such a signal requires careful consideration [137] and in any case this cannot be done in intact man except by oesophageal electrodes which have major drawbacks because their position relative to the phrenic nerve cannot be fixed. A similar approach is to take the diaphragmatic or intercostal EMG as an index of respiratory drive [138].

The measurement of inspiratory work might be thought appropriate, the idea being that the respiratory centre demands a certain work production, but the amount of ventilation produced by that work will depend on the mechanical coupling. Unfortunately the work of breathing is difficult to measure, and the best way of measuring it is not agreed.

Another possibility is to measure the tracheal or mouth pressure generated when the airway is suddenly occluded [139]. The magnitude of the pressure generated should then be a reflection of respiratory drive in the absence of ventilation. Unfortunately, while phasic vagal influences are probably abolished, we have seen that tracheal pressure in this circumstance is affected by intrinsic chest wall mechanisms, and in awake man also by cortical influences, and the pressure generated is not independent of experimental loading [140–142].

Probably the best idea so far involves the measurement of small pressure changes in a mouthpiece with a flap-valve [143, 144]. A very small opening pressure is required before the valve opens and inspiratory flow starts. Until the flap-valve opens, contraction of the chest wall muscles is isometric, and the change in lung volume due to expansion is negligible. Therefore no adjustment of response due to intrinsic chest wall mechanisms or vagal feedback occurs. Moreover this period of isometric contraction is too short for any cortical influence to take effect. The pressure in the mouth-piece is transduced and differentiated, and the maximum rate of pressure change $(dp/dt)_{max}$ is measured. It is found that $(dp/dt)_{max}$ occurs in the isometric period, and its value is taken as a direct reflection of the output of the respiratory centre.

PUTTING IT TOGETHER

It would seem reasonable that the respiratory control system should normally in the resting organism be set to maintain optimal metabolic conditions in the most important organ, namely the brain, and near-optimal conditions elsewhere. The respiratory centre in the brain stem appears to 'taste' the by-products of brain metabolism in much the same way that the carotid body 'tastes' the blood, as Heymans originally put it. Hierarchically, one would expect the brain control centre to dominate. The carotid body in any case sees the mixed result of metabolism in all the various tissues, and cannot detect mischief unless all tissues are malfunctioning (hypoxia) or the metabolic products of one tissue flood the mixed venous blood (exercise). There is no need for the brain centre to pay any attention to the carotid bodies except in these two emergencies, and there is doubt even then as to the exact contribution of peripheral chemoreceptors in exercise.

When rapid changes in metabolism occur, for example in exercise, the respiratory centre appears to sense $\dot{V}{CO_2}$ almost instantaneously, and $Pa,{CO_2}$ is kept normal. The peripheral chemoreceptors may play some part in this, but also in the maintenance of a normal $Pa,{CO_2}$ at rest, at least in some species. The carotid body is definitely responsible for the response to a most important and unusual emergency, namely hypoxia.

The respiratory centre puts out a neural signal which is transduced into a certain quantity of muscular effort, which is in turn transduced into ventilation. A certain value of ventilation may be represented by any number of pairs of values for frequency and tidal volume. A second function of the respiratory centre is to decide on suitable values for V_T, V_I, and T_E. This is done by generating a basic rhythm from the bulbopontine generator, and a respiratory drive in terms of rate of gas flow into the lung which sets the tidal volume. According to the inspiratory characteristic, the faster the inspiratory gas flow, the shorter T_I and the larger V_T. The shortening of T_I is achieved by phasic vagal feedback, which thus modifies the basic bulbopontine set rate. In many but not all circumstances T_E changes in the same direction as T_I. When the vagus is cut, or if its signals are ignored as in tidal breathing in man at rest, increased ventilation is achieved purely by increasing gas flows at the same rate, that is by increasing V_T at constant frequency. In these circumstances the output of the respiratory centre is represented purely by V_T and the basic set rate. In man, as V_T increases above a critical value of about twice normal, phasic vagal information is noted by the respiratory centre and T_I then shortens.

It would be attractive to believe that this complex secondary control mechanism which sets the respiratory rhythm for a given ventilation is designed to achieve that ventilation at a minimal energy expenditure, and there is evidence which suggests that this is so [145–147].

In addition to main metabolic control and secondary rhythm control, a tertiary defensive control mechanism appears to minimise the effects of superimposed resistive or elastic loads. Compensation for an elastic load is achieved mainly by an increase in chest wall stiffness supplemented by chemical feedback. Compensation for a resistive load is not so effective, is achieved at the expense of increasing FRC, and despite chemical feedback is less likely to result in normal blood gas tensions.

REFERENCES

1 MILHORN H.T. (1966). *The Application of Control Theory to Physiological Systems*. W.B. Saunders, Philadelphia.
2 PURVES M.J. (1966). Fluctuations of arterial oxygen tension which have the same period as respiration. *Resp. Physiol.* **1**, 281–296.
3 BAND D.M., CAMERON I.R. & SEMPLE S.J.G. (1969) Oscillations in arterial pH with breathing in the cat. *J. Appl. Physiol.* **26**, 261–7.
4 HORNBEIN T.F. (1965). Effect of respiratory oscillation of arterial pO_2 and pCO_2 on carotid chemoreceptor activity and phrenic nerve activity. *The Physiologist* **8**, (3), 197.
5 BISCOE T.J. & PURVES M.J. (1967). Observations on the rhythmic variation in the cat carotid body chemoreceptor activity which has the same period as respiration. *J. Physiol.* (*Lond.*) **190**, 389–412.
6 HORNBEIN T.F., GRIFFO E.J. & ROOS A. (1961). Quantitation of chemoreceptor activity: interrelation of hypoxia and hypercapnia. *J. Neurophysiol.* **24**, 561–8.

7 BISCOE T.J., PURVES M.J. & SAMPSON S.R. (1970). The frequency of nerve impulses in single carotid body chemoreceptor afferent fibres recorded in vivo with intact circulation. *J. Physiol.* (*Lond.*) **208**, 121–131.

8 FITZGERALD R.S. & PARKS D.C. (1971). Effect of hypoxia on carotid chemoreceptor response to carbon dioxide in cats. *Resp. Physiol.* **12**, 218–229.

9 BLACK A.M.S., MCCLOSKEY D.I. & TORRANCE R.W. (1971). The responses of peripheral chemoreceptors to sudden changes of hypercapnic and hypoxic stimuli. *Resp. Physiol.* **13**, 36–49.

10 BAND D.M., SAUNDERS K.B. & WOLFF C.B. (1971). The relation between chemoreceptor discharge and respiratory fluctuation of arterial pH in the anaesthetised cat. *J. Physiol.* (*Lond.*) **218**, 73–74P.

11 DUTTON R.E., HODSON W.A., DAVIES D.G. & CHERNICK V. (1967). Ventilatory adaptation to a step change in P_{CO_2} at the carotid bodies. *J. Appl. Physiol.*, **23**, 195–202.

12 DUTTON R.E., HODSON W.A. & DAVIES D.G. (1967). Effect of the rate of rise of carotid body P_{CO_2} on the time course of ventilation. *Resp. Physiol.* **3**, 367–79.

13 DUTTON R.E., FITZGERALD R.S. & GROSS N. (1968). Ventilatory response to square-wave forcing of carbon dioxide at the carotid bodies. *Resp. Physiol.* **4**, 101–108.

14 DUTTON R.E., SMITH E.J., GHATAK P.K. & DAVIES D.G. (1973). Dynamics of the respiratory controller during carotid body hypoxia. *J. Appl. Physiol.* **35**, 844–850.

15 FITZGERALD R.S., LEITNER L.M. & LIAUBET M.J. (1969). Carotid chemoreceptor response to intermittent or sustained stimulation in the cat. *Resp. Physiol.* **6**, 395–402.

16 BISCOE T.J. & SAMPSON S.R. (1968). Rhythmical and non-rhythmical spontaneous activity recorded from the central cut end of the sinus nerve. *J. Physiol.* (*Lond.*) **196**, 327–338.

17 SAMPSON S.R. & BISCOE T.J. (1970). Efferent control of the carotid body chemoreceptor. *Experientia.* **26**, 261–262.

18 NEIL E. & O'REGAN R.G. (1971a). The effects of electrical stimulation of the distal end of the cut sinus and aortic nerves on peripheral arterial chemoreceptor activity in the cat. *J. Physiol.* (*Lond.*) **215**, 15–32.

19 NEIL E. & O'REGAN R.G. (1971b). Efferent and afferent impulse activity recorded from few-fibre preparations of otherwise intact sinus and aortic nerves. *J. Physiol.* (*Lond.*) **215**, 33–47.

20 BAND D.M., CAMERON I.R. & SEMPLE S.J.G. (1969). Effect of different methods of CO_2 administration on oscillations of arterial pH in the cat. *J. Appl. Physiol.* **26**, 268–273.

21 BLACK A.M.S. & TORRANCE R.W. (1971). Respiratory oscillations in chemoreceptor discharge in the control of breathing. *Respir. Physiol.* **13**, 221–237.

22 CUNNINGHAM D.J.C. (1975). A model illustrating the importance of timing in the regulation of breathing. *Nature* **253**, 440–442.

23 CAMERON I.R. (1972). The central chemical regulation of breathing. *Modern Trends in Physiology* 1: pp. 268–291. Butterworths, London.

24 CUMMING G. & SEMPLE S.J.G. (1973). *Disorders of the Respiratory System.* pp. 140–150. Blackwell Scientific Publications, Oxford.

25 MITCHELL R.A., LOESCHKE H.H., MASSION W.H. & SEVERINGHAUS J.W. (1963). Respiratory responses mediated through superficial chemosensitive areas on the medulla. *J. Appl. Physiol.* **18**, 523–533.

26 LOESCHKE H.H. (1965). A concept of the role of intracranial chemosensitivity in respiratory control. In *Cerebrospinal Fluid and the Regulation of Ventilation* Ed. C.McC. Brooks, F.F. Kao and B.B. Lloyd. p. 183. Blackwell Scientific Publications, Oxford.

27 PAPPENHEIMER J.R. (1965). The ionic composition of cerebral extracellular fluid and its relation to control of breathing. *Harvey Lect.* **61**, 71–94.

28 FENCL V., MILLER T.B. & PAPPENHEIMER J.R. (1966). Studies on the respiratory response to disturbances of acid base balance, with deductions concerning the ionic composition of cerebral interstitial fluid. *Am. J. Physiol.* **210**, 459–472.

29 FENCL V., VALE J.R. & BROCH J.A. (1976). Respiration and cerebral blood flow in metabolic acidosis and alkalosis in humans. *J. Appl. Physiol.* **27**, 67–76.

30 WICHSER J. & KAZEMI H. (1975). C.S.F. bicarbonate regulation in respiratory acidosis and alkalosis. *J. Appl. Physiol.* **38**, 504–512.

31 HASAN F.M. & KAZEMI H. (1976). Dual contribution theory of regulation of C.S.F. HCO_3^- in respiratory acidosis. *J. Appl. Physiol.* **40**, 559–567.

32 DEMPSEY J.A., FORSTER H.V., GLEDHILL N. & DOPICO G.A. (1975). Effects of moderate hypoxaemia and hypocapnia on C.S.F. [H^+] and ventilation in man. *J. Appl. Physiol.* **38**, 665–674.

33 FORSTER H.V., DEMPSEY J.A. & CHOSY L.W. (1975). Incomplete compensation of C.S.F. [H^+] in man during acclimatisation to high altitude. *J. Appl. Physiol.* **38**, 1067–1072.

34 LLOYD B.B., JUKES M.G.M. & CUNNINGHAM D.J.C. (1958). The relation between alveolar oxygen pressure and the respiratory response to carbon dioxide in man. *Quart. J. Exp. Physiol.* **43**, 214–227.

35 REYNOLDS W.J., MILHORN H.T. Jr. & HOLLOMAN G.H. Jr. (1972). Transient ventilatory response to graded hypercapnia in man. *J. Appl. Physiol.* **33**, 47–54.

36 FENN W.O. & CRAIG A.B. (1963). Effect of CO_2 on respiration using a new method of administering CO_2. *J. Appl. Physiol.* **18**, 1023–1024.

37 CHAMBILLE B., GUENARD H. & LONCLE M. (1974). Time variations of $\dot{V}A$ and $PACO_2$ during inhalation of CO_2, either at constant fraction ($FICO_2$) or at constant flow rate ($\dot{V}ICO_2$) at rest and during muscular exercise. *Pfluger's Arch.* **352**, 69–80.

38 READ D.J.C. (1967). A clinical method for assessing the ventilatory response to carbon dioxide. *Austr. Ann. Med.* **16**, 20–32.

39 READ D.J.C. & LEIGH J. (1967). Blood-brain tissue PCO_2 relationships and ventilation during rebreathing. *J. Appl. Physiol.* **23**, 53–70.

40 LINTON R.A.F., POOLE-WILSON P.A., DAVIES R.J. & CAMERON I.R. (1973). A comparison of the ventilatory response to carbon dioxide by steady-state and rebreathing methods during metabolic acidosis and alkalosis. *Clin. Sci.* **45**, 239–249.

41 STOLL P.J. (1969). Respiratory system analysis based on sinusoidal variations of CO_2 in inspired air. *J. Appl. Physiol.* **27**, 389–399.

42 LAMBERTSEN C.J., GELFAND R. & KEMP R.A. (1965). Dynamic response characteristics of several CO_2-reactive components of the respiratory control system. In: *Cerebrospinal Fluid and the Regulation of Ventilation*, ed. C.McC. Brooks, F.F. Kao and B.B. Lloyd. Blackwell Scientific Publications, Oxford.

43 DAUBENSPECK J.A. (1973). Frequency analysis of CO_2 regulation: afferent influences on tidal volume control. *J. Appl. Physiol.* **35**, 662–672.

44 BORISON H.L. & MCCARTHY L.E. (1973). CO_2 ventilatory response time obtained by inhalation step forcing in decerebrate cats. *J. Appl. Physiol.* **34**, 1–7.

45 SWANSON G.D. & BELLVILLE J.W. (1975). Step changes in end-tidal CO_2: methods and implications. *J. Appl. Physiol.* **39**, 377–385.

46 CHAMBILLE B., GUENARD H., LONCLE M. & BARGETON D. (1975). Alveostat, an alveolar $PACO_2$ and PAO_2 control system. *J. Appl. Physiol.* **39**, 837–842.

47 BOUVEROT D., FLANDROIS R. & GRANDPIERRE R. (1961). A propos du mécanisme d'action chémoréflexe ou central due 'stimulus CO_2' de la ventilation. *Compt. Rend. Acad. Sci. Paris* **252**, 790–792.

48 GABEL R.A., KRONENBERG R.S. & SEVERINGHAUS J.W. Vital capacity breaths of 5% or 15% CO_2 in N_2 or O_2 to test carotid chemosensitivity. *Resp. Physiol.* **17**, 195–208.

49 ELDRIDGE F.L. (1973). Post hyperventilation breathing: different effects of active and passive hyperventilation. *J. Appl. Physiol.* **34**, 422–430.

50 TAWADROUS F.D. & ELDRIDGE F.L. (1974). Post hyperventilation breathing patterns after active hyperventilation in man. *J. Appl. Physiol.* **37**, 353–356.

51 ELDRIDGE F.L. (1974). Central neural respiratory stimulatory effect of active respiration. *J. Appl. Physiol.* **37**, 723–735.

52 ELDRIDGE F.L. (1976). Central neural stimulation of respiration in unanaesthetised decerebrate cats. *J. Appl. Physiol.* **40**, 23–28.

53 BERAL V. & READ D.J.C. (1971). Insensitivity of respiratory centre to carbon dioxide in the Euga people of New Guinea. *Lancet* **2**, 1290–1294.

54 ARKINSTALL W.W., NIRMEL K., KLISSOURAS V. & MILIC-EMILI J. (1974). Genetic differences in the ventilatory response to inhaled CO_2. *J. Appl. Physiol.* **36**, 6–11.

55 LEIGH J., WALKER W.L. & FOWLER K.T. (1973). Effect of hypnotic suggestions on the respiratory response to transient CO_2 breathing in man. *Resp. Physiol.* **19**, 210–220.

56 GEDDES D.M., RUDOLF M. & SAUNDERS K.B. (1976). The effect of nitrazepam and flurazepam on the ventilatory response to carbon dioxide. *Thorax*, in press.

57 LEITCH A.G., CLANCY L. & FLENLEY D.C. (1974). The effect of bendrofluazide and frusemide on the ventilatory response to carbon dioxide and hypoxia in normal man. *Clin. Sci Mol. Med.* **47**, 377–385.

58 LEITCH A.G., CLANCY L.J., COSTELLO J.F. & FLENLEY D.C. (1976). Effect of intravenous salbutamol on ventilatory response to carbon dioxide and hypoxia and on heart rate and plasma potassium in normal men. *Brit. Med. J.* **1**, 365–367.

59 WEIL J.V., BYRNE-QUINN E., SODAL I.E., FRIESEN W.O., UNDERHILL B., FILLEY G.F. & GROVER R.F. (1970). Hypoxic ventilatory drive in normal man. *J. Clin. Invest.* **49**, 1061–1072.

60 REBUCK A.S. & CAMPBELL E.J.M. (1974). A clinical method for assessing the ventilatory response to hypoxia. *Amer. Rev. Resp. Dis.* **109**, 345–350.

61 DEJOURS P. (1962). Chemoreflexes in breathing. *Physiol. Rev.* **42**, 335–358.

62 KRONENBERG R., HAMILTON F.N., GABEL R., HICKEY R., READ D.J.C. & SEVERINGHAUS J. (1972). Comparison of three methods for quantitating respiratory response to hypoxia in man. Resp. Physiol. **16**, 109–125.

63 REYNOLDS W.J. & MILHORN H.T. Jr. (1973). Transient ventilatory response to hypoxia with and without controlled alveolar P_{CO_2}. *J. Appl. Physiol.* **35**, 187–196.

64 GODFREY S., EDWARDS R.H.T., COPLAND G.M. & GROSS P.L. (1971). Chemosensitivity in normal subjects, athletes, and patients with chronic airways obstruction. *J. Appl. Physiol.* **30**, 193–199.

65 REBUCK A.S., KANGALEE M., PENGELLY L.D. & CAMPBELL E.J.M. (1973). Correlation of ventilatory responses to hypoxia and hypercapnia. *J. Appl. Physiol.* **35**, 173–178.

66 HIRSHMAN C.A., McCULLOUGH R.E. & WEIL J.V. (1975). Normals values for hypoxic and hypercapnic ventilatory drives in man. *J. Appl. Physiol.* **38**, 1095–1098.

67 WEIL J.V., BYRNE-QUINN E., SODAL I.E., KLINE J.S., McCULLOUGH R.E. & FILLEY G.F. (1972). Augmentation of chemosensitivity during mild exercise in normal man. *J. Appl. Physiol.* **33**, 813–819.

68 EISELE J.H., RITCHIE B.C. & SEVERINGHAUS J.W. (1967). Effect of stellate ganglion blockade on the hyperpnoea of exercise. *J. Appl. Physiol.* **22**, 966–969.

69 BYRNE-QUINN E., WEIL J.V., SODAL I.E., FILLEY G.F. & GROVER R.F. (1971). Ventilatory control in the athlete. *J. Appl. Physiol.* **30**, 91–98.

70 HUDGEL D.W. & WEIL J.V. (1974). Asthma associated with decreased hypoxic ventilatory drive. *Ann. Intern. Med.* **80**, 622–625.

71 FLENLEY D.C., FRANKLIN D.H. & MILLAR J.S. (1970). The hypoxic drive to breathing in chronic bronchitis and emphysema. *Clin. Sci.* **38**, 503–518.

72 EVANS R.J.C., BENSON M.K. & HUGHES D.T.D. (1971). Abnormal chemoreceptor response to hypoxia in patients with tabes dorsalis. *Brit. Med. J.* **1**, 530–531.

73 WEIL J.V., McCULLOUGH B.S., KLINE J.S. & SODAL I.E. (1975). Diminished ventilatory response to hypoxia and hypercarbia after morphine in normal man. *New Eng. J. Med.* **292**, 1103–1106.

74 MORRILL C.G., MEYER J.R. & WEIL J.V. (1975). Hypoxic ventilatory depression in dogs. *J. Appl. Physiol.* **38**, 143–146.

75 LEE L. & MILHORN H.T. (1975). Central ventilatory responses to O_2 and CO_2 at three levels of carotid chemoreceptor stimulation. *Resp. Physiol.* **25**, 319–333.

76 RIGATTO H., VERDUZCO R. de la T. & CATES D.B. (1975). Effects of O_2 on the ventilatory response to CO_2 in preterm infants. *J. Appl. Physiol.* **39**, 896–899.

77 WEISKOPF R.B. & GABEL R.A. (1975). Depression of ventilation during hypoxia in man. *J. Appl. Physiol.* **39**, 911–915.

78 MILLER M.J. & TENNEY S.M. (1975). Hypoxia-induced tachypnea in carotid-deafferented cats. *Resp. Physiol.* **23**, 31–39.

79 BARRATT-BOYES B.G. & WOOD E.H. (1958). Cardiac output and related measurements and pressure values in the right heart and associated vessels, together with an analysis of the haemodynamic response to the inhalation of high oxygen mixtures in healthy subjects. *J. Lab. Clin. Med.* **51**, 72–90.

80 MILLER M.J. & TENNEY S.M. (1975). Hyperoxic hyperventilation in carotid-deafferented cats. *Resp. Physiol.* **23**, 23–30.

81 ROSENSTEIN R., McCARTHY L.E. & BORISON H.L. (1975). Slow respiratory stimulant effect of hyperoxia in chemodenervated decerebrate cats. *J. Appl. Physiol.* **39**, 767–772.

82 SWANSON G.D. & BELLVILLE J.W. (1974). Hyperoxic-hypercapnic interaction in human respiratory control. *J. Appl. Physiol.* **36**, 480–487.

83 MILLER J.P., CUNNINGHAM D.J.C., LLOYD B.B. & YOUNG J.M. (1974). The transient respiratory effects in man of sudden changes in alveolar CO_2 in hypoxia and in high oxygen. *Resp. Physiol.* **20**, 17–32.

84 BERGER A.J., KRASNEY J.A. & DUTTON R.E. (1973). Respiratory recovery from CO_2 breathing in intact and chemodenervated awake dogs. *J. Appl. Physiol.* **35**, 35–41.

85 BISGARD G.E., FORSTER H.V., ORR J.A., BASS D.D., RAWLINGS C.A. & RASMUSSEN B. (1976). Hypoventilation in ponies after carotid body denervation. *J. Appl. Physiol.*, **40**, 184–190.

86 WASSERMAN K., WHIPP B.J., KOYAL S.N. & CLEARY M.G. (1975). Effect of carotid body resection on ventilatory and acid-base control during exercise. *J. Appl. Physiol.* **39**, 354–358.

87 GABEL R.A. & WEISKOPF R.B. (1975). Ventilatory interaction between hypoxia and $[H^+]$ at chemoreceptors of man. *J. Appl. Physiol.* **39**, 292–296.

88 BAINTON C.R. (1972). Effect of speed vs grade and shivering on ventilation in dogs during active exercise. *J. Appl. Physiol.* **33**, 778–787.

89 BALI H. & SAUNDERS K.B. (unpublished).

90 BISCOE T.J. & PURVES M.J. (1967). Factors affecting the cat carotid chemoreceptor and cervical sympathetic activity with special reference to passive hind-limb movements. *J. Physiol. (Lond.)* **190**, 425–441.

91 PARIDA B., SENAPATI J. & KALIA M. (1969). Role of carotid body in hyperpnoea due to stimulation of muscle receptors in the dog. *J. Appl. Physiol.* **27**, 519–522.

92 DAVIES R.O. & LAHIRI S. (1973). Absence of carotid chemoreceptor response during hypoxic exercise in the cat. *Resp. Physiol.* **18**, 92–100.

93 AGGARWAL, MILHORN H.T. & LEE L.Y. (1976). Role of the cartoid chemoreceptors in the hyperpnoea of exercise in the cat. *Resp. Physiol.* **26**, 147–155.

94 ASMUSSEN E. (1973). Ventilation at transition from rest to exercise. *Acta Physiol. Scand.* **89**, 68–78.

95 YAMAMOTO W.S. & EDWARDS M.W. (1960). Homeostasis of carbon dioxide during intravenous infusion of carbon dioxide. *J. Appl. Physiol.* **15**, 807–818.

96 LINTON R.A.F., MILLER R. & CAMERON I.R. (1976). Ventilatory response to CO_2 inhalation and intravenous infusion of hypercapnic blood. *Resp. Physiol.* **26**, 383–394.

97 SYLVESTER J.T., WHIPP B.J. & WASSERMAN K. (1973). Ventilatory control during brief infusions of CO_2-laden blood in the awake dog. *J. Appl. Physiol.* **35**, 178–186.

98 WASSERMAN K., WHIPP B.J., CASABURI R., HUNTSMAN D.J., CASTAGNA J. & LUGLIANI R. (1975). Regulation of arterial PCO_2 during intravenous CO_2 loading. *J. Appl. Physiol.* **38**, 651–656.

99 LEWIS S.M. (1975). Awake baboon's ventilatory response to venous and inhaled CO_2 loading. *J. Appl. Physiol.* **39**, 417–422.

100 YAMAMOTO W.S. (1960). Mathematical analysis of the time course of alveolar CO_2. *J. Appl. Physiol.* **15**, 215–219.

101 MARSH R.H.K., LYEN K.R., MCPHERSON G.A.D., PEARSON S.B. & CUNNINGHAM D.J.C. (1973). Breath-by-breath effects of imposed alternate-breath oscillations of alveolar CO_2. *Resp. Physiol.* **18**, 80–91.

102 WIDDICOME J.G. (1971). Breathing and breathlessness in lung diseases. *Sci. Basis Med. Ann. Rev.* 148–160.

103 GUZ A. (1976). Regulation of respiration in man. *Ann. Rev. Physiol.* **37**, 303–323.

104 YOUNES M., VAILLANCOURT P. & MILIC-EMILI J. (1974). Interaction between chemical factors and duration of apnoea following lung inflation. *J. Appl. Physiol.* **36**, 190–201.

105 GUZ A., NOBLE M.I.M., EISELE J.H. & TRENCHARD D. (1971). The effect of lung deflation on breathing in man. *Clin. Sci.* **40**, 451–461.

106 SELLICK H. & WIDDICOMBE J.G. (1971). Stimulation of lung irritant receptors by cigarette smoke, carbon dust, and histamine aerosol. *J. Appl. Physiol.* **31**, 15–19.

107 GLOGOWSKA M. & WIDDICOMBE J.G. (1973). The role of vagal reflexes in experimental lung oedema, bronchoconstriction and inhalation of halothane. *Resp. Physiol.* **18**, 116–128.

108 ARMSTRONG D.J., LUCK J.C. & MARTIN V.M. (1976). The effect of emboli upon intrapulmonary receptors in the cat. *Resp. Physiol.* **26**, 41–54.

109 TRENCHARD D., GARDNER D. & GUZ A. (1972). Role of pulmonary vagal afferent nerve fibres in the development of rapid shallow breathing in lung inflammation. *Clin. Sci.* **42**, 251–263.

110 PHILLIPSON E.A., MURPHY E., KOZAR L.F. & SCHULTZE R.K. (1975). Role of vagal stimuli in exercise ventilation in dogs with experimental pneumonitis. *J. Appl. Physiol.* **39**, 76–85.

111 JAIN S.K., TRENCHARD D., REYNOLDS F., NOBLE M.I.M. & GUZ A. (1973). The effect of local anaesthesia of the airway on respiratory reflexes in the rabbit. *Clin. Sci.* **44**, 519–538.

112 DAIN D.S., BOUSHEY H.A. & GOLD W.M. (1975). Inhibition of respiratory reflexes by local anaesthetic aerosols in dogs and rabbits. *J. Appl. Physiol.* **38**, 1045–1050.

113 EMPEY D.W., LAITINEN L.A., JACOBS L., GOLD W.M. & NADEL J.A. (1976). Mechanisms of bronchial hyperreactivity in normal subjects after upper respiratory tract infection. *Amer. Rev. Resp. Dis.* **113**, 131–139.

114 CAMPBELL E.J.M. (1974). *Clinical Physiology.* 4th Edn. Ed. Campbell, Dickinson and Slater, p. 126. Blackwell Scientific Publications, Oxford.

115 EISELE J., TRENCHARD D., BURKI N. & GUZ A. (1968). The effect of chest wall block on respiratory sensation and control in man. *Clin. Sci.* **35**, 23–34.

116 NOBLE M.I.M., EISELE J.H., FRANKEL H.L., ELSE W. & GUZ A. (1971). The role of the diaphragm in the sensation of holding the breath. *Clin. Sci.* **41**, 275–283.

117 NEWSON DAVIS J., GOLDMAN M., LOH L. & CASSON M. (1976). Diaphragm function and alveolar hypoventilation. *Quart. J. Med.* **45**, 87–100.

118 CLARK F.J. & VON EULER C. (1972). On the regulation of depth and rate of breathing. *J. Physiol. (Lond.)* **222**, 267–295.

119 GRUNSTEIN M.M., YOUNES M. & MILIC-EMILI J. (1973). Control of tidal volume and respiratory frequency in anaesthetised cats. *J. Appl. Physiol.* **35**, 463–476.

120 FISHMAN N.H., PHILLIPSON E.A. & NADEL J.A. (1973). Effect of differential cold blockade on breathing pattern in conscious dogs. *J. Appl. Physiol.* **34**, 754–758.

121 PHILLIPSON E.A., FISHMAN N.H., HICKEY R.F. & NADEL J.A. (1973). Effect of differential vagal blockade on ventilatory response to CO_2 in awake dogs. *J. Appl. Physiol.* **34**, 759–763.

122 PHILLIPSON E.A. (1974). Vagal control of breathing pattern independent of lung inflation in conscious dogs. *J. Appl. Physiol.* **37**, 183–189.

123 MISEROCCHI G. (1976). Role of peripheral and central chemosensitive afferents in the control of depth and frequency of breathing. *Resp. Physiol.* **26**, 101–111.

124 NEWSOM DAVIS J. & STAGG D. (1976). Interrelationships of the volume and time components of individual breaths in resting man. *J. Physiol. (Lond.)* **245**, 481–498.

125 LYNNE-DAVIES P., COUTURE J., PENGELLY L.D. & MILIC-EMILI J. (1971). Immediate ventilatory response to added inspiratory elastic loads in cats. *J. Appl. Physiol.* **30**, 512–516.

126 PENGELLY L.D., GRENNER J., BOWMER I., LUTERMAN A. & MILIC-EMILI J. (1975). Effect of added elastances on the first loaded breath in man. *J. Appl. Physiol.* **38**, 39–43.

127 YOUNES M., ARKINSTALL W. & MILIC-EMILI J. (1973). Mechanism of rapid ventilatory compensation in added elastic loads in cats. *J. Appl. Physiol.* **35**, 443–454.

128 ORTHNER F.H. & YAMAMOTO W.S. (1974). Transient respiratory response to mechanical loads at fixed blood gas levels in rats. *J. Appl. Physiol.* **36**, 280–287.

129 BRUCE E.N., SMITH J.D. & GRODINS E.S. (1974). Chemical and reflex drives to breathing during resistance loading in cats. *J. Appl. Physiol.* **37**, 176–182.

130 LYNNE-DAVIES P., BOWDEN J.A. & GILES W. (1975). Effect of hypoxia on immediate ventilatory load response in dogs. *J. Appl. Physiol.* **39**, 367–371.

131 REBUCK A.S., BETTS M. & SAUNDERS N.A. (1975). Effect of elastic loading on ventilatory response to hypoxia in conscious man. *J. Appl. Physiol.* **39**, 548–558.

132 ZECHMAN F.W., FRAZIER D.T. & LALLY D.A. (1976). Respiratory volume-time relationships during resistive loading in the cat. *J. Appl. Physiol.* **40**, 177–183.

133 REBUCK A.S. & JUNIPER E.F. (1975). Effect of resistive loading on ventilatory response to hypoxia. *J. Appl. Physiol.* **38**, 965–968.

134 GRUNSTEIN M.M., WYSZOGRODSKI I. & MILIC-EMILI J. (1975). Regulation of frequency and depth of breathing during expiratory threshold loading in cats. *J. Appl. Physiol.* **38**, 869–874.

135 CHERNIACK N.S., STANLEY N.N., TUTEUR P.G., ALTOSE M.D. & FISHMAN A.P. (1973). Effects of lung volume changes on respiratory drive during hypoxia and hypercapnia. *J. Appl. Physiol.* **35**, 635–641.

136 STANLEY N.N., ALTOSE M.D., CHERNIACK N.S. & FISHMAN A.P. (1975). Changes in strength of lung inflation reflex during prolonged inflation. *J. Appl. Physiol.* **38**, 474–480.

137 ELDRIDGE F.L. (1975). Relationship between respiratory nerve and muscle activity and muscle force output. *J. Appl. Physiol.* **39**, 567–574.

138 ALTOSE M.D., STANELY N.N., CHERNIACK N.S. & FISHMAN A.P. (1975). Effects of mechanical loading and hypercapnia on inspiratory muscle EMG. *J. Appl. Physiol.* **38**, 467–473.

139 WHITELAW W.A., DERENNE J.P. & MILIC-EMILI J. (1975). Occlusion pressure as a measure of respiratory centre output in conscious man. *Resp. Physiol.* **23**, 181–199.

140 ALTOSE M.D., KELSEN S.G., STANLEY N.N., LEVINSON R.S., CHERNIACK N.S. & FISHMAN A.P. (1976). Effects of hypercapnia on mouth pressure during airway occlusion in conscious man. *J. Appl. Physiol.* **40**, 338–344.

141 ALTOSE M.D., KELSEN S.G., STANLEY N.N., CHERNIACK N.S. & FISHMAN A.P. (1976). Effects of hypercapnia and flow-resistive loading on tracheal pressure during airway occlusion. *J. Appl. Physiol.* **40**, 345–351.

142 KELSEN S.G., ALTOSE M.D., STANLEY N.N., LEVINSON R.S., CHERNIACK N.S. & FISHMAN A.P. (1976). Effect of hypoxia on the pressure developed by inspiratory muscles during airway occlusion. *J. Appl. Physiol.* **40**, 372–378.

143 MATTHEWS A.W. & HOWELL J.B.L. (1975). The rate of isometric inspiratory pressure development as a measure of responsiveness to carbon dioxide in man. *Clin. Sci. Mol. Med.* **49**, 57–68.

144 MATTHEWS A.W. & HOWELL J.B.L. (1976). Assessment of responsiveness to carbon dioxide in patients with chronic airways obstruction by rate of isometric inspiratory pressure development. *Clin. Sci. Mol. Med.* **50**, 199–205.

145 YAMASHIRO S.M. & GRODINS E.S. (1971). Optimal regulation of respiratory airflow. *J. Appl. Physiol.* **30**, 597–602.

146 YAMASHIRO S.M. & GRODINS F.S. (1973). Respiratory cycle optimisation in exercise. *J. Appl. Physiol.* **35**, 522–525.

147 YAMASHIRO S.M., DAUBENSPECK J.A., LAURITSEN T.N. & GRODINS F.S. (1975). Total work rate of breathing optimisation in CO_2 inhalation and exercise. *J. Appl. Physiol.* **38**, 702–709.

Chapter 6. Asthma

Asthma may be described as a disease characterised by episodes of diffuse obstruction to airflow in the lungs. The hall-mark of the disease is lability. The airways obstruction is to a greater or lesser extent reversible either spontaneously or following treatment, although the time needed for obstruction to be alleviated varies from minutes to weeks. In mild asthma the lungs are clinically normal between attacks, but in severe forms of the disease airways resistance is abnormal even when the patient is in best health. The causes of airways obstruction are

1   inappropriate contraction of bronchial smooth muscle;
2   mucosal oedema;
3   the presence of respiratory secretions, often tenacious, sometimes inspissated; and
4   dynamic compression of airways on expiration.

The relative importance of these mechanisms varies from patient to patient, from time to time, and from lobe to lobe.

Immunology

Asthma may be classified as extrinsic where allergic mechanisms may be demonstrated, or intrinsic where such mechanisms cannot be demonstrated [1, 2]. Possibly fewer patients will be placed in the latter category as investigative expertise continues to improve.

Extrinsic asthmatics usually have a personal or family history of atopy, and their symptoms begin in childhood or adolescence. An immunological Type 1 reaction between cell-attached reagin (IgE, rarely IgG) and allergen is followed by the release of several pharmacologically active substances, including histamine, slow reacting substance of allergy (SRSA), serotonin, and prostaglandins. Histamine, SRSA, and prostaglandin $F_{2\alpha}$ are bronchoconstrictors. Sometimes a delayed Type 3 reaction mediated by precipitins (IgG) occurs a few hours later, as in allergic aspergillosis. Even in a non-atopic subject, intensive exposure to an antigen may cause asthma, when the reaction is usually of Type 3, but occasionally Type 1 as well.

The relevance of immunological mechanisms in intrinsic asthma is obscure. Caspary and colleagues [3] used lymphocyte sensitisation tests to show that lymphocytes from intrinsic asthmatics react to a broad spectrum of nonspecific antigens (e.g. Kveim antigen, PPD) whereas lymphocytes from extrinsic asthmatics tended to react only with specific antigens relevant to their disease (e.g. pollen, aspergillus). They postulate therefore a general and undefined immunity disorder in intrinsic asthma.

Immunopharmacology

Before discussing actions of individual substances, the following three precepts must be recognised.
1   Airways down to the terminal bronchiole are innervated by the vagus and perfused by the bronchial arteries.
2   Respiratory bronchioles and alveolar ducts contain smooth muscle, are not innervated by the vagus, and are perfused by the pulmonary circulation.
3   Many broncho-active substances, including prostaglandins E_1, E_2, and $F_{2\alpha}$, serotonin, acetyl choline and bradykinin are almost entirely removed from the venous blood by the lung in a single passage [4]. Histamine is not removed in this way.
    Thus the effect of experimentally applied substances may vary depending on whether they are inhaled, or delivered into mixed venous or bronchial blood, and none of these modes of administration will necessarily mimic the effect of the substance when locally released in the lung.

Histamine

Histamine is released after a Type 1 reaction, and whole blood histamine concentration was found to be raised in asthmatic children with symptoms but not in asymptomatic children or those on steroids [5]. Yet antihistamines which block H1 receptors, such as mepyramine, are of no use in the treatment of asthma. (H2 receptors have been found in airways of sheep and cat [6], but stimulation of these receptors leads to bronchodilatation.)
    De Kock, Colebatch, Nadel and others showed the following in the dog [7, 8, 9]
1   Injection of histamine into the bronchial arteries caused constriction of innervated trachea isolated from the circulation and of airways down to the terminal bronchiole. There was a large rise in airways resistance and a small fall in compliance. This effect could be blocked by cutting the vagus, and differential cooling studies showed that both afferent and efferent limbs of the reflex lay in the vagus nerve.
2   Injection of histamine into the pulmonary arteries caused an immediate constriction of respiratory bronchioles and alveolar ducts with a small rise in resistance (since these airways make up a small fraction of total resistance), and a large fall in compliance (presumably because alveolar ducts form part of the expansile lung parenchyma and their constriction diminishes lung volume), and this effect was not altered by vagal blockade.

3   This peripheral airways constriction on pulmonary artery injection of histamine was confirmed in vagotomised cats with histological verification.

4   The effect was closely mimicked by injection of 48/80, a histamine releaser, into the right ventricle.

5   The result of injecting 48/80 could not be blocked by mepyramine, whereas the result of injecting histamine intravenously could be. It appears that while H1 blockade would nullify the effect of circulating histamine it could not prevent the effect of histamine locally released in the lung. In clinical asthma it is still uncertain whether H1 blockers are ineffective because histamine is not important in the pathogenesis of the attack or because they cannot block locally released histamine.

Histamine not only causes contraction of smooth muscle, but oedema of the bronchial wall [10, 11]. In the dog, whether given by subpleural, intravenous or intracheal routes, the mechanism appears to be an increased permeability restricted to bronchial venules, in the endothelium of which holes of up to 5000 Å diameter appear.

Serotonin [8]

Colebatch and colleagues showed that serotonin in the vagotomised cat (where histamine caused peripheral bronchial and alveolar duct constriction) produced a large rise in airways resistance, a fall in dead space (suggesting constriction of large airways), and a small fall in compliance, and interpreted this as evidence of constriction in large as well as small airways. Note that some serotin must have got through the pulmonary filter in order to reach large airways via the bronchial arteries. Serotinin does not affect bronchial venular permeability.

Bradykinin [12]

When infused in man intravenously, bradykinin caused no change in resistance of large or small airways, but a fall in vital capacity suggesting alveolar duct constriction.

Slow-reacting substance of anaphylaxis

The relevance of this in clinical asthma is obscure.

Prostaglandins

Whereas asthmatics react to about one-hundredth of the dose of inhaled histamine required to cause measurable broncho-constriction in normals, they may react to about one-ten-thousandth of the dose of prostaglandin $F_{2\alpha}$ that gives a measurable reaction in normals [13]. While both prostaglandin $F_{2\alpha}$, a bronchoconstrictor, and prostaglandins E_1 and E_2, bronchodilators, are released by a Type 1 reaction, the relevant proportions of each are unknown and the overall effect thus unpredictable. Some patients' asthma is apparently improved by aspirin, which inhibits prostaglandin synthetase, but there is as yet no published information about prostaglandin metabolism in such patients.

Szentivanyi, cyclic AMP and the sympathetic system

It was Szentivanyi [14] who observed that asthmatics behave 'as if' they were affected by a continuous but partial state of β-adrenoceptor blockade. In that review he marshalled a great deal of evidence in favour of the theory, and subsequent work has almost invariably tended to confirm it. For example, adrenaline given to normal subjects causes hyperglycaemia and an increased output of cyclic AMP in the urine, but both of these effects occur to a lesser degree in asthmatic patients [15]. More recently Parker and colleagues [16, 17, 18] using in vitro preparations of white blood cells have shown

1   that leucocytes and lymphocytes from asthmatics have a significantly lower concentration of cyclic AMP than cells from normal subjects;

2   that these cells from asthmatics have a smaller cyclic AMP response to β-adrenoceptor agonists;

3   that this alteration was most marked in periods of severe asthma, but that episodes of bronchospasm could occur in the presence of a normal cyclic AMP response;

4   that cells from asthmatics with an abnormal cyclic AMP response respond normally to prostaglandin E_1 which activates cyclic AMP by a mechanism which does not involve β-adrenoceptors; and

5   that glucocorticoids stimulate cyclic AMP accumulation in both asthma and control white cells, this effect being potentiated by theophylline. Alston and Patel [19] in a similar preparation showed additionally that cyclic AMP response could be restored by α-adrenoceptor antagonists. Finally Lichtenstein and colleagues [20] found

1   that agents which increase intracellular concentration of cyclic AMP, such as catecholamines, methylxanthine and prostaglandins of the E series, inhibit IgE-type histamine release;

2   that histamine itself once released inhibits its further release by negative feedback; and

3   that this inhibition of its own further release is prevented not by H1 receptor antagonists such as mepyramine, but by H2 receptor antagonists such as burimamide. Thus drugs like burimamide if given for other clinical

reasons such as to decrease gastric acid secretion might be expected to cause deterioration in an asthmatic if his attacks were due to the direct local effect of histamine released by a Type 1 reaction. This does not seem to have occurred as yet, and, as will be discussed below, makes one wonder if the direct local effect of histamine on bronchi is really of importance in asthma.

LUNG MECHANICS IN CLINICAL ASTHMA

While it had long been known from clinical observation that the lungs of patients suffering from an asthmatic attack were hyperinflated, it was not until the first measurements of lung volumes were made in severe asthma that the degree of hyperinflation was appreciated. Woolcock and Read [21] found that in the severe attack not only were residual volume (RV) and total lung capacity (TLC) increased, but that in some cases RV was increased above the TLC of the patient when subsequently in good health. In other words all the patient's breathing was occurring at lung volumes greater than the maximum volume which he could achieve when fit—an astounding finding. It was soon found [22, 23] that this increase in lung volume was accompanied by a decrease in the lung elastic recoil at any given volume, the lung compliance curve being shifted up and to the left. We will not at this point explore the full implications of this finding, but shall do so below in the section on emphysema. For the moment note only that a severe asthmatic attack may be accompanied by a fundamental change in the mechanics of the lung such that the recoil pressure is less at any given lung volume. This might be due to a change in the character of the lung parenchyma or of the surfactant lining. If the former it suggests that, when subjected to an abnormally high distending pressure for a long time, the lung parenchyma either tends to 'creep', a word used to describe a slow increase in length of a material held at constant stress, or alternatively to show stress-strain relaxation, the implication here being that the lung is acutely exposed to a high distending pressure which hyperinflates it, and that subsequently the distending pressure required to maintain this hyperinflation falls. Either phenomenon would shift the compliance curve to the left (Fig. 7.1), with creep moving the operating point vertically and stress-strain relaxation moving it horizontally.

Initial results were from patients with severe asthma, and recovery from hyperinflation and return of the compliance curve to normal were slow. TLC can increase by 1–2 L within minutes, for example after exercise, and can be reversed equally rapidly following an inhalation of isoprenaline. We do not yet know the accompanying moment-to-moment changes in compliance over such a short period.

Could this change in lung mechanics be due to a surfactant effect? No applicable technique exists in man, but in dogs Buhain and colleagues [24] put an expiratory resistance into the trachea in experiments over 2–4 weeks and demonstrated progressive hyperinflation and shift of the compliance curve to the left, but the compliance curve of the excised fluid-filled lungs was the same in control and experimental animals, suggesting that the change in the pressure-volume relation is due to surface effects. Why hyperinflation should lead to a generally diminished surface tension is not easy to see, but the authors postulate either that the accompanying respiratory pattern of slow rate and high end-expiratory level decreases the rate of surfactant breakdown or that, less likely, on hyperinflation more surfactant was recruited from angles and crevices in the alveolar surface.

The third possible mechanism in the hyperinflation of severe asthma relates to the interaction of agonist and antagonist muscles of respiration and the diaphragm, a problem which is unexplored in this condition. Clearly it must be relevant when man breathes at a volume higher than that he could previously achieve by maximum voluntary full inspiration.

The site of airways obstruction within the bronchial tree during symptomatic asthma is not agreed. In one study [23] using body plethysmography and the Mead concept of upstream (peripheral) and downstream (central, large airway) resistance, it was concluded that although resistance was increased throughout the bronchial tree, the most important site was in the small peripheral airways, where resistance could remain abnormal even when FEV_1 was brought back to normal by a bronchodilator drug. In another study [25] it was found that some asthmatics could increase their maximum flow at any given lung volume by breathing a helium-oxygen mixture, and some could not, and that these findings were repeatable on different days. It was suggested (p. 29) that in the first group the important obstruction lay mainly in the larger airways, while in the second group it lay in peripheral small airways. While the technique used requires large assumptions about the nature of flow in the bronchial tree, there seems no prima facie reason why the distribution of resistance throughout the tree should be the same in all types of asthma in all patients.

Many asthmatics are clinically normal between attacks, with normal overall airways resistance. The more subtle tests of small airway function such as frequency dependence of compliance [26] and closing volume [27] will almost always be abnormal even if the patient seems entirely fit.

GAS EXCHANGE

Any lung disease which interferes with the distribution of ventilation may be expected to cause abnormal distribution of ventilation-perfusion ($\dot{V}/\dot{Q}$) ratios. Presence of abnormally low $\dot{V}/\dot{Q}$ areas will lead to arterial hypoxia and an increased alveolar-arterial gradient for oxygen. High $\dot{V}/\dot{Q}$ areas cause an abnormal proportion of wasted ventilation shown by a high V_D/V_T ratio, with the result that an abnormally large total ventilation is required to keep arterial P_{CO_2} normal. Both these abnormalities may be found even in asymptomatic asthma [28], and become more abnormal during the acute attack. In the latter state, however, despite a high V_D/V_T ratio arterial P_{CO_2} is typically lower than normal, which means that the patient is breathing more than is required to maintain a normal arterial P_{CO_2}. The added drive is derived partly from hypoxia and partly probably from impulses from irritant receptors in the bronchi conducted up the vagus nerve (p. 171). In a very severe attack the patient may become exhausted, unable any longer to meet the demands of his respiratory control system, and ventilation decreases with a rise in arterial P_{CO_2}, and if this trend is allowed to continue death may ensue in respiratory failure usually with a terminal arrhythmia. Thus arterial P_{CO_2} rising from below normal towards normal in severe asthma may mean that the patient is recovering or that he is becoming exhausted and is in danger of death, so that careful clinical observation and frequent measurements are needed to interpret blood gas results in this state.

Paradoxically, if a patient with asthma is given a bronchodilator drug, while airways obstruction may be relieved, arterial P_{O_2} tends to fall, and V_D/V_T to rise. The fall in P_{O_2} may be clinically significant with isoprenaline and aminophylline [29, 30, 31], and is less obvious or non-existent with β_2-adrenoceptor stimulators such as salbutamol.

The very fact that bronchodilators in asthma tend to worsen gas exchange suggests that local adaptive readjustments to abnormal $\dot{V}/\dot{Q}$ ratios have already been made in the lung and that widespread bronchodilation while essential for relieving the attack interferes with these local mechanisms. We should therefore consider the relation of alveolar P_{O_2} to the calibre of the local airways and pulmonary blood vessels. We know that breathing gases of low P_{O_2} tends to cause bronchoconstriction in normal subjects [32]. This does not help to explain the isoprenaline effect in hypoxic low $\dot{V}/\dot{Q}$ areas, for if some of the bronchoconstriction is due to hypoxia itself an increase in local ventilation by bronchodilation should relieve the hypoxia, if flow is unchanged. We also know that a low alveolar P_{O_2} causes pulmonary vasoconstriction which tend to restore P_{O_2} towards normal [33]. Isoprenaline, which has both β_1 and β_2 actions will not only bronchodilate but will also cause an increase in pulmonary blood flow and pulmonary blood volume, due either to vasodilation or to recruitment of new vessels [34]. If this is so, we may speculate that the local effect of isoprenaline in low $\dot{V}/\dot{Q}$ areas might be to increase $\dot{Q}$ proportionally more than $\dot{V}$, thus improving airways resistance while making $\dot{V}/\dot{Q}$ matching worse. This view is supported by the finding that practolol, a relatively selective β_1-adrenoceptor antagonist, prevents the fall in arterial P_{O_2} caused by isoprenaline [35].

MODELS OF ASTHMA

Allergic dogs [36, 37, 38]

Gold and colleagues have used dogs sensitised to common allergens such as round-worms or pollen to produce controlled asthmatic attacks by bronchial challenge. They showed by tantalum bronchography that narrowing of the airways occurred down to bronchi of 0·5 mm diameter but the maximum narrowing was in the 1–8 mm range. Compliance fell, but could be restored to normal by a single full inspiratory manoeuvre suggesting initial deterioration of surfactant properties restored by full expansion of the surface film.

Bronchoconstriction produced by antigen challenge could be abolished by vagal blockade either efferent (atropine) or afferent (differential cooling). Antigen introduced into one lung caused bronchoconstriction on both sides; but this bilateral bronchoconstriction could be prevented by unilateral vagal blockade on the side of antigen challenge. Thus in dogs asthma caused by antigen inhalation is reflexly mediated, both limbs of the reflex lying in the vagus nerve.

The same group also showed that, in a small series of extrinsic asthmatics, intravenous or inhaled atropine would completely block asthma caused by antigen inhalation [39].

Provoked asthma in humans

An episode of wheezing apparently similar to a clinical attack of asthma may be provoked in susceptible subjects by inhalation of histamine, methacholine, prostaglandin $F_{2\alpha}$, or a relevant allergen, and such episodes are easier to study than naturally occurring attacks. It is reasonable to believe that the information obtained from them applies also to the very early stages of a clinical attack.

A rise in RV and fall in FEV_1 and VC, and a rise in airways resistance measured by any technique, are constant findings. TLC may also increase but this is infrequent. The most marked effects occur on flows in the effort-independent part of the MEFV curve (p. 23) [40, 41], and in some patients this may be the only observable change, suggesting obstruction to small airways. After methacholine inhalation [42] the change in pulmonary resistance (which includes airways resistance) occurred more quickly and was of shorter duration than the change in FEV_1, suggesting that there were independent time-courses for large and small airways respectively. FEV_1 however is a very impure measure of small airways resistance. Olive and Hyatt [41] commented on the frequent finding of a parallel shift in the descending portion of the MEFV curve pointing out that this could in theory be accounted for by pure loss of vital capacity by air trapping, some airways being shut with the remainder having normal calibre. While it is known from xenon and ^{131}I-albumen lung scans that $\dot{V}/\dot{Q}$ disturbances are patchily distributed over the lung, it seems unlikely that the distinction between normal and abnormal airways would be so discrete. Nevertheless this possible effect of air trapping on the MEFV curve should be noted.

Exercise asthma

In susceptible subjects, a period of exercise may be followed by an episode of wheezing which may be totally abolished by isoprenaline. This episode is accompanied in young extrinsic asthmatics by a fall in PEFR of up to 60% control, and large changes in RV and TLC (1–3 L), these changes being highly reproducible from day to day [43]. Different sorts of exercise produce different degrees of post-exercise asthma, even when the differing types of exercise are graded to cause a similar oxygen uptake [44]. Running produces a larger effect than bicycling, while swimming causes little change. The reason for this is quite obscure.

Equally obscure are the mechanisms of exercise asthma. Paterson and colleagues [45] found evidence of minor narrowing of airways after exercise even in normal subjects, suggesting that in asthmatics exercise asthma is an exaggeration of a normal response. These authors give full reference to previous work on the cause of the phenomenon which will be briefly summarised here.

One possibility is that broncho-active substances are released. If so they may be released in the peripheral tissues after exercise, in which case they must pass the lung filter to reach large airways by the bronchial circulation. Histamine could do this, but blood levels are normal during exercise asthma and variation in blood level does not correlate with variation in measures of airways resistance. Exercise asthma is not blocked by H1 antihistamines, and the time course of response which follows inhalation of histamine is dissimilar.

If catecholamines of the type which stimulate α-adrenoceptors were responsible, α-blockade should prevent the bronchoconstriction, but it does not.

If the responsible agents were locally released, blood levels need not necessarily be raised. Attempts to prevent exercise asthma by previous administration of methysergide, aspirin [46] and indomethacin [47] have failed, suggesting that serotonin and prostaglandin $F_{2\alpha}$ are not responsible. The roles of bradykinin and SRSA have not been explored.

Voluntary hyperventilation without exercise is followed by bronchoconstriction, but to a lesser degree than that found after exercise with the same increase in ventilation. This bronchoconstriction seems to be caused by hypocapnia, for isocapnic voluntary hyperventilation has no effect. Yet hypocapnia cannot be responsible for exercise asthma, for hypocapnia does not always follow exercise.

A metabolic acidosis has been observed during the period of broncho-spasm by some workers, but this has not been confirmed by others.

The role of the vagus has been explored by giving atropine, and in some cases the exercise asthma has been prevented, but in most cases it is not.

The increased ventilation could present to the lungs an increased load of inhaled irritants, but the phenomenon occurs even when breathing filtered air.

Three drugs *will* prevent exercise asthma. The first two, isoprenaline and steroids, give us no clue to the primary mechanism. During the period of bronchospasm there is no correlation between the effect and simultaneous plasm cortisol levels [48]. The success of the third drug, sodium cromoglycate, merely adds to the confusion, for it is thought to act by preventing the release of pharmacological agents, none of which can be incriminated by the evidence described above.

Possibly the most likely answer to exercise asthma is that such agents are indeed released locally, but that relevant blocking drugs when given systematically do not reach the site of release in sufficient concentration to take effect, and that the bronchoconstriction may be mediated by the vagus nerve, but that in those experiments where atropine failed to prevent the bronchoconstriction, the dose was insufficient to achieve complete efferent blockade.

CONCLUSIONS

There are at the moment two main streams of thought about the patho-physiology of extrinsic asthma.

First, following Szentivanyi's concept, it appears that extrinsic asthmatics possess a sympathetic system which is abnormally tuned at the cellular level, with low cyclic AMP levels, so that they tend to release potentially active substances such as histamine and prostaglandins, either in normal amounts to less than normal stimuli, or in increased amounts to normal stimuli. The basic question here is whether this abnormal tuning is innate or whether it is produced secondarily as a result of overstimulation by frequent allergic reactions, or by drugs.

Second, if Gold's work with allergic dogs can be assumed to apply to humans, it appears that the role of substances locally released by the immunological reaction is not one of direct bronchoconstriction. On the contrary, they must act if at all by stimulating afferent fibres in the vagus nerve. Even if broncho-active substances are released into the systemic venous blood from the tissues, they cannot be expected to play an important part, for with the exception of histamine they should be filtered out by the lung and will not reach the bronchial circulation, so that they should act only on airways peripheral to the terminal bronchiole causing a fall in compliance with a minor rise in resistance, contrary to the findings in clinical asthma. It is perhaps more probable that these substances are more importantly concerned with the fine regulation of bronchomotor tone in health, and indeed in vasomotor tone control as occurs elsewhere in the body [49, 50, 51, 52].

It is possible to reconcile these two points of view if we regard the abnormality in the sympathetic system as primary, with the vagus responding normally to abnormal stimuli.

It may now be useful to construct a speculative account of what happens in an acute attack of extrinsic asthma. A similar account is given by Orange [53].

1   Allergen and reagin combine.

2   Bronchoconstrictor and tissue-inflammatory substances are released.

3   Immediate bronchostriction is mediated probably by the vagus, less likely by direct local action, possibly by both. Initially the constriction is mainly in larger airways of more than 2 mm diameter.

4   The lung becomes acutely hyperinflated. At this stage the episode may be abruptly terminated by a bronchodilator drug, with rapid subsidence of the hyperinflation, or it may resolve spontaneously.

5   If the attack continues, mucosal oedema and increased respiratory secretions, mediated by tissue-inflammatory substances, contribute to the airways obstruction, which may now affect the smaller airways as well. The constriction is now unresponsive to β_2-adrenoceptor agonists, for

(a) the hindrance to gas flow due to oedema and secretions is fixed;

(b) the adenyl cyclase system is less easily activated; and

(c) continuous treatment with catecholamines may itself lead to decreased responsiveness to bronchodilator drugs [54].

At this stage corticosteroids are usually given. They may

(a) decrease oedema and secretions by a direct anti-inflammatory effect;

(b) interfere with the further release of tissue-inflammatory substances by their membrane-stabilising properties; and

(c) restore towards normal the cyclic AMP response to catecholamines of cyclic AMP-depleted cells.

Finally we should note that almost nothing is known of the comparative pathophysiology of intrinsic asthma, and that it may well be very different.

LUNG FUNCTION TESTS IN THE MANAGEMENT OF ASTHMA

There are five main uses:

1   to assess immediate response to bronchodilator drugs;

2   to assess response to therapy over days or weeks, for example in a trial of sodium cromoglycate or steroids;

3   to assess gradual progression or regression of the disease over the years;

4   to assess recovery from a severe asthmatic attack; and

5   in the diagnosis of asthma.

First and above all, remember that asthma is a labile disease. In a patient living a normal life, peak expiratory flow rate (PEFR) may vary from say 500 to 250 L/min over the course of a normal day, and may drop even lower following a bout of moderate exercise.

In the assessment of bronchodilator effect, significant improvement will usually be shown by the simplest measures (PEFR or FEV_1) five minutes after an inhalation of isoprenaline. If for clinical reasons isoprenaline is contra-indicated, give a β_2-selective drug such as salbutamol and wait thirty minutes for peak effect. If the effect of the bronchodilator is doubtful by simple measurements, it is reasonable to try further tests, either airways resistance by plethysmography or flow measurements at 50% VC from MEFV curves. This is rarely necessary, and in any case if a positive bronchodilator effect can only be shown by a highly sensitive measurement, one should always wonder whether the prescription of that drug is anything more than an academic exercise. When interpreting results, remember that an absent or poor bronchodilator response may mean merely that the patient happens at that moment to be at his best. It is therefore more than useful to have some knowledge of the extent of the lability of his disease.

This is not only important but essential in assessing response to treatment over a period of days or weeks. Since any measurement or index of airways resistance may vary spontaneously and widely throughout the day, single measurements of any sort made at infrequent intervals, such as once a week, are irrelevant and serve only to impress the ignorant. (This may sometimes be useful, but is not science.) It was thought until recently that measurements of the degree of hyperinflation such as RV/TLC ratio tended to change much more slowly, and were therefore relatively free from this objection, but we now know that in young labile asthmatics RV and TLC may change by 1–3 L within a few minutes of exercise.

There is only one available technique which can conveniently be performed several times a day for a period of weeks, and that is the measurement of PEFR by the Wright peak-flow meter. The instrument is easily portable, can be taken to work, and measurements take only a few seconds to make. Following the practice of Fletcher and of Morrow Brown's group, we usually advise the patient to make three blows four times a day, namely on rising, at mid-day, on returning from work, and before retiring. Each day therefore four sets of three numbers are recorded, and from each set of three the highest reading is selected. A useful way of handling the information is to plot the highest and lowest of the four selected readings for each day. The within-day variability or lability of the disease is then reflected in the vertical distance between 'best' and 'worst' readings. Often the effect of a drug is shown not so much by an increase in the highest measurement of the day, but in the lowest, with a gradual decrease in lability.

While it is practical to supply a peak-flow meter to patients for the three to four weeks required for a relevant drug trial, this cannot be done for years. It is reasonable therefore in assessing disease progress on that time scale to measure at perhaps 6-monthly intervals lung gas volumes before and after a bronchodilator, and transfer factor as a general measure of gas exchange.

When the patient is admitted to hospital with acute severe asthma the most important initial measurements to be made are of the blood gases, both immediately on admission, and after an hour on oxygen, which should be given routinely in the first instance and continued if the arterial Po_2 is less than 65 mmHg (8·7 kPa). Without going into details of therapy [55], we may note that arterial Pco_2 is usually low and rises to normal with recovery, that in severer cases arterial Pco_2 may be high at first falling to normal with successful treatment, and that the danger sign of exhaustion and impending respiratory failure and death is a rising arterial Pco_2 in a patient clinically deteriorating despite energetic treatment. The frequency of blood gas analysis required depends on the complexity and severity of the case.

The only tests of ventilatory function possible in acute severe asthma are PEFR and FEV_1. We prefer the former since it requires less effort from an already tired and frightened patient, and use the paediatric instrument for patients who cannot achieve the minimum reading of 60 L/min on the adult meter. In interpreting serial PEFR measurements in this state, two factors must be remembered. First, if deflation with gradual fall of RV and TLC is taking place, PEFR may not necessarily improve very much even though the patient is obviously doing so. We do not find it necessary to resort to plethysmography or helium dilution in these very sick patients to prove that deflation is taking place. Second, PEFR is effort-dependent (p. 23), but this is now no disadvantage, for a falling PEFR means either increasing airways obstruction or increasing exhaustion despite treatment, and demands careful clinical reappraisal and frequent blood gas measurements. In summary, in a patient with acute severe asthma, expect the PEFR to rise with treatment, but do not be surprised if it rises more slowly than you would expect from the degree of clinical improvement. Pay the closest attention to any patient where PEFR is falling despite treatment.

Since asthma is defined in terms of reversibility or variability of airways obstruction, it is essential in diagnosis to be certain that abnormal airways resistance is present during an attack, and varies. While in the young asthmatic the history of episodes of wheezing and the physical signs during the attack are diagnostic, in the elderly with chronic cough and sputum the distinction from chronic bronchitis with wheezing may be difficult. Lability of airways obstruction suggesting asthma may be sought by giving a broncho-dilator, or by exercising the patient, although the latter procedure is often impractical. Any type of measurement or index of airways resistance may be used. There is a group of elderly patients whose symptoms initially consist of wheezing at night sufficient to interfere with sleep, and in whom measurement of airways resistance during the day may be normal or almost so, with little bronchodilator effect. (The clinical differential diagnosis from left ventricular failure will not be discussed here.) A peak-flow meter supplied to the patient for making measurements during the wheezing attacks will often show a marked fall, and this will not only prove the diagnosis but save the patient from a hospital admission for observation.

It will be apparent from the above discussion that almost all the measurements required for managing clinical asthma in or out of hospital can be obtained from blood gas electrodes and peak flow meters. While 50 peak-flow meters are much more useful to a chest department than a whole body plethysmograph, and cost about £10,000 less, it is ironic that it would certainly be easier to raise money for the latter than for the former.

REFERENCES

1 Pepys J. (1967) Hypersensitivity to inhaled organic antigens. *J. R. Coll. Physns. Lond.* **2**, 42–56.

2 Turner-Warwick M. (1973) Immunology of the respiratory tract. *Brit. J. Hosp. Med.* **9**, 19–26.

3 Caspary E.A., Feinmann E.L. & Field E.J. (1972) Lymphocyte sensitisation in asthma with special reference to nature and identity of intrinsic form. *Brit. Med. J.* **1**, 15–16.

4 Vane J.R. (1969) The release and fate of vaso-active hormones in the circulation. *Brit. J. Pharmacol.* **35**, 209–242.

5 Porter J.F. & Mitchell R.G. (1970) The distribution of histamine in the blood of healthy and asthmatic children. *Clin. Sci.* **38**, 135–143.

6 Eyre P. (1973) Histamine H_2-receptors in the sheep bronchus and cat trachea: the action of burimamide. *Brit. J. Pharmacol.* **48**, 321–323.

7 De Kock M.A., Nadel J.A., Zwi S., Colebatch H.J.H. & Olsen C.R. (1966) New method for perfusing bronchial arteries: histamine bronchoconstriction and apnoea. *J. Appl. Physiol.* **21**, 185–194.

8 Colebatch H.J.H., Olsen C.R. & Nadel J.A. (1966) Effect of histamine, serotonin and acetylcholine on the peripheral airways. *J. Appl. Physiol.* **21**, 217–226.

9 Colebatch H.J.H., Olsen C.R. & Nadel J.A. (1966) Effects of 48/80 on the mechanical properties of the lungs. *J. Appl. Physiol.* **21**, 379–382.

10 Majno G., Gilmore V. & Leventhal M. (1967) On the mechanism of vascular leakage caused by histamine-type mediators: a microscopic study in vivo. *Circ. Res.* **21**, 833–847.

11 Pietra G.G., Szidon J.P., Leventhal M.M. & Fishman A.P. (1971) Histamine and interstitial pulmonary oedema in the dog. *Circ. Res.* **29**, 323–337.

12 Newball H.H. & Kaiser H.R. (1973) Relative effects of bradykinin and histamine on the respiratory system of man. *J. Appl. Physiol.* **35**, 552–556.

13 Mathé A.R., Hedquist P., Holmgren A. & Svanborg N. (1973) Bronchial hyperreactivity to prostaglandin $F_{2\alpha}$ and histamine in patients with asthma. *Brit. Med. J.* **1**, 193–196.

14 Szentivanyi A. (1968) The beta adrenergic theory of the atopic abnormality in bronchial asthma. *J. Allerg.* **42**, 203–232.

15 Bernstein R.A., Linarelli L., Facktor M.A., Friday G.A., Drash A.L. & Fireman P. (1972) Decreased urinary adenosine 3′, 5′ monophosphate (cyclic AMP) in asthmatics. *J. Lab. Clin. Med.* **80**, 772–779.

16 PARKER C.W. & SMITH J.W. (1973) Alterations in cyclic adenosine monophosphate metabolism in human bronchial asthma. I Leucocyte responsiveness to β-adrenergic agents. *J. Clin. Invest.* **52**, 48–59.

17 PARKER C.W., BAUMANN M.L. & HUBER M.G. (1973) Alterations in cyclic AMP metabolism in human bronchial asthma. II Leukocyte and Lymphocyte responses to prostaglandins. *J. Clin. Invest.* **52**, 1336–1341.

18 PARKER C.W., HUBER M.G. & BAUMANN M.L. (1973) Alterations in cyclic AMP metabolism in human bronchial asthma. III Leukocyte and lymphocyte responses to steroids. *J. Clin. Invest.* **52**, 1342–1348.

19 ALSTON W.C., PATEL K.R. & KERR J.W. (1974) Response of leucocyte adenyl cyclase to isoprenaline and effect of alpha-blocking drugs in extrinsic bronchial asthma. *Brit. Med. J.* **1**, 90–94.

20 LICHENSTEIN L.M. & GILLESPIE E. (1973) Inhibition of histamine release by histamine controlled by H_2 receptor. *Nature* **244**, 287–288.

21 WOOLCOCK A. & READ J. (1965) Improvement in bronchial asthma not reflected in forced expiratory volume. *Lancet* **2**, 1323–1325.

22 GOLD W.M., KAUFFMAN H.S. & NADEL J.A. (1967) Elastic recoil of the lungs in chronic asthmatic patients before and after therapy. *J. Appl. Physiol.* **23**, 433–438.

23 McFADDEN E.R., Jr. & LYONS H.A. (1969) Serial studies of factors influencing airway dynamics during recovery from acute asthma attacks. *J. Appl. Physiol.* **27**, 452–459.

24 BUHAIN W.J., BRODY J.S. & FISHER A.B. (1972) Effect of artificial airways obstruction on elastic properties of lung. *J. Appl. Physiol.* **33**, 589–594.

25 DESPAS P.J., LEROUX M. & MACKLEM P.T. (1972) Site of airways obstruction in asthma as determined by measuring maximal expiratory flow breathing air and a helium-oxygen mixture. *J. Clin. Invest.* **51**, 3235–3242.

26 HILL D.J., LANDAU L.I. & PHELAN P.D. (1972) Small airway disease in asymptomatic asthmatic adolescents. *Amer. Rev. Resp. Dis.* **106**, 873–880.

27 McCARTHY D. & MILIC-EMILI J. (1973) Closing volume in asymptomatic asthma. *Amer. Rev. Resp. Dis.* **107**, 559–570.

28 LEVINE G., HOUSLEY E., MacLEOD P. & MACKLEM P.T. (1970) Gas exchange abnormalities in mild bronchitis and asymptomatic asthma. *New Eng. J. Med.* **282**, 1277–1282.

29 KNUDSON R.J. & CONSTANTINE H.P. (1967) An effect of isoproterenol on ventilation perfusion in asthmatic versus normal subjects. *J. Appl. Physiol.* **22**, 402–406.

30 PALMER K.N.V. & DIAMENT M.L. (1967) Effect of aerosol isoprenaline on blood gas tensions in severe bronchial asthma. *Lancet* **2**, 1232–1233.

31 REES H.A., BORTHWICK R.C., MILLAR J.S. & DONALD K.W. (1967) Aminophylline in bronchial asthma. *Lancet* **2**, 1167–1169.

32 STERLING G.M. (1968) The mechanism of broncho-constriction due to hypoxia in man. *Clin. Sci.* **35**, 105–114.

33 HUGHES J.M.B., GRANT B.J.B., JONES H.A. & DAVIES E.E. (1974) Local regulation of alveolar gas tensions in lungs of coati mundi. *Scand. J. Resp. Dis. Supp.* **86**.

34 PIERSON R.N. & GRIECO M.H. (1972) Pulmonary blood volume in asthma. *J. Appl. Physiol.* **32**, 391–396.

35 PALMER K.N.V., LEGGE J.S., HAMILTON J.S. & DIAMENT M.L. (1969) Effect of a selective beta-adrenergic blocker in preventing falls in arterial oxygen tension following isoprenaline in asthmatic subjects. *Lancet* **2**, 1092–1094.

36 GOLD W.M., KESSLER G.-F., YU D.Y.C. & FRICK O.L. (1972) Pulmonary physiologic abnormalities in experimental asthma in dogs. *J. Appl. Physiol.* **33**, 496–501.

37 KESSLER G.-F., AUSTIN J.H.M., GRAF P.D., GAMSU G. & GOLD W.M. (1973) Airway constriction in experimental asthma in dogs: tantalum bronchographic studies. *J. Appl. Physiol.* **35**, 703–708.

38 GOLD W.M., KESSLER G.-F., & YU D.Y.C. (1972) Role of vagal nerves in experimental asthma in allergic dogs. *J. Appl. Physiol.* **33**, 719–725.
39 YU D.Y.C., GALANT S.P. & GOLD W.M. (1972) Inhibition of antigen-induced broncho-constriction by atropine in asthmatic patients. *J. Appl. Physiol.* **32**, 823–828.
40 CHAN-YEUNG M. (1973) Maximal expiratory flow and airway resistance during induced bronchoconstriction in patients with asthma due to western red cedar. *Amer. Rev. Resp. Dis.* **108**, 1103–1110.
41 OLIVE J.T. & HYATT R.E. (1972) Maximal expiratory flow and total respiratory resistance during induced bronchoconstriction in asthmatic subjects. *Amer. Rev. Resp. Dis.* **106**, 366–376.
42 CADE J.F., WOOLCOCK A.J., REBUCK A.S. & PAIN M.C.F. (1971) Lung mechanics during provocation of asthma. *Clin. Sci.* **40**, 381–391.
43 RUDOLF M.R. & SAUNDERS K.B. (1977) *Clin. Sci. Mol. Med.* In press.
44 GODFREY S., SILVERMAN M. & ANDERSON S.D. (1973) Problems of interpreting exercise-induced asthma. *J. Allerg. Clin. Immunol.* **52**, 199–209.
45 PATERSON N.A.M., AHMAN D. & LEFCORZ N.M. (1973) Airways narrowing in exercise in normal subjects and the effect of disodium cromoglycate. *Brit. J. Dis. Chest.* **67**, 197–207.
46 RUDOLF M.R. & SAUNDERS K.B. (1975) Aspirin in exercise-induced asthma. *Lancet* **1**, 450.
47 CUTHBERT M. Personal communication.
48 JAFFE P., KONIG P., IJADUOLA O., WALKER S. & GODFREY S. (1973) Relation between plasma cortisol and peak expiratory flow rate in exercise-induced asthma and the effect of sodium cromoglycate. *Clin. Sci. Mol. Med.* **45**, 533–541.
49 HAUGE A. (1969) Hypoxia and pulmonary vascular resistance. The relative effects of pulmonary arterial and alveolar P_{O_2}. *Acta Physiol. Scand.* **76**, 121–130.
50 COLEBATCH H.J.H. (1970) Adrenergic mechanisms in the effects of histamine in the pulmonary circulation of the cat. *Circ. Res.* **26**, 379–396.
51 McGIFF J.C. & ITSKOVITZ H.D. (1973) Prostaglandins and the kidney. *Circ. Res.* **33**, 479–488.
52 PICKARD J.D. & MACKENZIE E.T. (1973) Inhibition of prostaglandin synthesis and the response of cerebral circulation to carbon dioxide. *Nature New Biol.* **245**, 187–189.
53 ORANGE R.P. (1973) Immunopharmacological aspects of bronchial asthma. *Clin. Allergy* **3**, Supplement, 521–537.
54 BRITISH MEDICAL JOURNAL (1972) Leading Article **1**, 127.
55 SAUNDERS K.B. (1974) The management of asthma. *Brit. J. Hosp. Med.* **11**, 917–932.

Chapter 7. Chronic Bronchitis and Emphysema

DESCRIPTIONS

These conditions occur in combination so frequently that it is difficult to separate the individual contributions to disordered function. Without entering into semantic details we shall describe chronic bronchitis as a disease characterised by productive cough, on most days for at least three months in the year, for at least two years, in the absence of other diseases known to cause chronic cough with sputum (notably tuberculosis, bronchiectasis, pneumoconiosis, carcinoma of the bronchus, and heart failure). Emphysema is described as a disease characterised by hyperinflation of the lung, with destruction of lung parenchyma leading to coalescence of alveolar spaces and destruction of the alveolar-capillary bed. It is essential to include a mention of parenchymal damage, for simple reversible hyperinflation may occur in acute asthma without permanent structural changes.

The immediate implications are that in chronic bronchitis one might expect

1 excess mucous secretion and hypertrophy of goblet cells,
2 a tendency for abnormal secretions to become infected,
3 inflammatory damage to bronchial walls,
4 fixed airways obstruction, and
5 secondary abnormalities in gas exchange.
   In emphysema one might expect
1 destruction of the alveolar-capillary bed,
2 a primary defect in gas exchange,
3 secondarily a tendency for airways to collapse due to loss of elastic recoil following parenchymal destruction,
4 hyperinflation to overcome the tendency of the airways to collapse, and
5 perhaps an additional reason for abnormal gas exchange on account of hyperinflation.

This short schema begs many questions. For example does hyperinflation follow the initial parenchymal damage or is some of the parenchymal damage due to hyperinflation? It is intended merely as an intuitive framework on which we will attempt to fit the observed findings.

Although many patients with chronic fixed airways obstruction have both emphysema and chronic bronchitis, it is possible to recognise a continuous spectrum of disease with at one end patients with 'pure' emphysema and at the other patients with 'pure' chronic bronchitis [1]. The distinction is perhaps not as useful as originally supposed [2] but the differences are summarised in Table 7.1.

Table 7.1. Pink puffers and blue bloaters

Type A (*pure emphysema*)	Type B (*pure chronic bronchitis*)
Chest film: loss of peripheral vascular markings suggesting parenchymal destruction.	Preservation of peripheral vascular markings. Chronic inflammatory changes.
Sputum: none or minimal.	Persistent expectoration of more than 10 ml daily.
Total lung capacity: more than 100 % predicted normal.	Normal or low.
Transfer factor: low, especially when allowance made for high lung volume.	Normal.
Blood gases: often normal.	Abnormal with high Pa,co_2.
Right ventricular hypertrophy: Absent.	Present.
Heart failure: only as terminal event.	Recurrent episodes of cor pulmonale.
Dyspnoea: severe.	None.

It was the difference in the incidence of cyanosis, heart failure (oedema), and breathlessness which led Dornhurst to categorise them as pink puffers (Type A) and blue bloaters (Type B).

It is obvious that our original argument about what should be expected is already sadly askew. The patient with pure emphysema and a primary defect in gas exchange suggested by a low transfer factor may maintain a normal Pa,co_2 at the price of severe breathlessness. We unfortunately forgot to consider what the respiratory control system might do, and for the moment will leave that question and consider the disorder of lung function in more detail.

MECHANISMS OF AIRWAYS OBSTRUCTION

The possible mechanisms are:

1   intrinsic narrowing of airways due to disease, for example inflammatory mucosal oedema or chronic fibrotic constriction,
2   blockage by secretions,
3   narrowing of airways under static conditions due to loss of parenchymal elastic recoil,

4   inappropriate contraction of smooth muscle, and
5   abnormal narrowing of airways during forced expiration due to either (a) loss of parenchymal elastic recoil or (b) increased collapsibility due to intrinsic airways disease.

SITES OF AIRWAYS OBSTRUCTION

In patients with chronic airways obstruction, abnormal resistance to flow may be found at two levels [3];
A, in small airways, peripheral to the segmental bronchi, where the resistance tends to be fixed, occurs both in inspiration and expiration, and is largely independent of lung volume. This is presumptively due to mechanisms (1) and (2) above, with perhaps some contribution from (3) and (4).
B, in larger central airways, where the abnormal resistance is variable, occurring only on expiration, and due to mechanism 5, abnormal dynamic compression.

COMPLIANCE AND ELASTIC RECOIL

At this point it is helpful to distinguish between these two widely confused terms. In Fig. 7.1, take compliance curve AB, drawn linear for simplicity. The slope of the curve, θ, defines the compliance. The term elastic recoil pressure refers to the pressure required to produce any defined volume on the curve. Thus at volume X the recoil pressure is Z. There are therefore an infinite number of elastic recoil points on every compliance curve. A statement that elastic recoil pressure at a certain volume is a certain value says nothing about compliance. In Fig. 7.1 the elastic recoil pressure at point Y is common to both compliance curves AB and CD. A general statement that the compliance curve is left-shifted curiously tells us a lot about elastic recoil pressure (for example if curve AB is normal, elastic recoil pressures in curves EF, EG, and EH are all abnormally low for all volumes) but again nothing about compliance, for compliance of EG is normal, EF is low and EH is high. The words stiff and floppy are often applied in this context and can be seriously confusing. The lung represented by compliance curve EF requires smaller distending pressures to reach any common volume than lung AB. On the other hand any common pressure change will produce a smaller volume change in lung EF than in lung AB. If AB is normal is EF stiff or floppy? It is clear that a full description of the static elastic properties of the lung requires a statement of both the slope and the position of the compliance curve.

Studies of the elastic behaviour of the lung in patients with airways obstruction [4, 5] showed that in asthma the compliance curve was left-

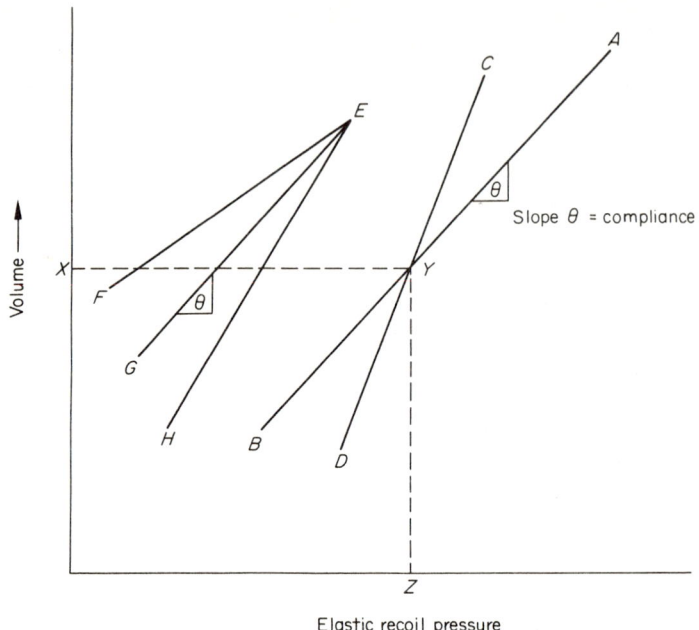

Fig. 7.1. Various compliance curves, all drawn linear for simplicity. The slope defines the compliance of the 'normal' volume-pressure relation *AB*. Line *EG* has the same slope and compliance, but is not a normal volume-pressure relation. See text.

shifted but that its slope was normal (Fig. 7.2). In emphysema the curve was shifted further to the left and its slope was increased, so that not only was elastic recoil pressure diminished at all lung volumes, but increases in lung volume could be achieved by smaller than normal increments in pressure.

    There are several possible reasons for a decreased elastic recoil pressure at all lung volumes

1   Elastic tissue components may be destroyed, for example by the degenerative emphysematous process.

2   There might be creep or stress-strain relaxation (p. 197) following the continuous exposure of lung tissue to abnormally great stresses or strains.

3   There might be a change in the influence of surfactant.

4   There might be closure of airways during deflation, when measurements of static compliance are usually made. This implies that as the lung deflates air-containing units become blocked off and, since they deflate no further, play no further part in the volume pressure relation. Thus the actual volume corresponding to the measured pressure is less than the volume measured. To correct for this the compliance curve must be shifted down to lower volumes, or contrariwise the effect of airway closure is to shift the curve upwards. Since

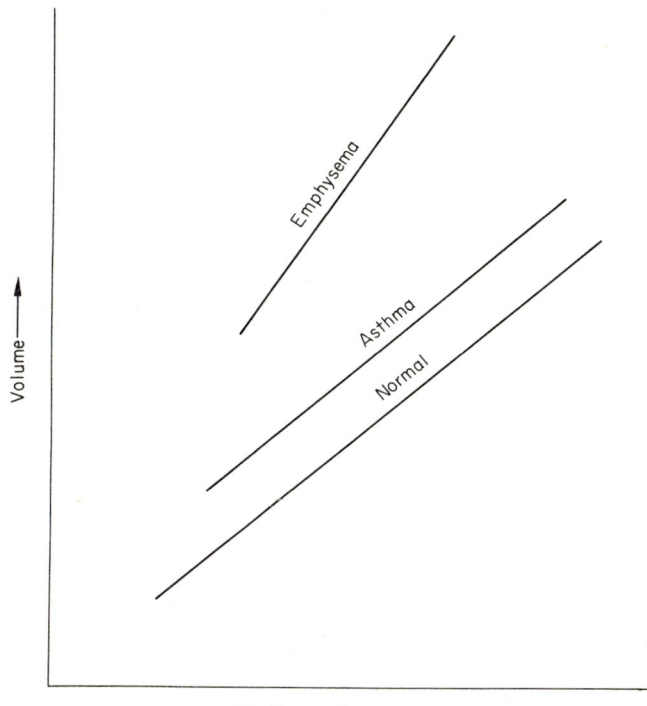

Fig. 7.2. Schematic representation of compliance curves from normal subjects, patients with emphysema, and patients with asthma.

compliance curves slope upwards and to the right, the abnormal closure of airways during deflation might appear to cause a leftwards shift of the compliance curve compared with the normal.

If we consider these four mechanisms in order

1   It is very reasonable and intuitively easy to believe that the leftward shift and increased compliance seen in emphysema is due to destruction of elastic tissue components.

2   There might be creep or stress-strain relaxation (p. 197) following the cularly over long periods of time.

3   An interesting paper by Buhain and colleagues [6] showed that when dogs were caused to breathe through an expiratory resistance, the pressure volume relation of the excised lung was shifted to the left, but that the pressure-volume relation of the fluid-filled lung was normal, suggestion that the abnormal compliance curve was due to altered surfactant properties. It is difficult to extrapolate these findings to the emphysematous lung in man.

4   We believe that airways do close, even in normal lungs, as deflation

approaches residual volume. Presumably airway closure may occur not only at the bases but elsewhere in highly abnormal emphysematous lungs. In general one would expect that the displacement effect of airway closure on the compliance curve would increase as the lung approached residual volume, and that the left-hand end of the curve would be raised more than the right-hand end, tending to produce a decrease in slope rather than the increase seen in emphysema.

Probably in emphysema the major cause of the abnormal volume-pressure relation is simple destruction of the lung parenchyma. In severe obstructive bronchitis with minimal emphysema, and particularly in asthma without emphysema, one or more of the other mechanisms presumably contributes, but their relative importance is unknown.

LOSS OF ELASTIC RECOIL AND AIRWAY COLLAPSIBILITY

Assessment of the contribution of these two factors to increased airways resistance in patients with chronic airways obstruction is a complicated problem. Two papers [7, 8] illustrate some possible approaches. It is again emphasised that loss of elastic recoil affects airway calibre in two ways, first under static conditions and second by increasing dynamic compression during forced expiration.

Three graphical plots are useful for considering the effect of recoil pressure on the static (no-flow) dimensions of airways. The first (Fig. 7.3a) is the volume-pressure relation of the lung and we have already considered reasons why it might be left-shifted in chronic airways obstruction. The second is the airways conductance-volume plot (Fig. 7.3b) where conductance is the reciprocal of resistance measured by the Dubois plethysmographic technique (p. 15). Since conductance measurements are made with the subject panting shallowly volume changes and flow rates are very small, and dynamic compression does not occur, at least in normal subjects. Hence it is considered that these conductance measurements reflect the static dimensions of the airways at the panting volume, which may be varied by the subject to obtain the conductance-volume plot. Of all varieties of respiratory acrobatics, this is possibly the most difficult, especially for patients. The third plot is obtained by combining the information from the first two to obtain the relation between conductance and elastic recoil pressure (Fig. 7.3c). Note that if conductance is thought to reflect the overall dimensions of the airways under quasi-static conditions, and recoil pressure to reflect the static distending pressure acting on the airways, the slope of this plot is closely related to airways compliance.

If in a diseased lung the airways were intrinsically normal but narrowed

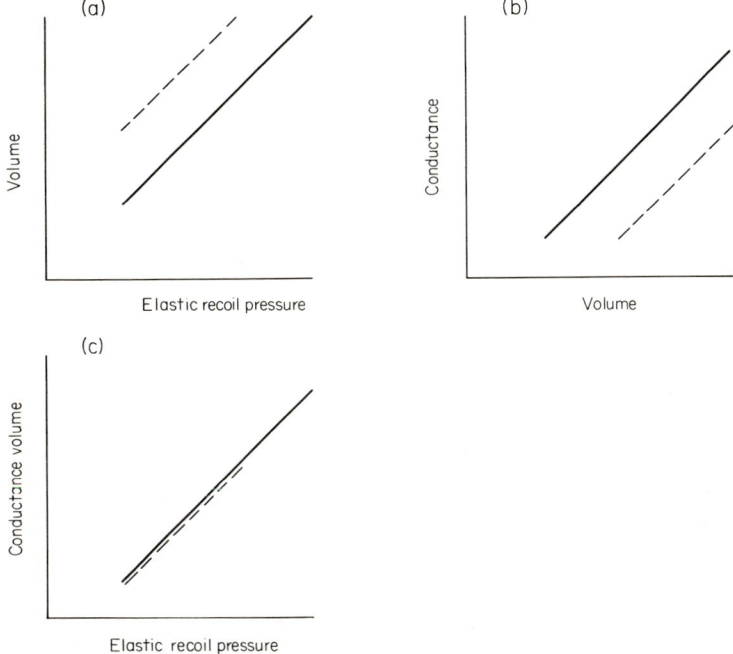

Fig. 7.3. Solid lines show normal relations. Dotted lines show a hypothetical lung where (a) the compliance curve is left shifted, and (b) the airways are narrower at any volume because of loss of elastic recoil pressure, but (c) the relation between conductance and recoil pressure is normal.

due to loss of parenchymal elastic recoil properties, one would expect, under static or quasi-static conditions, that

1 The overall compliance curve of the lung would be left-shifted (Fig. 7.3a).

2 The conductance-volume plot would be abnormal, with conductance low for any given volume (Fig. 7.3b).

3 The conductance-elastic recoil plot would be normal, with the obtained measurements lying over the lower end of a normal 'airways compliance' curve. This implies only that, although the airways are narrow, their calibre is appropriate to their distending pressure. This is exactly what Gelb and colleagues [7] found in some patients with bullous lung disease, and what Leaver [8] and colleagues found in seven of 17 patients with chronic airways obstruction. In these cases the loss of elastic recoil appeared to account entirely for the abnormally high airways resistance under static conditions.

To understand what happens to resistance or conductance under dynamic conditions of forced expiratory flow consider the isovolume pressure-flow curve of Fig. 7.4. Since conductance measured by plethysmography is derived from shallow panting manoeuvres with very low flows, the slope of the line

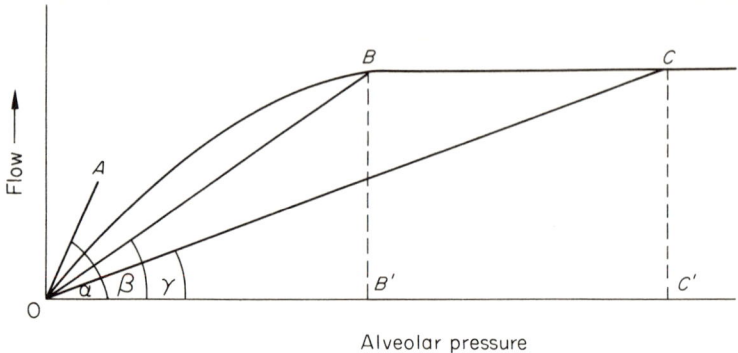

Fig. 7.4. An iso-volume pressure-flow curve; the lung volume is constant. See text.

AO, α, represents airways conductance as measured by plethysmography. The slope of the line OB, β, represents airways conductance with driving pressure minimum for producing maximum or plateau flow conditions (p. 24). As driving pressure is increased from B' to C' no increase in flow occurs, but obviously conductance (e.g. slope γ of line OC) decreases as dynamic compression increases. Thus from Fig. 7.4, for a given lung volume, conductance for expiratory flow is maximum at low flows, and decreases as flow increases, at first gradually, then more rapidly as the maximum flow plateau is reached, where Ptm' is the critical transmural pressure (intrabronchial minus extrabronchial) at which flow-limiting airways narrow sufficiently to restrict flow, and Gs is the conductance of airways upstream to this point during forced expiration. Differences in collapsibility are signified by differences in Ptm'.

We can make useful deductions about the effect of loss of elastic recoil and of collapsibility from the maximum expiratory flow-elastic recoil pressure plot (Fig. 7.5). The elastic recoil pressure on the abscissa is as usual measured under static conditions at varying lung volumes. Maximum flow measurements on the ordinate are made under plateau conditions except at high lung volumes, where there is no flow plateau.

Take now the Mead concept of the equal pressure point (EPP) where resistance upstream of the EPP (Rus) is equal to elastic recoil pressure (Pel) at that volume divided by maximum flow under plateau conditions ($\dot{V}e_{max}$). Taking upstream conductance (Gus) as reciprocal to resistance.

$$Gus = \dot{V}e_{max}/Pel \qquad (7.1)$$

from which we can see that Gus is the slope of the $\dot{V}e_{max}$-Pel plot provided that the line passes through zero.

If during maximum expiratory flow airway dimensions are altered by loss of lung elastic recoil pressure alone, then $\dot{V}e_{max}$ at a given lung volume will be low, but $\dot{V}e_{max}$ should still be normal for the recorded Pel at that volume, and the $\dot{V}e_{max}$-Pel line should overlie the lower part of the normal relation (Fig. 7.4a). This is what Gelb and colleagues [7] found in their patients with bullous lung disease, and they concluded that in those patients both the decrease in airways dimensions under static conditions and the decrease in conductance during maximum expiratory flow could be accounted for by loss of elastic recoil pressure alone, and that no intrinsic abnormality of airways need be postulated.

Leaver and colleagues [8] extended the analysis of this $\dot{V}e_{max}$-Pel plot to include the previous theoretical considerations of Pride *et al.* [9] Mead's EPP theory merely states that there is a point at which pressure inside and outside the airway are equal, and therefore does not allow any treatment of collapsibility. Pride *et al.* derived a rather similar relation to Mead's equation 7.1, namely

$$\dot{V}e_{max} = (Pel - Ptm').Gs \qquad (7.2)$$

This equation when plotted (Fig. 7.5b) has an intercept on the abscissa which is equal to Ptm' and is negative in normal subjects. Negative Ptm' implies that pressure outside the airway must be higher by a certain critical amount than pressure within it before the bronchus narrows.

If airways were abnormally collapsible, Ptm' should be less negative, and the $\dot{V}e_{max}$-Pel line should be shifted to the right, but the slope, which is Gs, should be unchanged. In three of the 7 subjects who had a normal conductance-recoil pressure relation (Fig. 7.3c), and the static decrease in conductance was entirely accounted for by decreased Pel, the $\dot{V}e_{max}$-Pel line was indeed shifted to the right with unchanged slope, and the authors concluded that in these three patients both decrease in static airways dimensions and decrease in maximum flow during forced expiration could be entirely explained by loss of elastic recoil and increased collapsibility without any intrinsic airway narrowing.

However the $\dot{V}e_{max}$-Pel lines in these three cases were shifted to the right so far that they gave a *positive* Ptm' (Fig. 7.5b) that is critical transmural pressure occurred when pressure inside the airways was greater than pressure outside, and the authors were unable to explain this. Possibly the difficulty arises from the extrapolation of the relation to zero flow, which is equivalent to assuming that at unmeasured low flow values close to residual volume the relation between $\dot{V}e_{max}$ and Pel would be unchanged, whereas for all we know the slope might in fact decrease and intercept the abscissa at an intuitively reasonable negative value.

This technically difficult study, despite difficulties in interpretation, is important in stressing that in some patients with chronic airways obstruction

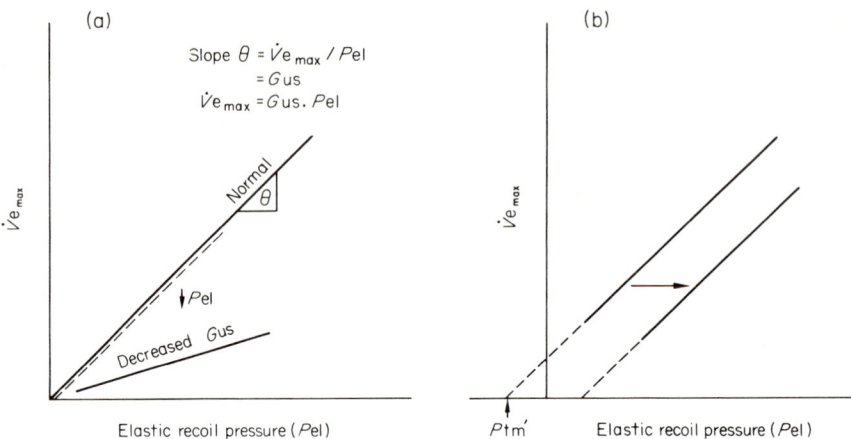

Fig. 7.5. (a) The relation between maximum expiratory flow ($\dot{V}e_{max}$) and elastic recoil pressure (Pel), the slope of which is the upstream conductance (Gus) according to the Mead concept of the equal pressure point. $\dot{V}e_{max}$ may be low (for a given volume) because Pel is low (dotted line) or because Gus is decreased.
Fig. 7.5. (b) The concept of critical transmural pressure Ptm' as applied by Pride et al. See text.

loss of elastic recoil and increased collapsibility of airways may be the major if not the sole reason for increased airway resistance.

It is worth repeating that Mead's concept of the EPP leads inexorably to equation 2.10 where it can be seen that the determinants of $\dot{V}e_{max}$ are the elastic recoil pressure of the lung and the dimensions of the airways upstream to the EPP (Fig. 7.5a). A change in collapsibility of the airways in the downstream section cannot be considered. The approach of Pride and colleagues [8, 9] attempts to take account of collapsibility by postulating a critical transmural pressure at which flow-limiting narrowing occurs, and which might change with increased collapsibility, but as we have seen this approach leads to further difficulties in interpretation. Detailed investigation of the point in patients is obviously extremely difficult but in excised dog lungs Jones and colleagues [10] have shown conclusively that $\dot{V}e_{max}$ is indeed dependent on the compliance of the flow limiting airways, and were able to predict $\dot{V}e_{max}$ with some accuracy from measurement of the relation between transmural pressure and cross-sectional area.

Obvious pathological reasons for increased collapsibility may be found on microscopy in emphysematous lungs. However Thurlbeck and colleagues [11] found most cartilage loss to occur in segmental and first or second order subsegmental bronchi, whereas expiratory flow limitation, as assessed by cinebronchography and intrabronchial pressure measurements [12], appeared to occur at lobar level.

Interest in bronchial wall mechanics has been stimulated by the gross abnormalities found in chronic airways obstruction. Apart from the influence of structural pathological changes such as cartilage loss we should briefly consider further the influence of surrounding pulmonary parenchyma and of the state of contraction of bronchial smooth muscle.

Since in the intra-parenchymal airways any decrease in volume of airways must tend to cause an increase in volume of surrounding airspaces, two general principles of interdependence apply (p. 37). First, if any lung unit, either airway or alveolus, decreases in volume out of phase with volume changes in surrounding units, its collapse will tend to be diminished by the increased distending forces generated by the compensatory dilatation of surrounding units. Second, these distending forces will be distributed over a smaller surface area of the collapsing unit, thus automatically increasing the distending pressure, for pressure is force per unit area. Certainly in dog lungs bronchi behave as if they were much stiffer when surrounded by parenchyma than when excised [13].

SMOOTH MUSCLE AND STABILITY OF AIRWAYS

At first sight bronchoconstriction should increase and bronchodilatation decrease airways resistance. No-one who has seen the effect of a bronchodilator drug in an asthmatic attack will doubt it. Changes in smooth muscle tone however alter not only bronchial calibre but also the compliance of the bronchial wall, and as we have seen changes in bronchial compliance or collapsibility will in turn affect events associated with dynamic compression [10]. Therefore one might suspect that changes in smooth muscle tone in normal subjects, or in patients with airways obstruction but without the gross bronchoconstriction of acute asthma, might have rather complex effects on maximum expiratory flow, and this proves to be the case.

In general, bronchoconstriction makes the airways narrower but stiffer; bronchodilatation makes the airways wider but more collapsible.

In a normal subject given an inhalation of isoprenaline, airways conductance frequently increases with no change or even a small fall in PEFR or FEV_1. One challenging hypothesis [14] is that after bronchodilatation the increase in conductance measured during panting without dynamic compression is offset during forced expiration by increased collapsibility of flow-limiting airways. Certainly in the isolated canine trachea smooth muscle constriction decreases conductance but increases maximum flow [15] when dynamically compressed. However it is vital to distinguish between events affecting a part as opposed to the whole of the bronchial system, as a second important paper by Jones and colleagues [16] shows.

They used an isolated dog lung-tracheal preparation, where they could control transmural pressure in the extrapulmonary airway and perform

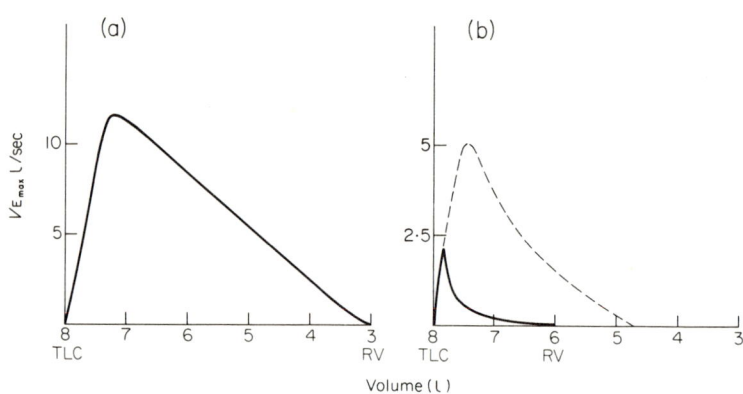

Fig. 7.6. Maximum expiratory flow-volume curves from a normal subject (a), a patient with severe emphysema (b, solid line) and a patient with moderate airways obstruction (b, dotted line).

forced expiratory manoeuvres, at the same time measuring diameter of the flow limiting segment, and flow. They could decrease the compliance of the trachea without affecting the smaller airways by treating it with acetylcholine. They could make the trachea completely rigid by inserting into it a metal tube. They could increase the compliance of the trachea by treating it with a protease. Finally they could decrease the compliance of the trachea and all airways down to the terminal bronchiole by vagal stimulation. The most spectacular finding was that the protease-treated preparation gave a highly abnormal MEFV curve very similar in shape to those found in patients with severe emphysema (Fig. 7.6). The implications are startling. One of the great advantages of the MEFV curve was that changes in flow in the descending limb were thought to reflect changes in calibre of upstream airways, if elastic recoil properties were normal, that is in the small airways of the lung which were the site of early disease. Yet in this preparation a grossly abnormal MEFV curve was obtained when elastic recoil and conductance of the bronchi were entirely normal. If the trachea was made stiffer with acetylcholine or rigid with a supporting tube within the lumen, the MEFV curve showed greater than normal flows at high lung volumes, but lower than normal flows at low lung volumes, and the explanation given is a complicated one. Referring to the rigid tracheal preparation they found that the EPP was within the tracheal segment at high lung volumes. Obviously no flow-limiting segment could be formed since the trachea could not narrow. Therefore flows were higher than normal. As the lung volume decreased during the forced expiration, Pel and Gus (from the Mead model) also fell with volume and the EPP moved peripherally, since the upstream driving pressure (Pel) decreased, and was dissipated over a shorter distance because of decreased Gus. When the EPP moved out of the splinted trachea into the main bronchi, one would have expected flow-limiting collapse to occur, and indeed lower than normal flows, for the compliance just upstream to the carina is much higher than in the trachea, and they had already shown that maximum flow was dependent on airway compliance. This did not occur for the flow-limiting segment was very short due to the splinting action of the end of the tracheal supporting tube on the airway immediately distal to it. When however the EPP moved upstream from the end of the trachea far enough for the flow limiting segment to be unconstrained by the tracheal support, the flow limiting segment lengthened and maximum flows were indeed less than normal. When the entire tracheo-bronchial system was constricted by vagal stimulation, the resulting MEFV curve was abnormal with low flows at all lung volumes, the descending limb being concave up like curves obtained from patients with moderate airways obstruction (Fig. 7.6). Any splinting effect of bronchoconstriction which might have given increased flows at high lung volumes was presumably disguised by the overall decrease in conductance in all but the most peripheral airways.

Thus there is really no confirmation here for the original hypothesis that after a bronchodilator in normal subjects conductance may be increased but PEFR unchanged because of the effect of a simultaneously increased airways compliance during forced expiration. A simpler explanation is that if the lungs are fully inflated, bronchial muscle tone is abolished [16]. Thus in the normal subject no increase in PEFR is to be expected after a bronchodilator drug, since the full inspiration preceding the PEFR manoeuvre causes complete bronchodilatation in any case.

CONCLUSIONS AND IMPLICATIONS

The consideration of mechanical events during forced expiration in patients with abnormal airways compliance has led us to revise radically the simple interpretation of the MEFV loop given in Chapter 2.

Conclusions related to maximum expiratory flow

1   As Mead postulated, the position of the EPP is determined by elastic recoil pressure Pel and upstream conductance Gus. Pel is the driving pressure across the upstream airways, and Gus determines the distance down the airways over which Pel is dissipated: at the end of that distance the EPP is located.

2   The actual plateau value for $\dot{V}e_{max}$ (Fig. 7.4) is determined by the compliance of the downstream flow-limiting segment, which determines its cross-sectional area, and to some extent by the nature of longitudinal attachments which determine its length.

3   The compliance of the airways varies in different sites. Therefore, Pel and

Gus can be considered to determine $\dot{V}e_{max}$ to the extent that they determine the site of the flow-limiting segment, which relates to $\dot{V}e_{max}$ by the particular compliance characteristics of that site.

One practical implication lies in the possibility that there exist patients with normal lungs but abnormally compliant tracheas and main bronchi. They might have apparently severe airways obstruction (cf. the protease experiment) which could be ameliorated by some surgical splinting procedure, to the trachea.

Such operations have been performed for this very reason [17], but the assessment of preoperative function and post-operative result was not thorough. As Jones and colleagues point out [16], ideally before such surgery is contemplated, it should be shown that the lung elastic recoil pressure and small airways resistance are normal, that flow is decreased, that the trachea is abnormally compliant, and that it is the site of the flow-limiting segment during the greater part of expiration.

It should also be noted that Jones et al particularly selected the dog as experimental animal because the length of the extrathoracic airways is such that for most experimental procedures the flow-limiting segment was extrapulmonary, experimentally a great advantage. In man the extrapulmonary airways are relatively short, and the flow-limiting segments are most frequently intrapulmonary. This means first that when considering the compliance characteristics of the bronchial wall which determine $\dot{V}e_{max}$, we must consider not only the intrinsic collapsibility and bronchial tone as they did, but also the supportive effect of the pulmonary parenchyma due to interdependence. Second, the possibly beneficial effects of tracheal splinting might be lost because of the long intrapulmonary collapsible segments between the trachea and the EPPs in various bronchi, which are probably inaccessible surgically.

Conclusions relating to bronchial muscle

1   Bronchial muscle tone is an important determinant of bronchial compliance. However the results of bronchoconstriction vary markedly depending on the site of narrowing. Narrowing in the trachea alone produces complex changes in the MEFV curve. If the entire bronchial tree is narrowed the overall effect in decreasing conductance at all lung volumes is probably more important than any supportive effect decreasing dynamic compression by decreasing bronchial compliance.

2   A full inspiration abolishes vagal tone in bronchial smooth muscle. Therefore when looking for small effects of drugs on bronchial muscle, it is better to perform a partial expiratory flow-volume curve [18], where the subject inspires only to 70–80% vital capacity before forced expiration, rather than an MEFV curve which starts from total lung capacity, in order to avoid the abolishment of vagal tone which accompanies full inspiration.

THE EFFECT OF BRONCHODILATOR DRUGS IN CHRONIC AIRWAYS OBSTRUCTION

Classically, we attempt to distinguish asthma from chronic bronchitis and emphysema by the finding that in the former airways obstruction is 'reversible' in the sense that it is decreased by giving a bronchodilator drug, while in the latter conditions airways obstruction is 'fixed' in that there is no response to a bronchodilator drug.

In fact it is often found that measurements of airways resistance by plethysmography decrease after a bronchodilator in patients with airways obstruction which is fixed as judged by change in PEFR or FEV_1 [19–21]. It is often said that this is because Raw is a more 'sensitive' measurement than PEFR or FEV_1 but it should now be clear that this is a misleading statement—it is rather an entirely different measurement, made under quasistatic conditions without dynamic compression (Fig. 7.4).

In normal subjects, similar small decreases in Raw are caused by a bronchodilator drug, due to the abolishment of normal vagal tone, and possibly this also occurs in patients with chronic airways obstruction. Clinically, the question is whether a demonstration of a change in Raw justifies the prescription of bronchodilator therapy in such patients. This may be approached in several ways, but a satisfactory answer will not be obtained. First, it might be thought that a bronchodilator should be prescribed if smooth muscle contraction is inappropriate, giving constriction in excess of that produced by normal vagal tone. However if airways resistance is high, and a bronchodilator causes a small decrease, we cannot know if this is due to a small change in inappropriate constriction or to a 'normal' effect on vagal tone which is superimposed on truly fixed structural narrowing of the airways. Second, if we accept that in normal subjects a small decrease in Raw follows a bronchodilator drug, it would be reasonable to prescribe only if the change were greater than normal. However the normal range for magnitude of bronchodilator effect is not defined, and one would suspect that normal vagal tone would vary markedly with time. Third, many physicians will take the view that in an intractable disorder any objective change for the better provides a rationale for giving a bronchodilator drug. This implies that almost all those tested will receive bronchodilators. Fourth, the reason for giving a drug to such patients is to improve symptoms, namely to decrease breathlessness and to increase exercise tolerance. Objectively demonstration of such an effect in every patient is quite impracticable. It would be of the greatest use to know what degree of changes in the various indices of lung function are usually accompanied by objective improvement in exercise tolerance, but this has not been done. Complete reliance on the patient's subjective account of drug effect is notoriously unreliable.

Thus no clear policy emerges. It is the author's practice to prescribe a bronchodilator only if a decrease in Raw is accompanied by repeatable, perhaps small, increases in PEFR or FEV_1. At least then one can be reasonably sure that any bronchodilatation is not causing increased resistance during forced expiration due to changes in airways compliance. In which case, why bother to measure Raw at all? By this argument, there is no need, although the measurement conveniently falls out during measurement of lung volume by plethysmography.

GAS EXCHANGE

General abnormalities

The lesions of both chronic bronchitis and emphysema are irregularly distributed. They affect the distribution of ventilation by causing airways obstruction, and the distribution of perfusion by destruction of the alveolar-capillary bed or hypoxic vasoconstriction. In addition we expect some difficulties in efficient transport of gas molecules down the airways if the terminal airways are deformed and widened, for the terminal distance over which gas molecules must be transported by diffusion will thereby be increased (p. 89).

Mismatch of ventilation and perfusion is expected to cause hypoxia with little or no hypercarbia. Hypercarbia does occur in some patients and the reasons for this and its implications are considered in Chapter 8.

Turning to experimental results, we know that abnormalities in distribution of ventilation can be found in bronchitics [22, 23], most of whom can be shown by radio-active xenon techniques to have areas with depressed $\dot{V}/\dot{Q}$ ratios, particularly at the bases. In the xenon method, each counter examines a section of lung containing about a million alveoli and many thousands of airways, and gives an overall result for that region. Wide variations in $\dot{V}/\dot{Q}$ ratios occurring within that section will be averaged out by this technique. Examination of the distribution of inspired gas at slow (compliance dependent) and fast (resistance dependent) inspiration rates (p. 83) suggests that the compliance of basal lung segments may be reduced in simple bronchitis when there is little or no emphysema, and this implies that there are lesions in the peripheral airways, that is alveolar ducts and respiratory bronchioles. Abnormalities of $\dot{V}/\dot{Q}$ distribution may be found in patients whose spirometric measurements are normal.

In normal subjects there has been considerable dispute about the relative importance of series and parallel inhomogeneity (p. 88) as causes of uneven ventilation and determinants of the shape of the alveolar plateau. In emphysema, particularly of the centrilobular variety, it might be thought that series inhomogeneity would be of great importance, since the pathological changes may lengthen the terminal diffusion distance. Since the dispute is unsettled in normal subjects, it can hardly be expected to be easier to settle in patients. Indeed either single breath tests examining the alveolar plateau (p. 90) or multibreath 'washout' procedures, will show abnormalities but we cannot as yet apportion these abnormalities to series or parallel inhomogeneity.

Collateral ventilation

The implications on pathogenesis are considerable. First, if there is airways obstruction, it would be expected that gas exchange would be more efficient if ventilation by collateral channels could be easily recruited, that is if the time constants of such channels were short. Thus the progression of lung disease in an individual patient may depend on the adequacy of his collateral channels. If a number of subjects are exposed to the same pollutant load for a period of years, some will develop chronic airways obstruction with parenchymal destruction and some will not. One factor known to be involved is alpha$_1$-antitrypsin deficiency. A second may be anatomical variation between subjects in the efficiency of collateral ventilation.

Second, collateral channels will be expected to expand with hyperinflation of the lung. We have seen that hyperinflation will widen airways. In the presence of airways obstruction it may also be expected to improve collateral ventilation.

Diffusing capacity (transfer factor)

Diffusing capacity measured by the single breath method tends to be reduced in patients with chronic airways obstruction, more so in Type A ('pure emphysema') than Type B [24]. A better separation may be obtained if the value for transfer factor is divided by the lung volume at which it was obtained to give the so-called 'diffusion constant', K. The result, D_{LCO}/V_A, actually occurs in the solution to the basic equation of motion (equation 3.30). Patients with emphysema tend to have low values of K, for they are generally markedly hyperinflated. This low value of diffusing capacity per unit lung volume reflects the destruction of the pulmonary capillary bed which accompanies the hyperinflation. A low value of K suggests, but does not prove, the presence of clinically important emphysema. A normal K value argues against the presence of severe emphysema.

Gas exchange in exercise

N.L. Jones [25] studied Type A and Type B patients during exercise, with the following mean findings.

1   At rest in Type A, Pa,o_2 was 12 mmHg (1·6 kPa) higher than in Type B.
2   During exercise Pa,o_2 in Type A fell by 11 mmHg (1·5 kPa), but rose by 6 mmHg (0·8 kPa) in Type B.
3   At rest the physiologic shunt (judged by $A-aDo_2$) was less in Type A than Type B.
4   During exercise the physiologic shunt increased (got worse) in Type A, but decreased in Type B.

These findings could be interpreted by postulating a very poorly ventilated area at rest in Type B, accounting for the lower Pao_2 and larger physiologic shunt, which low $\dot{V}/\dot{Q}$ area received a relatively large amount of ventilation during exercise, thus improving overall $\dot{V}/\dot{Q}$ matching, increasing Pa,o_2 and decreasing the shunt. Contrastingly in Type A, it was thought that the $\dot{V}/\dot{Q}$ mismatch was more widespread and relatively fixed, with increasing proportion of low $\dot{V}/\dot{Q}$ areas as cardiac output increased with exercise. Jones noted also that the greater hypoxaemia occurring on exercise in Type A patients gave them, during ordinary life, a drive to breathe which might be lacking in Type B patients. It should be stressed that in real life the relative '24 h blood gas experience' of patients in these two groups might be quite opposite to that supposed if only measurements at rest were considered. On the average Type A patients might be subjected to more hypoxia than Type B, despite a higher Pa,o_2 at rest.

Arterial hypoxaemia

Most patients with chronic airways obstruction have a low Pa,o_2. We have previously argued that a diffusion block due to thickened alveolar-capillary membrane is highly unlikely to be an important mechanism (p. 72). When $DLco$ is abnormally low, this is probably due to destruction of large areas of the alveolar-capillary bed. It might be thought that parenchymal destruction would lead to abnormally large anatomic or true shunts of venous blood past gas-exchanging areas. This surprisingly does not seem to occur, the proportion of blood thus shunted being less than 5% [26, 27]. Therefore almost all the arterial hypoxaemia is due to mismatch of $\dot{V}/\dot{Q}$ ratios.

THE PULMONARY CIRCULATION

In patients with chronic airways obstruction, particularly those with severe bronchitic symptoms, high Pa,co_2 and severe hypoxia, there may be pulmonary hypertension with right ventricular hypertrophy.

The hypertension may be attributed to
1   destruction of the capillary bed,
2   hypoxic vasoconstriction,

3 permanent narrowing of arterioles by medial hypertrophy secondary to long-standing vasoconstriction, or

4 increased blood viscosity due to polycythaemia associated with prolonged hypoxia.

Of these possible mechanisms, the second is of the greatest practical importance since relief of the vasoconstriction by O_2 breathing might in turn be followed by gradual resolution of the arterial wall thickening. The increased viscosity due to polycythaemia might also be diminished if oxygen therapy could be continued for long enough.

The difficulties of such treatment are first that O_2 must not be given in concentrations sufficient to depress ventilation (Chapter 8) and second that it must be given for sufficiently long periods of time to reverse long-standing pathologic changes. Obviously this might place severe restriction on the patient's mobility.

It has long been known that if a subject with this type of pulmonary hypertension is given a high concentration of oxygen to breathe, there will be a fall in pulmonary artery pressure, though not to normal levels, due in part to a small fall in cardiac output, but mainly to pulmonary vasodilatation [28, 29].

Acute venesection [30] is followed by a small fall in pulmonary artery pressure, but this may be due to a decreased total and central blood volume rather than a decrease in viscosity.

If a chronic bronchitic goes into acute respiratory failure there is a sudden fall in Pa,O_2 and rise in pulmonary artery pressure, which latter may be diminished either by breathing 24–28% O_2 or by infusion of acetylcholine, suggesting an acute hypoxic pulmonary vasoconstriction in these patients on top of their chronic pulmonary hypertension [31]. In subjects with chronic respiratory failure but without an acute exacerbation, continuous administration of oxygen for 4–8 weeks will cause a gradual decrease in pulmonary artery pressure, with no change in cardiac output, and a decrease in haematocrit, suggesting a regression in the muscular hypertrophy of the small pulmonary vessels [32]. It may not be necessary to give oxygen continuously to achieve a beneficial effect [33]. If it can be given mainly at night, say for 15 hours in every 24, the patient's life can be improved in quality. Present trials are designed to determine which patients may benefit, what the most convenient mode and most appropriate duration of oxygen therapy may be, and what, if any, is the effect on the overall prognosis.

Left ventricular function

It seems established that in patients dying of cor pulmonale, the left ventricle is hypertrophied as well as the right [34], although it is always difficult completely to exclude concomitant ischaemic heart disease or previous mild hypertension. The reasons for this are obscure [35], but it has been suggested that the hypertrophied right ventricle may impede left ventricular function, which seems unlikely, or that the left-sided hypertrophy is due to chronic coronary arterial hypoxia, which seems reasonable.

MUCOCILIARY FUNCTION AND COUGH

Ciliated cells are found in all airways as far peripherally as the respiratory bronchioles. Goblet cells secrete mucus, normally 10–100 ml per day. The mucous layer which immediately overlies the ciliated cells has a thin watery consistency, and is covered by a thicker sticky layer in which inhaled particles impact. When the cilia beat, they move through the thin watery later except at maximum velocity on the forward stroke, when they connect with the superficial layer and move it forward towards the upper airways.

Mucociliary function is impaired by irritants such as tobacco smoke, by inflammation, and by inhalation of dry air. In chronic bronchitis mucus production is increased by definition, and the excess secretions are prone to infection, which may itself interfere with mucociliary clearance. In patients dying in severe asthmatic attacks, or even in patients with asthma who die from some other cause, an important finding is the blockage of small airways by inspissated secretions. Why this should occur particularly in asthma is not known. Bronchial lavage in patients with severe asthma will remove many such mucous plugs.

In order to cough, the glottis is closed and the gas in the lungs compressed to high pressures (100–200 cmH$_2$O). The glottis being suddenly opened, air is expelled at high linear velocity, calculated to approach the speed of sound. At the moment of glottal release, the stage is set for marked dynamic compression, and dynamic compression is the mechanism whereby sufficient gas velocity is achieved to 'scrub' the secretions out of the large airways, since narrowing of these large airways causes larger linear velocity for a given flow. If in some part of the lungs dynamic compression occurs more peripherally, because of increased upstream resistance or diminished elastic recoil pressure, the large central airways may not narrow sufficiently to provide a satisfactory 'scrubbing' velocity, thus diminishing the efficacy of the cough.

THE AETIOLOGY OF EMPHYSEMA

There is considerable difficulty in the pathological classification of emphysema, particularly considering the significance of the centrilobular and panlobular variants [36]. Without attempting to distinguish the mechanisms which might lead to these differing patterns, we may recognise three observations of which we may be reasonably certain.

1   Emphysema is associated with cigarette smoking.

2   It may be closely mimicked in the experimental animal by placing proteolytic enzymes in the alveoli, either papain [37–40], or proteases derived from white cells [41, 42]. The changes in morphology are accompanied by striking alterations in lung function, particularly diminution in expiratory flows secondary to loss of elastic recoil properties.

3   Severe emphysema is commonly found in subjects homozygous for alpha$_1$-antitrypsin deficiency [43–45].

If one postulates the existence of defences normally present against lung breakdown by proteases, emphysema might then occur because the defences were abnormal (3, above), or because of the effect of an abnormal insult on normal defences (1). Nevertheless not all heavy smokers have severe emphysema, nor do all subjects homozygous for alpha$_1$-antitrypsin deficiency. Kilburn [46] has pointed out other questions which require attention, namely,

1   Is emphysema a developmental defect of bronchial subdivision?

2   Is there a structural or biochemical abnormality of the interstitial space or its basal laminae?

3   Are blood or lymph vessels primarily involved, in the sense that damage to capillary endothelium might lead to subsequent alveolar wall destruction?

DETECTION OF EARLY DISEASE IN SMALL AIRWAYS

In normal subjects airways of less than 2 mm diameter account for only a small proportion (say 0.2 cmH$_2$O/(L/sec)) of the total airways resistance, which has a wide normal range (0.5–2.0 cmH$_2$O/(L/sec) or 0.05–0.2 kPa/(L/sec)). Therefore a large increase in resistance, even four or five-fold, may occur in the small airways without taking the total airways resistance out of the normal range.

Since chronic bronchitis and emphysema are an important cause of debility, with large economic implications, much effort has been expended in trying to devise tests which will detect disease in small airways at an early stage, before symptoms. This does not imply, unfortunately, that we would know how to treat such subjects when found and improve their prognosis, other than advising them not to smoke. Nevertheless it is a reasonable view that we are unlikely ever to devise such treatment if the subjects requiring it cannot be identified.

Initially it seemed that the finding of frequency dependence of compliance [47] would provide the answers, but that technique is time-consuming and unpleasant for the patient, requires tedious analysis, and the records of oesophageal pressure are sufficiently noisy to make repeatability of the test exceedingly unsatisfactory, unless possibly computer averaging is used.

Closing volume (p. 86) and the use of flows from the MEFV curve have also been recommended, and both these tests have the advantages of being simple, relatively cheap, rapid to perform, acceptable to the patient, and uncomplicated to analyse.

With closing volume, the exact position of transition to Phase 4 may be hard to determine, and while the presence of a high closing volume probably indicates abnormal small airways, it seems to be abnormal in an ever-increasing proportion of lung diseases, and gradually increases with ageing, with a relatively wide normal range even allowing for age. There is no guarantee that a normal closing volume indicates completely normal airways.

The MEFV curve shows rather wide variation between apparently normal non-smoking individuals [48], again making the definition of abnormality difficult. Moreover the concept that abnormally low flows in the lower two-thirds of the vital capacity reflect abnormalities in small airways has been shaken, as we have seen, by the findings of Jones et al [16] when highly abnormal MEFV curves were found in an experimental preparation with normal intrapulmonary airways.

In summary neither closing volume nor the MEFV loop can be regarded as satisfactory screening procedures. In particular we need more details of day-to-day variability, which in normal subjects may be due to actual physiologic variation as well as to technical problems. One may confidently predict that the detection of early disease in small airways will continue to occupy the attention of a possibly excessive proportion of applied respiratory physiologists.

REFERENCES

1 BURROWS B., NIDEN A.H., FLETCHER C.M. & JONES N.L. (1964) Clinical types of chronic obstructive lung disease in London and in Chicago. *Amer. Rev. Resp. Dis.* **90**, 14–27.

2 THURLBECK W.M., HENDERSON J.A., FRASER R.G. & BATES D.V. (1970) Chronic obstructive lung disease. *Medicine (Baltimore)*, **49**, 81–145.

3 MACKLEM P.T., FRASER R.G. & BROWN W.G. (1965) Bronchial pressure measurements in emphysema and bronchitis. *J. Clin. Invest.* **44**, 897–905.

4 FINUCANE K.E. & COLEBATCH H.J.H. (1969) Elastic behaviour of the lung in patients with with airway obstruction. *J. Appl. Physiol.* **26**, 330–338.

5 COLEBATCH H.J.H., FINUCANE K.E. & SMITH M.M. (1973) Pulmonary conductance and elastic recoil relationships in asthma and emphysema. *J. Appl. Physiol.* **34**, 143–153.

6 BUHAIN W.J., BRODY J.S. & FISHER A.B. (1972) Effect of artificial airways obstruction on elastic properties of lung. *J. Appl. Physiol.* **33**, 589–594.

7 GELB A.F., GOLD W.M. & NADEL J.A. (1973). Mechanisms limiting airflow in bullous lung disease. *Amer. Rev. Resp. Dis.* **107**, 571–578.

8 LEAVER D.G., TATTERSFIELD A.E. & PRIDE N.B. (1973) Contribution of loss of lung recoil and of enhanced airways collapsibility to the airflow obstruction of chronic bronchitis and emphysema. *J. Clin. Invest.* **52**, 2117–2128.

9 PRIDE N.B.,PERMUTT S., RILEY R.L. & BROMBERGER-BARNEA B. (1967) Determinants of maximum expiratory flow in the lungs. *J. Appl. Physiol.* **23**, 646–662.

10 JONES J.G., FRASER R.B. & NADEL J.A. (1975) Prediction of maximum expiratory flow rate from area-transmural pressure curve of compressed airway. *J. Appl. Physiol.* **38**, 1002–1011.

11 THURLBECK W.M., PUN R., TOTH J. & FRASER R.G. (1974) Bronchial cartilage in chronic obstructive lung disease. *Amer. Rev. Resp. Dis.* **109**, 73–80.

12 MACKLEM P.T., FRASER R.G. & BROWN W.G. (1965) Bronchial pressure measurements in emphysema and bronchitis. *J. Clin. Invest.* **44**, 897–905.

13 TAKISHIMA T., SASAKI H. & SASAKI T. (1975) Influence of lung parenchyma on collapsibility of dog bronchi. *J. Appl. Physiol.* **38**, 875–881.

14 BOUHUYS A. & VAN DE WOESTIJNE K.P. (1971) Mechanical consequences of airway smooth muscle relaxation. *J. Appl. Physiol.* **30**, 670–676.

15 KNUDSON R.J. & KNUDSON D.W. (1975) Effect of muscle constriction on flow-limiting collapse of isolated canine trachea. *J. Appl. Physiol.* **38**, 125–131.

16 JONES J.G., FRASER R.B. & NADEL J.A. (1975) Effect of changing airway mechanics on maximum expiratory flow. *J. Appl. Physiol.* **38**, 1012–1021.

17 HERZOG H. (1963) Expiratory stenosis of the trachea and main bronchi in cases of obstructive pulmonary emphysema. *Triangle (Sandoz)* **6**, 85–90.

18 ZUSKIN E., MITCHELL C.A. & BOUHUYS A. (1974) Interaction between effects of β-blockade and cigarette smoke on airways. *J. Appl. Physiol.* **36**, 449–452.

19 ISHIKAWA S. & CHERNIACK R.M. (1969). The effect of nebulised bronchodilators on air flow resistance in chronic airways obstruction. *Amer. Rev. Resp. Dis.* **99**, 703–710.

20 ASTIN T.W. (1972) Reversibility of airways obstruction in chronic bronchitis. *Clin. Sci.* **42**, 725–733.

21 AYRES S.M., GRIESBACH S.J., REIMOLD F. & EVANS R.G. (1974) Bronchial component in chronic obstructive lung disease. *Am. J. Med.* **57**, 183–191.

22 ANTHONISEN N.R., BASS H., ORIOL A., PLACE R.E.G. & BATES D.V. (1968) Regional lung function in patients with chronic bronchitis. *Clin. Sci.* **35**, 495–511.

23 HUGHES J.M.B., GRANT B.J.B., GREENE R.E., ILIFF L.D. & MILIC-EMILI J. (1972) Inspiratory flow rate and ventilation distribution in normal subjects and in patients with simple chronic bronchitis. *Clin. Sci.* **43**, 583–595.

24 BEDELL G.N. & OSTIGUY G.L. (1967) Transfer factor for carbon monoxide in patients with airways obstruction. *Clin. Sci.* **32**, 239–248.

25 JONES N.L. (1966) Pulmonary gas exchange during exercise in patients with chronic airway obstruction. *Clin. Sci.* **31**, 39–50.

26 WILSON R.H., EBERT R.V., BORDEN C.W., PEARSON R.T., JOHNSON R.S., FALK A. & DEMPSEY M.E. (1953) The determination of bloodflow through non-ventilated portions of the normal and diseased lung. *Amer. Rev. Tuberc.* **68**, 177–187.

27 FRITTS H.W. Jr., HARDEWIG A., ROCHESTER D.F., DURAUD J. & COURNAND A. (1960) Estimation of pulmonary arteriovenous shunt-flow using intravenous injections of T-1824 dye and $Kr.^{85}$. *J. Clin. Invest.* **39**, 1841–1850.

28 WILSON R.H., HOSETH W. & DEMPSEY M.E. (1955) The effect of breathing 99·6% oxygen on pulmonary vascular resistance and cardiac output in patients with pulmonary emphysema and chronic hypoxia. *Ann. Int. Med.* **42**, 629–637.

29 HOLT J.H. & BRANSCOMB B.V. (1965) Haemodynamic responses to controlled 100% O_2 breathing in emphysema. *J. Appl. Physiol.* **20**, 215–220.

30 SEGEL N. & BISHOP J.M. (1966) The circulation in patients with chronic bronchitis and emphysema at rest and during exercise, with special reference to the influence of changes in blood viscosity and blood volume on the pulmonary circulation. *J. Clin. Invest.* **45**, 1555–1568.

31 ABRAHAM A.S., COLE R.B., GREEN I. D., HEDWORTH-WHITTY R.B., CLARKE S.W. & BISHOP J.M. (1969) Factors contributing to the reversible pulmonary hypertension of patients with acute respiratory failure studied by serial observation during recovery. *Circulation Res.* **24**, 51–60.

32 ABRAHAM A.S., COLE R.B. & BISHOP J.M. (1968) Reversal of pulmonary hypertension by prolonged oxygen administration to patients with chronic bronchitis. *Circulation Res.* **23**, 147–157.

33 STARK R.D., FINNEGAN P. & BISHOP J.M. (1972) Daily requirement of oxygen to reverse pulmonary hypertension in patients with chronic bronchitis. *Brit. Med. J.* **3**, 724–728.

34 EDWARDS C.W. (1974) Left ventricular hypertrophy in emphysema. *Thorax* **29**, 75–80.

35 BAUM G.L., SCHWARTZ A., LLAMAS R. & CASTILLO C. (1971) Left ventricular function in chronic obstructive lung disease. *New Eng. J. Med.* **285**, 361–365.

36 Leading Article (1974) Types of emphysema. *Brit. Med. J.* **2**, 571–572.

37 PARK S.S., GOLDRING J.P., SHIM C.S. & WILLIAMS M.H. Jr. (1969) Mechanical properties of the lung in experimental pulmonary emphysema. *J. Appl. Physiol.* **26**, 738–744.

38 CALDWELL E.J. (1971) Physiologic and anatomic effects of papain on the rabbit lung. *J. Appl. Physiol.* **31**, 458–465.

39 MARCO V., MERANZE D.R., YOSHIDA M. & KIMBELL P. (1972) Papain-induced experimental emphysema in the dog. *J. Appl. Physiol.* **33**, 293–299.

40 NIEWOENNER D.E. & KLEINERMAN J. (1973) Effects of experimental emphysema and bronchiolitis on lung mechanics and morphometry. *J. Appl. Physiol.* **35**, 25–31.

41 MASS B., IKEDA T., MERANZE D.R., WEINBAUM G. & KIMBEL, P. (1972) Induction of experimental emphysema: cellular and species specificity. *Amer. Rev. Resp. Dis.* **106**, 384–391.

42 WEINBAUM G., MARCO V., IKEDA T., MASS B., MERANZE D.R. & KIMBEL P. (1974) Enzymatic production of experimental emphysema in the dog. Route of exposure. *Amer. Rev. Resp. Dis.* **109**, 351–357.

43 HUTCHINSON D.C.S. (1973) Alpha-1-antitrypsin deficiency and pulmonary emphysema: the role of proteolytic enzymes and their inhibitors. *Brit. J. Dis. Chest* **67**, 171–196.

44 Leading Article (1973) Enzymes and Emphysema. *Brit. Med. J.* **1**, 1–2.

45 Leading Article (1974) Pathogenesis of emphysema. *Brit. Med. J.* **1**, 527–528.

46 KILBURN K.H. (1975) New clues for the emphysemas. *Am. J. Med.* **58**, 591–600.

47 WOOLCOCK A.J., VINCENT N.J. & MACKLEM P.T. (1969) Frequency dependence of compliance as a test for obstruction of small airways. *J. Clin. Invest.* **48**, 1097–1106.

48 GREEN M., MEAD J. & TURNER J.M. (1974) Variability of maximum expiratory flow-volume curves. *J. Appl. Physiol.* **37**, 67–74.

Chapter 8. Respiratory Failure

Much of the necessary groundwork has already been covered by previous considerations of the effect of interacting abnormalities in lung mechanics and gas exchange, and of the response of the respiratory controller to hypercapnia and hypoxia. This chapter is intended to summarise the basic concepts, to provide a simple functional classification of the types of respiratory failure, to highlight certain problems of present interest, and to underline the principles of rational therapy.

DEFINITIONS

Failure to do what? Respiratory failure can be defined only if the purpose of the respiratory system is defined. What is it for? Here some possibilities.

1   To allow gas transport without discomfort. Then anyone with dyspnoea is in respiratory failure, including the quarter-miler most of the way, and most of us at the top of four flights of stairs.

2   To maintain critical levels of Po_2, Pco_2 and pH at the mitochondrion. Unfortunately we cannot measure these variables, and in any case, which mitochondrion? It seems improbable that every single mitochondrion in the body is maintained at optimal metabolic condition at all times, and also unnecessary.

3   To adjust ventilation instantaneously to match metabolic output of CO_2. This sounds reasonable and there is much evidence to suggest that the system does that very well, but it is not a purpose which lends itself easily to the inverse definition of failure, since the demonstration of failure would require measurement of transient changes in ventilation and CO_2 output.

4   To adjust ventilation so that *in the steady state* ventilation is matched to metabolic CO_2 output. If this were so Pa,co_2 would be kept constant, in the steady state, and that can be measured. But what about oxygen?

5   To maintain blood gases normal, let us say Pa,co_2 35–45 mmHg (4·7–6 kPa), and Pa,o_2 80–100 mmHg (10·7–13·3 kPa). But the respiratory system of a subject with Pa,co_2 25 (3·3 kPa), Pa,o_2 110 (14·7 kPa) is not failing, but hyperventilating.

6   To maintain $Pa,co_2 < 45$ mmHg (6 kPa) and $Pa,o_2 > 80$ mmHg (10·7 kPa). But is a patient with Pa,co_2 46 mmHg and Pa,o_2 79 mmHg actually in trouble? Would you consider admitting him to hospital on those grounds? It might be practical to take rather more abnormal values, say $Pa,co_2 < 49$ mmHg (6·5 kPa), $Pa,o_2 > 60$ mmHg (8 kPa), and this is what most people do [1].

RESPIRATORY FAILURE IS PRESENT WHEN Pa,CO_2 IS
MORE THAN 49 mmHg (6·6 kPa), OR Pa,O_2 IS LESS THAN
60 mmHg (8 kPa), OR BOTH, AND THE SUBJECT IS
BREATHING AIR.

This is a simple operational definition of failure with no deep implications, and its major advantage is that both variables can be measured. The inverse purpose from which it arises is fairly naive.

TYPES OF RESPIRATORY FAILURE

Classification on blood gases

The simple definition above allows three possible combinations of blood gases.
1   High Pa,CO_2, normal Pa,O_2, breathing air. This is rare, for any rise in Pa,CO_2 must be accompanied by some fall in Pa,O_2, and in patients with hypercarbia for any reason there is almost always sufficient disturbance of ventilation-perfusion matching to bring Pa,O_2 down below normal.
2   Pa,O_2 low, Pa,CO_2 normal (or low). 'Hypoxic (hypocapnic) failure.'
3   Pa,O_2 low, Pa,CO_2 high. 'Hypoxic hypercapnic failure.'
Both these combinations are common.

Functional classification

It is usual to classify such causes anatomically, siting the primary problem in brain, spinal cord, nerves, thoracic cage, muscle, pulmonary circulation or lung. From the previous discussion of respiratory control, it may be now more useful to classify causes as due to malfunction in the controller, by which we mean the entire brainstem mechanism plus the carotid bodies; or in the controlled system, hereafter for brevity called the system.

The concept of controller failure is simple—a primary malfunction results in inappropriate signals to the system, which does not therefore maintain blood gases at correct levels. The signals to the controller are correct, but the signals from the controller are wrong. The system is shouting, but the controller is not listening.

In primary system failure, the abnormalities caused by disease are so great the controller cannot compensate by adjusting ventilation. The signals to the controller are correct, and the signals from the controller are appropriate, but the disturbance of system function dominates, so that blood gases are abnormal. The design of the regulator is insufficiently robust.

The only complication lies in the fact that certain diseases in the lung are associated with additional abnormal signals to the controller (e.g. from J- or irritant receptors); the results of such signals are not necessarily beneficial. Thus system failure may be divided into failure with appropriate signals and failure with additional abnormal signals.

Summary of classification

CONTROLLER FAILURE: correct input to controller, incorrect output from controller.

SYSTEM FAILURE: TYPE 1 correct input to controller, correct output from controller.

TYPE 2 same with additional abnormal inputs.

This functional classification is given because it will probably adapt to future research findings more easily than present anatomic or pathologic classifications.

CONTROLLER FAILURE

The classic example is primary alveolar hypoventilation, originally described as the Pickwickian syndrome. Subjects with this rare condition are obese. Alveolar ventilation is abnormally low, resulting in hypoxia and hypercapnia. Pulmonary hypertension follows longstanding hypoxia. Obesity in itself causes minor abnormalities in lung function, in particular a modest decrease in arterial Po_2 which may well be accounted for by the finding that closing volume occurs in the tidal range, and therefore some basal airways are closed for a part of the respiratory cycle. Nevertheless very few obese patients go into respiratory failure, and therefore it is most likely that in patients with true primary alveolar hypoventilation, both the obesity and the hypoventilation are caused by a primary medullary abnormality.

SYSTEM FAILURE

Neurological disturbances of spinal cord function (trauma) or of motor nerves to the muscles of respiration (poliomyelitis) are obvious examples. Deformity of the thoracic cage loads the respiratory system abnormally, and it is noteworthy that a generalised symmetrical deformity (ankylosing spondylitis) rarely causes respiratory failure, but a contortional deformity (kyphoscoliosis) more frequently does so.

Turning to the lungs and pulmonary circulation, we find four conditions which frequently cause hypocapnic hypoxic failure, namely pulmonary embolism, acute left ventricular failure, pneumonia and asthma. The primary insult in each case will plainly cause ventilation-perfusion abnormalities and Pa,O_2 will tend to fall and PA,CO_2 to rise. The controller responds by increasing ventilation, and may settle for a normal Pa,CO_2 with a low Pa,O_2. Frequently however Pa,CO_2 is low, say 30 mmHg (4 kPa), and Pa,O_2 also low, say 55 mmHg (7·3 kPa). It is often thought that Pa,CO_2 is low because of hypoxia, that the controller is hyperventilating the system to alleviate hypoxia. That this is rarely true is shown by the effect of giving a high inspired concentration of O_2 when Pa,O_2 may well rise to over 100 mmHg (13 kPa), but Pa,CO_2 usually remains low. Here the experimental evidence (p. 172) suggests that the controller is being driven by an abnormal input derived from irritant or J-receptors and transmitted by the vagus nerve. This is what is meant by system failure Type 2.

The end-point of severe lung disease

If there is widespread destruction of the lung parenchyma for any reason but particularly from long-standing chronic airways obstruction, chronic hypoxia is eventually followed by carbon dioxide retention. If in addition there is fluid retention with oedema, hepatomegaly and raised jugular venous pressure, we recognise the picture of cor pulmonale. What type of respiratory failure is this?

Clearly there might be System Failure Type 1, but it is often found that the apparent sensitivity to carbon dioxide and hypoxia is low. This might also be due to System Failure in that the output of the controller might be appropriate, but the mechanical defect so severe that appropriate levels of ventilation cannot be sustained. Alternatively there may be Controller Failure, possibly because the respiratory centre has adapted to continuous exposure to hypercapnia and hypoxia, and is reset to a level of output which is inappropriately low by normal standards.

To determine this some measure of controller output independent of loading is required. Initial attempts to assess this included the measurement of inspiratory work. In an abnormal system, an appropriate work demand by the controller would not produce an appropriate ventilatory response. The measurement is difficult and tedious and the best methodology not agreed. Further attempts to assess output by pressure generated during complete airway occlusion will probably be superseded by the measurement of maximum dp/dt during isometric contraction again a low-resistance flap valve (p. 183).

At the moment, it seems likely that at least some patients with cor pulmonale who are apparently insensitive to CO_2 have Controller Failure. We have no idea what the lung receptors may be doing in these circumstances.

PROBLEMS, PROBLEMS

Pink puffers and blue bloaters

Some patients with chronic airways obstruction are apparently insensitive to CO_2 and have recurrent episodes of cor pulmonale. Others have severe airways obstruction but keep Pa,CO_2 normal or even low with only mild hypoxia, at the expense of distressing breathlessness. The reason for this differential behaviour is one of the most intriguing clinical problems in respiratory physiology.

Much recent work has focussed on the fact that apparently normal people have a wide range of responses to hypoxia and CO_2. Possibly the subjects with inborn low sensitivity will develop into blue bloaters if they develop chronic airways obstruction, while subjects at the other end of the scale will become pink puffers.

The most interesting group are those who despite severe airways obstruction have a low Pa,CO_2 and a slightly low Pa,O_2. They are breathing in fact more than they need to, for the ventilation decrease required to lift Pa,CO_2 to normal would not cause dangerous hypoxia. The parallel between this picture and that of System Failure Type 2 as defined here allows speculation that these patients have abnormal vagal traffic from lung receptors, and it is noticeable that they tend to be at the emphysematous rather than at the bronchitic end of the spectrum. Possibly the differing responses to chronic airways obstruction are caused by differing sensitivities of lung receptors, or of the controller to impulses from those receptors. A very few patients seem to have been made more comfortable by cutting the vagus nerve [2].

Sensitivity to oxygen

If high concentrations of oxygen are given to a patient with cor pulmonale, ventilation usually decreases and Pa,CO_2 rises, and the patient may even become unconscious, stop breathing and die.

The usual explanation is that the patient is insensitive to CO_2, and is therefore relying on hypoxic drive. We have seen that in normal subjects hypoxic drive probably arises purely from the peripheral chemoreceptors. The removal of this drive kills the patient.

I suspect that this explanation is naive. Most of these patients are severely hypoxic. If there is hypoxic metabolic acidosis in the brain with formation of lactic acid, hypoxia may in a sense be driving ventilation centrally in these highly pathological circumstances. Then the cessation of lactic acid production following oxygen breathing may cut off not only a peripheral but also a central drive. This hypothesis is due to S.J.G. Semple, and is appallingly difficult to test in intact sick humans.

If on the one hand the decrease in ventilation following oxygen breathing were due to abolition of a normal hypoxic drive in the presence of a diminished CO_2 response, then one might expect the rise and rate of rise of Pa,co_2 to correlate with the initial Pa,co_2, which should be higher for a lower CO_2 drive. On the other hand, if the decrease in ventilation were due to abolishing a hypoxic drive produced at the central chemoreceptor by severe lactic acidosis, then one might expect the rise and rate of rise of Pa,co_2 to correlate inversely with the initial Pa,o_2, in so far as this reflects the magnitude of the central hypoxia. There is not sufficient information in the literature to test the approach.

Why do patients with cor pulmonale have oedema?

Initially it was thought that cor pulmonale was right heart failure. Patients with heart failure are oedematous, so there was no problem peculiar to cor pulmonale. This begs two questions, first on the definition of heart failure, and second on the reason why patients with heart failure get oedema, which we certainly will not go into here.

In general the presence of raised venous pressure and peripheral oedema does not necessarily imply that the heart is behaving abnormally either at rest or, more critically, on exercise [3]. Cardiac output in cor pulmonale is normal or a little high. Fluid retention here appears to be associated with abnormal blood gases, rather than to follow impairment of cardiac function caused by those blood gas abnormalities. Nevertheless, the oedema itself may impair lung function, if we accept evidence that diuretics per se improve blood gas tensions without any other form of treatment [4].

Campbell and colleagues [5] made serial weight measurements on patients with chronic bronchitis and hypoxia. As peripheral oedema and raised jugular venous pressure appeared, weight increased, but very little. Diuretic therapy decreased body weight markedly and oedema disappeared, but during convalescence weight rose gradually to or above the weight found on admission to hospital, without any reappearance of oedema. Measurements of total exchangeable sodium did not consistently suggest that sodium retention accompanied oedema. It was proposed that much of the oedema fluid was derived from the intracellular water of cells destroyed by hypoxia, and that the lost tissue mass was subsequently restored during convalescence.

In patients with lung disease and $\dot{V}/\dot{Q}$ mismatch, why does Pa,o_2 fall before Pa,co_2 rises?

It is commonly said that this depends on the relatively linear form of the CO_2 dissociation curve compared with that for O_2. Thus in Fig. 8.1a there are two 'normal lungs' each with ventilation 1 unit, blood flow 1 unit, producing blood

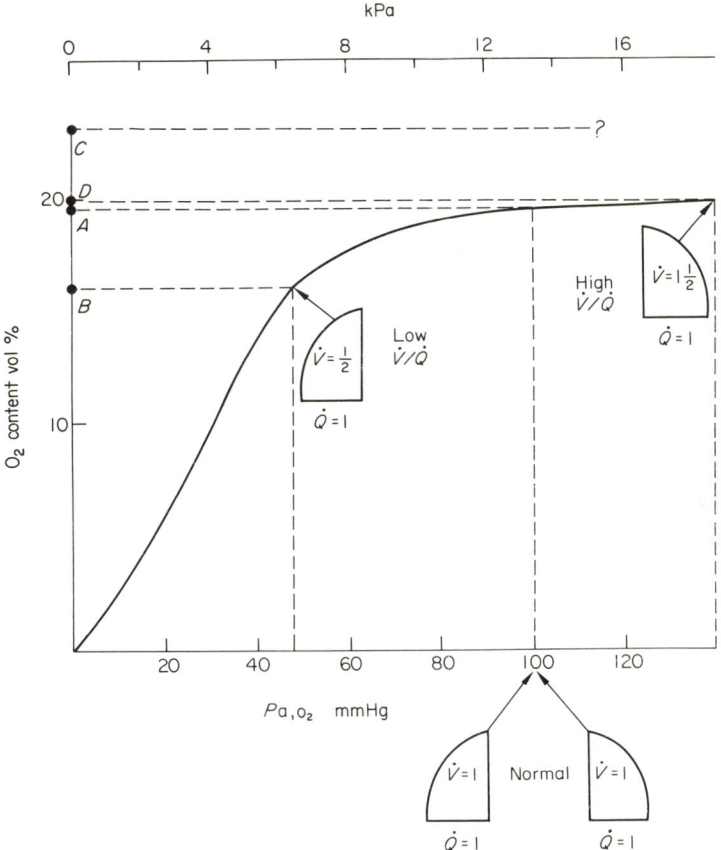

Fig. 8.1. See text.
(a) Two normal lungs give an arterial Po_2 of 100 mmHg, and content of 19·5 Vol%. If one lung is hypoventilated to give content B, the other cannot be hyperventilated to content C. Increasing the ventilation to keep total $\dot{V}$ at 2 produces a very small increase in content D, and when blood from both lungs is mixed, Pa,o_2 will be low for O_2 content will be half-way between D and B.

with Pa,o_2 100 mmHg (13·3 kPa), O_2 saturation 95%. If $\dot{V}$ to one lung is decreased to 0·5, O_2 content in blood from that lung falls by the distance AB. If the other lung is to compensate, it must raise the O_2 content in blood from that lung by the equal distance AC—but this is impossible because of the upper limit on the O_2 dissociation curve. In fact if $\dot{V}$ is increased to $1\frac{1}{2}$, thus keeping total $\dot{V}$ equal to 2, only a small increase in content AD is achieved. The mixture of blood from both lungs must have a lower than normal O_2 content and Pa,o_2. On the other hand, for a hypothetical linear dissociation curve for CO_2 (Fig. 8.1b), if one lung is hypoventilated so that Pco_2 in blood

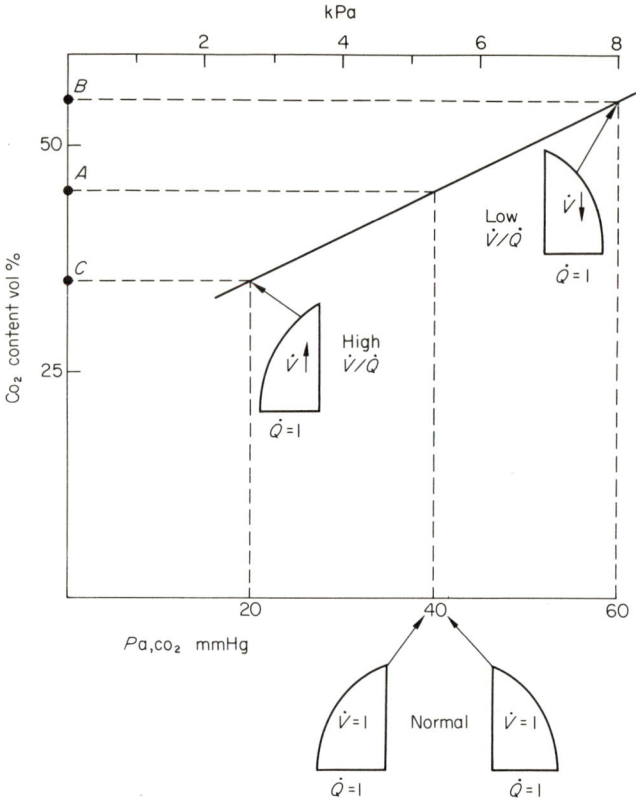

Fig. 8.1. See text.
(b) In contrast, with a linear CO_2 dissociation curve, it seems that hyperventilation of one lung can compensate for hyperventilation of the other.

leaving it is 60 mmHg (8 kPa), then the other lung can be hyperventilated to 20 mmHg (2·7 kPa), and the mixture of blood from both will still have P_{CO_2} 40 mmHg (5·3 kPa), since blood flow is equal to both lungs, and AB = AC.

It was Haldane who first implied that this could be done without increasing total ventilation from normal. Thus it seemed that $Pa,_{CO_2}$ was less sensitive to $\dot{V}/\dot{Q}$ mismatch than $Pa,_{O_2}$, and a further assumption was made that $\dot{V}/\dot{Q}$ mismatch impeded O_2 uptake but not CO_2 elimination. West and colleagues have shown this is to be untrue in a series of difficult mathematical papers (references in [6]).

We may get quite a long way on that road without much mathematics by the simple process of putting some numbers on Fig. 8.1b. Thus (Fig. 8.1c) we know that $Pa,_{CO_2} = K \cdot \dot{V}_{CO_2}/\dot{V}$ (equation 3.11, 3.13b), where K is a constant to convert fractional concentration to partial pressure. We hold $\dot{V}_{CO_2}$

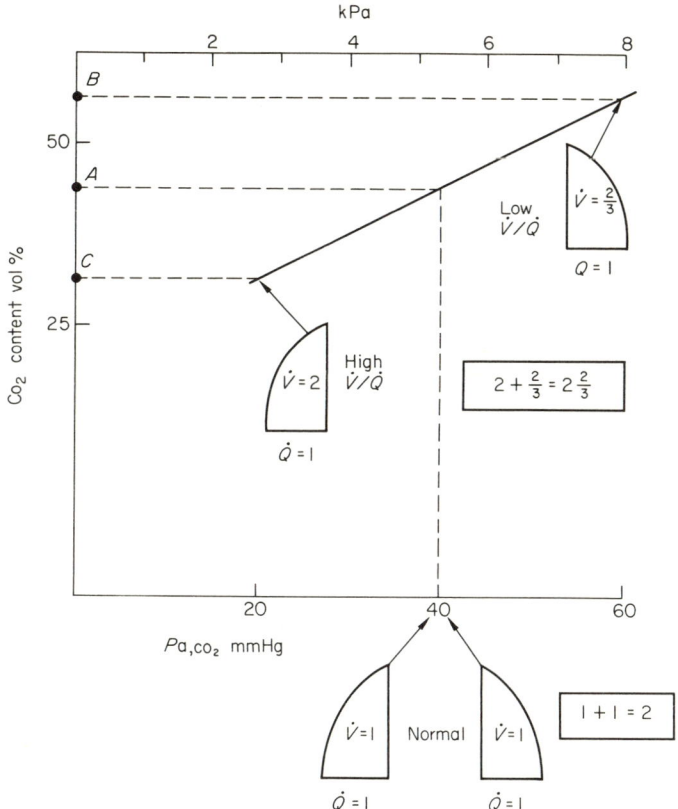

Fig. 8.1. See text.
(c) But when we put the numbers in for ventilation, we find it can only be done at the cost of increased total ventilation.

constant and equal in both lungs. Then if one lung is hypoventilated to produce Pa,co_2 60 mmHg (8 kPa), from the above equation $\dot{V}$ will be $\frac{2}{3}$. To compensate for this the other lung must be hyperventilated to Pa,co_2 20 mmHg (2·7 kPa). Then $\dot{V} = 2$ for the second lung. Now $2 + \frac{2}{3} = 2\frac{2}{3}$, but original normal ventilation was 2. Therefore we cannot compensate for the low $\dot{V}/\dot{Q}$ lung by hyperventilating the other, and still keep the same total ventilation, even when the CO_2 dissociation curve is perfectly linear. On the contrary (Fig. 8.1d) let us take an alinear dissociation curve. Again take a low $\dot{V}/\dot{Q}$ lung with Pa,co_2 60 mmHg, $\dot{V}\frac{2}{3}$. Hyperventilate the other lung down the dissociation curve to the Pa,co_2 where AC = AB. This now occurs at Pa,co_2 30 mmHg (4 kPa). The ventilation required to hyperventilate from Pa,co_2 40 to Pa,co_2 30 mmHg (5·3 to 4 kPa) is $1\frac{1}{3}$. $1\frac{1}{3} + \frac{2}{3} = 2$, which is our original

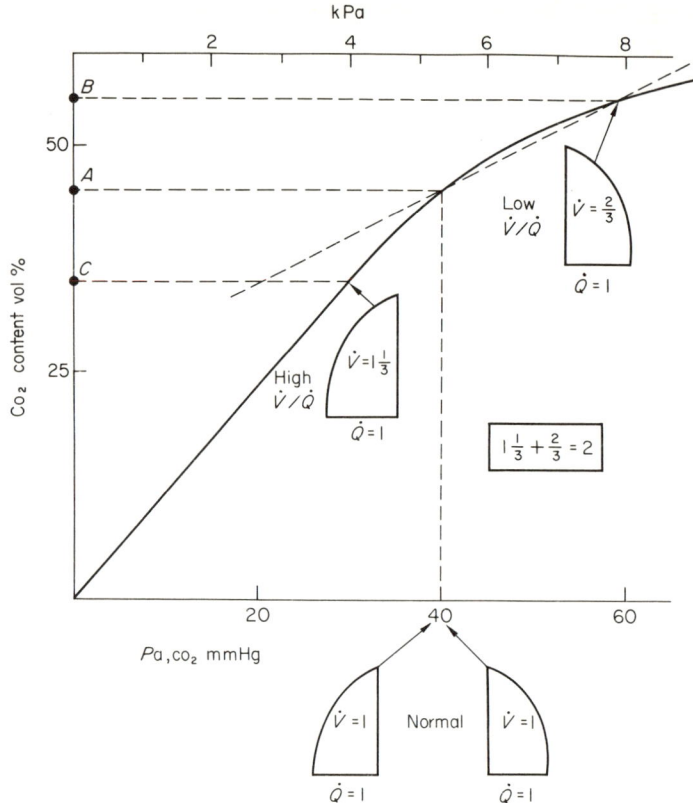

Fig. 8.1. See text.
(d) With a concave-down alinear dissociation curve, it can be done for the same total ventilation.

normal ventilation. We have now compensated for the low $\dot{V}/\dot{Q}$ lung without increasing the total ventilation, *not* because the CO_2 dissociation curve is 'comparatively linear', but because it is fortunately alinear, but concave down.

In this simple example $\dot{V}CO_2$ and $\dot{Q}$ are kept constant and equal for both lungs, and no notice is taken of Haldane or Bohr effects, among other assumptions. Evans and colleagues [6] examined the whole question in terms of $\dot{V}/\dot{Q}$ ratios rather than $\dot{V}$, and concluded that complete compensation for low $\dot{V}/\dot{Q}$ areas could not be attained by hyperventilating other areas down any *linear* dissociation curve at constant total $\dot{V}$, that the concave down shape of the CO_2 dissociation curve was favourable towards such compensation (as in Fig. 8.1d), but that even so complete compensation could never quite be achieved.

Thus we conclude that it is true that hyperventilation of one part of the lung to compensate for other low $\dot{V}/\dot{Q}$ areas will compensate more efficiently for Pa,CO_2 than for Pa,O_2. The primary reason for this is that hyperventilation can increase O_2 content very little over the normal value, whatever the ventilation. Additionally the curvilinear concave-down shape of the CO_2 dissociation curve favours compensation for Pa,CO_2 with very little increase in total ventilation.

What happens in acute exacerbations of chronic respiratory failure?

This is dark mystery. We are familiar with the patient with chronic airways obstruction who runs a Pa,CO_2 of 60 mmHg (8 kPa) and a Pa,O_2 of 45 mmHg (6 kPa), and lives on this basis a disabled but reasonably satisfactory life, at least for a year or two. Occasionally he will become for no apparent reason very ill indeed. We usually attribute this to a superadded infection, yet there may be no fever, no purulence of sputum, no new opacity on the chest film, and no virological or bacteriological evidence for that assumption.

At any rate Pa,CO_2 rises, Pa,O_2 falls, the patient becomes stuporose, cannot clear secretions, and is in danger of death. What caused this? Here is a list of information which we do not have.

(a) We have no good criteria for identifying an infection. Virological studies are frequently negative, and take too long. Blood culture is usually negative. Sputum culture may reflect only the result of recent antibiotic consumption. Organisms grown may be normal commensals, or if abnormal may be colonising the upper respiratory tract but not infecting, that is invading, the patient. Possibly recent attempts to identify infection by serology will prove successful [7].

If there is no infection, there is no present hypothesis to explain the cause of the exacerbation.

(b) We do not know if these acute exacerbations are preceded by a deterioration in the mechanical or gas-exchanging function of the lung. We do know that during recovery from acute on chronic respiratory failure, Pa,CO_2 returns towards normal, and Pa,O_2 during airbreathing rises, and there is usually some improvement in simple indices of airways obstruction, which are usually all that can be measured in the acutely ill patient. We do not know how much of this improvement is due to change in lung function and how much to change in controller function. Present evidence cannot disprove the hypothesis that in patients with chronic airways obstruction, some episodes of acute on chronic respiratory failure are due primarily to a brain-stem disturbance which causes further hypercapnia and hypoxia, and impairment of consciousness, with secondary deterioration in pulmonary function due to retained secretions.

(c) We do not know whether patients respond differently to increasing the inspired fraction of O_2 when they are in chronic stable respiratory failure, as opposed to during the acute exacerbation.

Chronic hypoxia and 2-3-diphosphoglycerate [8, 9]

In chronic anaemic hypoxia, or chronic hypoxia at altitude, the haemoglobin dissociation curve is right-shifted due to an increase in red-cell 2-3-diphosphoglycerate (2-3-DPG). This occurs first because increasing concentrations of 2-3-DPG directly decrease the affinity of haemoglobin for O_2 and second because there is a decrease in pH within the red cell relative to plasma pH, with a right shift of the curve by the Bohr effect, and Fig. 8.2 shows that with normal gas exchange, for the same mixed venous Po_2 more O_2 is unloaded to the tissue (distance AB). Since mixed venous Po_2 reflects the driving pressure for O_2 across the alveolar-capillary membrane, the efficiency of O_2 delivery to the tissues is increased in the sense that more O_2 goes across for the same driving pressure.

For parallel reasons a right shift in the curve impedes O_2 uptake at the lung, but because of the shape of the curves the magnitude of this disadvantageous effect (distance CD, Fig. 8.2) is much less. In the patient with chronic respiratory failure, a right-shifted curve would again assist unloading at the tissues (distance EF, Fig. 8.2), but now with a low arterial Po_2 there is an approximately equal disadvantageous effect on loading at the lung (distance GH, Fig. 8.2). Thus what is gained on the swings in the tissues is lost on the roundabouts at the lung, and in fact in such patients consistent changes in the dissociation curve have not been demonstrated [9].

Blood viscosity

Dintenfass [10] calculated that, with haematocrit greater than 60%, Pa,o_2 less than 40 mmHg (5·3 kPa), and pH approaching 7·0, if the aggregation of red blood cells was increased due to pulmonary infection (high ESR), the viscosity of blood in small pulmonary vessels would approximate to that of a thick concrete sludge. This challenging metaphor has not been proved fallacious.

THERAPY OF ACUTE RESPIRATORY FAILURE IN PATIENTS WITH CHRONIC AIRWAYS OBSTRUCTION

The primary aims are
1 to treat the cause of the exacerbation. Antibiotics are required if there is objective evidence of infection (fever, purulent sputum, or consolidation on

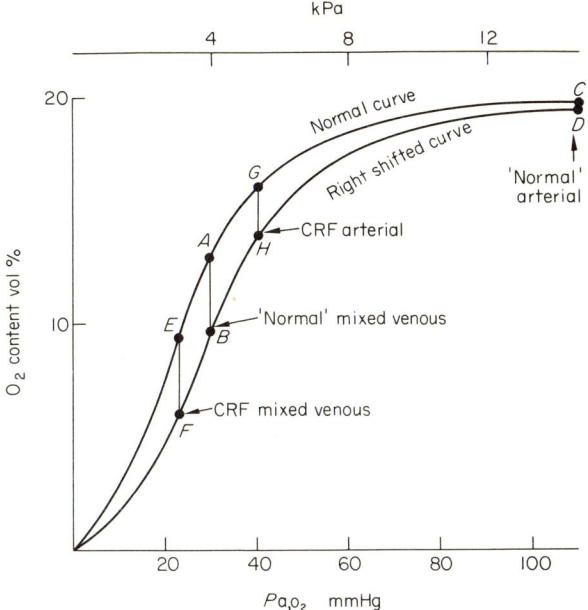

Fig. 8.2. Schematic effect of a right-shift in the O_2 dissociation curve with 'normal' Pa,o_2, and in chronic respiratory failure (CRF). See text.

the chest X-ray film), and are usually given even if such evidence is not present;
2 to maintain a 'safe' level of Pa,o_2;
3 to clear respiratory secretions.

Controlled oxygen therapy is started with low concentrations of inspired O_2 (24 or 28%) by a suitable mask (e.g. Ventimask). Since the Pa,o_2 lies on the steep part of the dissociation curve in these hypoxic patients, an increase of only a few mmHg in Pa,o_2 will be accompanied by a useful increase in arterial oxygen saturation. A 'safety value' of 50 mmHg (6·7 kPa) is frequently assumed for Pa,o_2. It may be better to settle for 45 mmHg (6 kPa) if artificial ventilation is thereby avoided. It is the author's prejudice that more patients have perished from an increase in the concentration of inspired O_2 than have been saved by this method from stroke, myocardial infarction or terminal arrhythmia.

It has been long known that in such patients if O_2 therapy is stopped, Pa,o_2 may subsequently fall below the level found before O_2 therapy. Originally it was supposed that this related to the different sizes of the O_2 and CO_2 stores with a relatively slow washout for CO_2, or possibly to a continuing hypoventilation following the cessation of O_2 therapy. Systematic measurement [11] shows that in fact when the undershoot in Pa,o_2 occurs, Pa,co_2 has returned to control levels, excluding both the above hypotheses. A similar phenomenon can be shown in hypoxic patients with asthma or myocardial infarction with normal Pa,CO_2 which does not increase with O_2 breathing. Probably O_2 breathing produces the shunt like effect of increased venous admixture which persists when the subject returns to air breathing [12].

Obviously O_2 administration should be at the lowest concentration necessary to produce a 'safe' Pa,O_2, and it should be continuous, although this is a counsel of perfection. After stopping O_2 therapy in these patients, Pa,O_2 falls to the level seen before O_2 therapy in about 20 minutes, then undershoots to about 45 minutes [11]. Therefore brief periods of interruption (say less than 10 minutes) will not be accompanied by lethal hypoxia.

The level of Pa,CO_2 reached during O_2 therapy is of less importance than the level of consciousness. The primary requirement is that the patient must be capable of co-operating with the physiotherapist in clearing his secretions. If a 'safe' Sa,O_2 cannot be attained without impairment of level of consciousness beyond this point, then intubation with intermittent positive pressure respiration is required. There is little point in using artificial ventilation if the patient has been a respiratory cripple before the acute exacerbation (e.g. bed-bound) since subsequent weaning is then unlikely to be successful.

In borderline cases, where it is felt that given a little extra stimulation the use of artificial ventilation could be postponed or even made unnecessary, it is reasonable to use so-called respiratory stimulants [13, 14, 15]. It is often found that the dosage required for clinical benefit is very close to that which will produce severe toxic effects such as epileptic fits. Certainly continuous infusions require close personal supervision. Of the available preparations doxapram appears the most satisfactory. The main benefit of these drugs, when given as slug doses, may be to arouse the patient to cough up secretions, rather than to decrease Pa,CO_2.

Apart from antibiotics, physiotherapy and oxygen, it is reasonable to prescribe a diuretic [4]. A definite benefit from digoxin has never been obvious unless there is atrial fibrillation. Bronchodilators are usually given, even in the absence of demonstrable effect.

CHEYNE-STOKES RESPIRATION
(PERIODIC BREATHING)

It is an old observation that some patients have alternating periods of apnoea and hyperpnoea. Such patients may have heart failure, with long circulation times, when the cycle length of this periodic phenomenon is rather long, 45 seconds or more, or some form of cerebral damage such as stroke or head injury, when the cycle length is usually shorter.

This is not necessarily, by our previous definition, an example of respiratory failure, but it is a very curious abnormality of respiratory control,

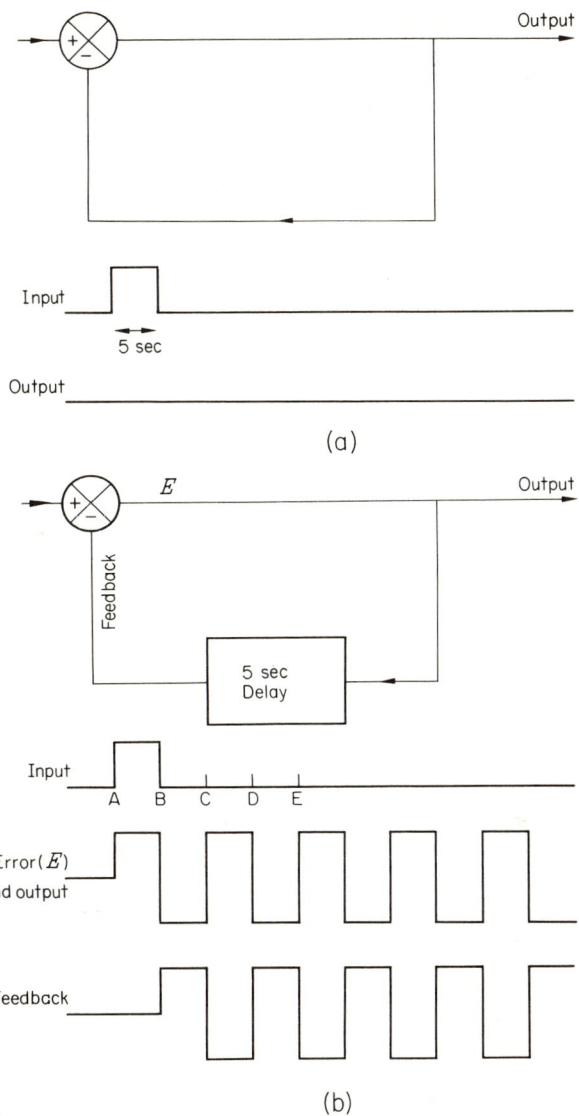

Fig. 8.3. (a) The nothing-happens machine, which by the addition of a 5 second delay is converted (b) at a stroke into the it-happens-for-ever machine. See text.

and as such a suitable point to conclude this book. Consider the simplest possible feedback loop of Fig. 8.3a. There are no dynamics and no time delays. If a square-wave pulse is the input, it will instantaneously subtract itself via negative feedback. The output is always zero. We have invented the original nothing-happens machine.

Now include a simple pure time delay of 5 seconds (Fig. 8.3b). The input is a square wave pulse 5 seconds lung. During period AB, the 5 second signal is transmitted to the output. No feedback gets through the delay till point B, when it is subtracted to form a negative error and output pulse AB, lasting 5 seconds. This in turn is fed back and subtracted from the input, now zero, to give positive error and output pulse CD, and so on. Why does it not return to zero? During period BC the comparator, here the controller, sees a positive feedback pulse. Essentially the controller makes a bad assumption, that because the feedback pulse is positive, the output is positive. The output is not positive during BC, though it was during AB. The controller is misled by outdated information.

This is a simple example of how time delays may produce instability. This instability may take the form of sustained oscillation, as here with ventilation, or oscillations of ever-increasing amplitude which in the electronics workshop may end in a small fire, or oscillations which die away. The conditions which determine the presence and nature of the instability have been mathematically determined for linear systems. For our purposes the conditions for sustained oscillations are that the phase lag produced by the system, including lag due to pure time delays, for a sine wave input, must be half a cycle (180°) or more, and that the loop gain must be greater than one.

Under such conditions, a sudden disturbance imposed on a steady state may produce sustained oscillatory output. The larger the lags and the higher the gain the more likely this form of instability becomes, and the smaller the disturbance required to produce it.

The parallels between the systems theory and the pathological findings in Cheyne-Stokes breathing are particularly illuminating, since it is indeed those patients with increased circulation delays who tend to show this instability. In patients with increased controller gain due to central nervous system damage, or due to hypoxia (altitude) periodic breathing may also be observed.

In summary, ventilatory instability of the Cheyne-Stokes type may be produced by increasing delays within the feedback loop, when the controller acts on out-dated and directionally misleading information, or by increasing controller gain, when the controller over-reacts to a possibly more appropriate signal.

REFERENCES

1 CAMPBELL E.J.M. (1965) Respiratory failure. *Brit. Med. J.* **1**, 1451–1460.
2 GUZ A. (1976) Regulation of respiration in man. *Ann. Rev. Physiol.* **37**, 303–323.
3 GUZ A., NOBLE M.I.M., TRENCHARD D., GARNETT E.S., CLARKSON E.M., McDONALD S.J. & DE WARDENER H.E. (1966) The significance of a raised central venous pressure during sodium and water retention. *Clin. Sci.* **30**, 295–303.

4 NOBLE M.I.M., TRENCHARD D. & GUZ A. (1966) The value of diuretics in respiratory failure. *Lancet* 2, 257–260.

5 CAMPBELL R.H.A., BRAND H.L., COX J.R. & HOWARD P. (1975) Body weight and body water in chronic cor pulmonale. *Clin. Sci. Mol. Med.* 49, 323–335.

6 EVANS J.W., WAGNER P.D. & WEST J.B. (1974) Conditions for reduction of pulmonary gas transfer by ventilation-perfusion inequality. *J. Appl. Physiol.* 36, 533–538.

7 NICHOLLS A.C., PEASE P.E. & GREEN I.D. (1976) A study of the agglutinin response in 40 cases of bacterial pneumonia. *J. Clin. Path.* 28, 453–456.

8 THOMAS H.M., LEFRAK S.S., IRWIN R.S., FRITTS H.W. & CALDWELL P.R.B. (1974) The oxyhaemoglobin dissociation curve in health and disease. Role of 2,3-Diphosphoglycerate. *Am. J. Med.* 57, 331–348.

9 FAIRWEATHER L.J., WALKER J. & FLENLEY D.C. (1974) 2,3-Diphosphoglycerate concentrations and the dissociation of oxyhaemoglobin in ventilatory failure. *Clin. Sci. Mol. Med.* 47, 577–588.

10 DINTENFASS L. & READ J. (1968) Pathogenesis of heart failure in acute-on-chronic respiratory failure. *Lancet* 1, 570–572.

11 RUDOLF M., HARRISON B.D.W., RIORDAN J.F. & SAUNDERS K.B. (1975) Changes in arterial blood gases after cessation of oxygen breathing in patients with chronic respiratory failure. *Clin. Sci. Mol. Med.* 49, 10P.

12 DANTZKER D.R., WAGNER P.D. & WEST J.B. (1975) Instability of lung units with low $\dot{V}_A/\dot{Q}$ ratios during O_2 breathing. *J. Appl. Physiol.* 38, 886–895.

13 EDWARDS G. & LESZCZYNSKI S.O. (1967) A doubleblind trial of five respiratory stimulants in patients in acute ventilatory failure. *Lancet* 2, 226–229.

14 BREWIS R.A.L. & HODGES N.G. (1970) Long-term and short-term effects of oral prethcamide in chronic ventilatory failure. *Brit. Med. J.* 2, 764–766.

15 RIORDAN J.F., SILLETT R.W. & McNICOL M.W. (1975) A controlled trial of doxapram in acute respiratory failure. *Brit. J. Dis. Chest* 69, 57–62.

Index